THE BUSY VET'S GUIDE TO CYTOLOGY

THE BUSY VET'S GUIDE TO
CYTOLOGY

What Do All the Blobs Mean?

Nicholas Marsh
BVSc Dip. ACVP (Clin. Path) MRCVS

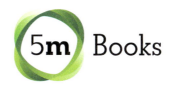

First published 2024

Copyright © Nick Marsh 2024

The right of Nick Marsh to be identified as author of this Work has been asserted by him/her in accordance with sections 77 and 78 of the Copyright, Designs and Patents Act 1988.

All rights reserved. No part of this publication may be reproduced, stored in a retrieval system, or transmitted, in any form or by any means, electronic, mechanical, photocopying, recording or otherwise, without prior permission of the copyright holder.

Published by
5M Books Ltd
Lings, Great Easton
Essex CM6 2HH, UK
Tel: +44 (0)330 1333 580
www.5mbooks.com

Follow us on
Twitter @5m_Books
Instagram 5m_books
Facebook @5mBooks
LinkedIn @5mbooks

A Catalogue record for this book is available from the British Library

ISBN 9781789183474
eISBN 9781789183627
DOI 10.52517/9781789183627

Book layout by Cheshire Typesetting Ltd, Cuddington, Cheshire
Printed by Hobbs the Printers
Photos by the author courtesy of the Veterinary Pathology Group (VPG Exeter) unless otherwise indicated
Illustrations by Elaine Leggett

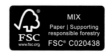

Contents

Preface viii
Note on magnification, staining, percentages and differential counts x
Textbook format xi

PART ONE – CYTOLOGICAL BASICS

1 **Cytology explained** 3
   Introduction to cytology 3
   Equipment for cytology 6

2 **Sampling and preparation** 14
   Choice of sampling technique 14
   Sampling techniques 16

3 **The basics of cytology** 29
   What is all this stuff? 29
   What am I actually looking at? 29
   Nucleated cells 29
   Non-nucleated cells 47
   Other useful cytological concepts 52

4 **General principles of cytology** 55
   Stepwise approach to evaluating cytology smears 55
   Cytology of inflammation 59
   Cytology of neoplasia 70
   Cytology of non-inflammatory and non-neoplastic lesions 96
   Some final points on general cytology 104

5 **Infectious agents** 106
   Bacteria 107
   Fungi 116
   Protozoa 119
   Multicellular parasites 122

PART TWO – CYTOLOGY OF SPECIFIC LOCATIONS

6 Skin and subcutaneous lesions — 129
  Neoplasia of the skin and subcutis — 134
  Inflammatory lesions of the skin and subcutis — 171

7 Gastrointestinal system — 182
  Oral cavity — 182
  Liver — 186

8 Genitourinary system — 204
  Kidney — 204
  Urine — 209
  Bladder — 212
  Prostate — 213

9 Respiratory system — 217
  Nose — 217
  Broncho-alveolar lavage (BAL) and trans-tracheal wash (TTW) — 219
  Lung — 227

10 Lymph nodes, spleen and thymus — 231
  Lymph nodes — 231
  Spleen — 248
  Thymus — 257

11 Muscle, bone and synovial fluid — 259
  Muscle — 259
  Bone — 261
  Synovial fluid — 265

12 Cavity effusions — 269
  Fluid analysis — 269
  Fluid classification — 274

13 Blood films — 282
  Blood film preparation — 282
  Blood film evaluation — 285
  Some 'classic' patterns — 310

PART THREE – FURTHER THOUGHTS ON CYTOLOGY

14	'Edge cases'	317
	Specific edge cases	318
15	Submitting to an external lab	331
16	Digital and remote cytology	335

APPENDICES

A.	Summary of cell examination and description	337
B.	Decoding pathology reports – a cytological glossary	338
C.	Backgrounds	340
D.	Common crystals	341
E.	Species/sex/breed predispositions	343
F.	Further staining and extra tests	344
G.	Mitotic figures	345
H.	Pathology jokes	347

Bibliography	348
Index	352

Preface

My first encounter with a microscope was in my first year at veterinary school. I wasn't in the best place for a new scientific relationship at the time; I'd gone from being at the top of all my classes in high school and college to the bottom third at university. Imposter syndrome was my new companion and I was desperately trying to look as confident and relaxed with the tonnes of new information being piled upon us as everyone else around me seemed to be. One of our first classes was histology, and it was in a nervous and frazzled state of mind that I sat down in front of the pale beige microscope on my desk, and peered myopically down to get my first view of the internal mechanisms of the body.

It was not love at first sight.

Those now-distant histology lessons still retain their flavour of misery and boredom in my memory. Lessons comprised flicking through the heavy sheaf of notes we had alongside *Wheater's Functional Histology* and utterly failing to connect the images in the textbook with the bizarre cubist mess of purple and blue splats I could see down the microscope. It was enough to put me off microscopes for life – or so I thought.

In my career in general practice, I only used the microscope to search for skin mites, but the thrill of seeing them waving up at me from their tiny hidden world always evoked a sense of wonder that those interminable histology lessons years before never came close to. Every time I saw a mite, I yearned to learn more about the mysterious realm they inhabited, but the everyday stresses and tragedies of practice had a way of hammering away notions of self-improvement. When the mood took me and when the practice was (whisper it) *quiet*, I sometimes dusted off the mysterious bottles of *Diff-Quik* and stained up a slide, only to be almost immediately disheartened peering at the bluish blobs in front of me. These slides didn't look like the ordered but incomprehensible preparations from the histology class. They were splats of chaotic nonsense. I couldn't even begin to understand what I was looking at, let alone do something as lofty as reach a diagnosis. I barely knew a neutrophil from a macrophage, let alone an inflammatory lesion from a neoplastic one.

I remember general practice very well. I remember the lack of time, the lack of energy, the attempts at self-improvement which rarely survived exposure to the next barrage of clients and conundrums. I have written this book with general practice in mind. If even tiny parts of my story above seem familiar to you, then I am here to assure you that sense can be made of those slides. I have come to appreciate not only the power of cytology as a screening and diagnostic tool, but also the strange beauty of that hidden inner world that lives within each of us, highlighted in striking azure and magenta tones. I am going to try to prove to you that if someone like me can learn to understand the mysteries of this subject then, without question, you can too. With some patience and time I suspect you will soon feel, as I do, privileged to be offered such a rare and exquisite insight into how these amazing millennia-honed biological machines we heal, help and inhabit actually work. It has been a source of great pleasure for me to be given a window onto this incredible miniature universe, and when those blobs coalesce into meaning for you, as I promise they will, I suspect they will bring you great joy too.

Welcome to cytology.

Nick Marsh

Notes

A note on images (magnification)

The images in this book are labelled with their magnification; this includes the x10 magnification provided by most ocular lenses in the head of the microscope, as well as the magnification from the objective lens. For example, images labelled '×100' will have been attained using the ×10 objective and the ×10 ocular lens, images labelled '×1000' with the ×100 objective and the ×10 ocular lens, and so on.

A note on images (staining)

The majority of samples photographed within this book have been stained with Wright-Giemsa stain. This is a methanol Romanowsky stain (MR), whereas many in-practice stains (such as *Diff-Quik*) are aqueous Romanowsky stains (AR). Although the stains produce similar results, there are some notable differences. Firstly, AR stains often accentuate nuclear features, increasing the contrast within the nucleus – principally nucleoli are often more prominent than displayed in many of the pictures in this textbook, and care must be taken not to over interpret this finding as atypical.

Secondly, AR stains tend to not reliably stain many cytoplasmic granules, most notably mast cell granules, but also granules within basophils and lymphocytes, and this should again be considered when examining samples in house. Another effect of the poor staining of cytoplasmic granules is to make the cytoplasm of neutrophils appear paler on AR preparations than the images in this book (it appears as clear white rather than pale grey).

A note on percentages and differential counts

Cytology specimens are not standardised, and consequently have a very varied appearance. One method for applying order to sometimes chaotic specimens is by differential counting of certain cells or features, to estimate proportions or percentages (i.e. the percentage of neutrophils within joints, or the number of mitotic figures present in a group of lymphocytes). Whilst this is often extremely valuable, such figures should be interpreted with caution and always in context. For example, applying a rigid rule such as 'any joint aspirate containing over 10% neutrophils has neutrophilic inflammation' fails to take into account the amount of blood which may or may not be present, and will lead to over diagnosis of inflammation. Where percentages of cells or features are mentioned in this book, they are <u>always</u> guidelines rather than rigid rules, and the context of every specimen must be considered before applying them.

Textbook format

This textbook is divided into three main parts. Part I, Cytological Basics, deals with general cytology – what it is, basic cytological features, general features of neoplasia and inflammation etc. Part II, Cytology of Specific Locations, forms the bulk of the textbook. It takes the basics from part one and applies them to specific locations – the skin, liver, cavity fluids, blood film etc. Part III, Further Thoughts on Cytology, contains wider thoughts about cytology – what to do with cases that don't fit into the neat boxes provided by Part II, how to submit material to external labs, and so on.

The book is designed for vets in general practice – this means consideration has been given to those under time pressure. Part II – the section most likely to be flipped through in a hurry – lists conditions in rough order of commonality, so that the most frequently found lesions are towards the start of most sections. In order to avoid too much searching, many terms are defined whenever they are used, and references to other related conditions are present within the text, as well as in the index.

Part one

Cytological basics

Chapter 1

Cytology explained

The principal use of cytology is as a screening test: 'Is this lesion neoplastic?' 'Is it inflammatory?' 'Are infectious agents present?' 'Are further tests needed?' – but it is possible to extract far more information from a needle full of cells than that. Cytology is a nuanced and initially bewildering subject, but with practice those blue and purple blobs cohere into a fuller picture of our patient's health than we have any right to reasonably expect.

Simple and cheap to perform, with patience, time and study, cytology can also function as a powerful diagnostic tool – indeed, it is one of the most cost-effective diagnostic tests available, perhaps second only to comprehensive physical examination and detailed history. It has the added advantages of being quick, comparatively safe, minimally invasive and, in the opinion of the author, fascinating, rewarding, and extremely beautiful.

Introduction to cytology

Why this book?

Whilst rewarding, cytology can also be confusing and frustrating, especially initially. There are many excellent textbooks and other material on the subject (see references). This textbook is not an exhaustive list of all cytological possibilities but has been written with less experienced cytologists in mind. Consequently, throughout this book the author has adhered to several principles.

- **Common things occur commonly** – the focus of this material is on the lesions most often encountered, and how to recognise differences from these common lesions which require more detailed examination, further tests, or referral to experienced pathologists; the lists of possibilities for each location always start with common lesions first, progressing to rarer lesions.
- **Free time in general practice is rare, short and unpredictable** – the chapters are organised in a way to make the most relevant material rapidly accessible, with key points highlighted so they are not lost within the remainder of the text, and take home messages at the end of every chapter.
- **There are many traps and pitfalls in cytology** – the textbook will show the most frequent errors made by inexperienced cytologists, how to recognise and avoid them, and what questions it is reasonable to expect to answer with the samples taken.

This book is intended for those taking their first steps into the eerily beautiful field of cytology. It will be valuable for vets and veterinary nurses in practice, as well as early clinical pathology residents and interns, and late veterinary students (that is, veterinary students toward the end of their course, rather than dead).

Clinical pathology versus anatomic pathology (and cytology versus histology)

For most of my career in practice, I was only dimly aware of what a pathologist was. They were a black box from my perspective. I sent samples in, and the results came back – the bit in the middle was arcane, unknowable. This section will probably be stating the obvious for most of you, but it may be helpful to some.

Pathology is the study of disease and is divided into two broad categories for our purposes: *clinical pathology* and *anatomic pathology*.

Anatomic pathologists are who most people think of when they hear the word 'pathology' – they study whole bodies, organs, and larger specimens with a variety of techniques, stains, and they keep manufacturers of formaldehyde in business. Their reports take longer but are usually definitive.

Clinical pathologists, in contrast, are the first responders of the pathology world. They study smaller samples – needle aspirates, blood and other fluids – and offer a more rapid opinion. Perhaps the simplest, albeit somewhat facetious, definition of what clinical pathology does is this: If you can fit it through a needle, then a clinical pathologist will have a look at it for you.

This may seem obvious, but it is a point worth remembering: anatomic and clinical pathology, whilst related, are different disciplines, with different exams for their qualifications and *very* different day jobs – as different, if not more so, than endocrinology and cardiology, or any other two medical or surgical specialities.

Both anatomic and clinical pathologists study the microscopic structure of the body – for anatomic pathologists, the discipline is *histopathology*. They examine larger formalin-fixed specimens. The anatomy of the tissues remains intact, although the process of fixing fixes and somewhat homogenises the cellular structure. The clarity of the tissue architecture comes with the slight price of making the individual cellular details less distinct (Fig 1.1).

Conversely, *cytology*, studied by clinical pathologists, removes the cells from their immediate surroundings. Cells are directly aspirated via needle biopsy or observed within tissue fluids. Cells and other structures are more detailed on cytological specimens, at the expense of loss of context and surrounding detail. This loss of context for cytological specimens means that, even more so than for histopathology, the history of the lesion, the gross appearance and the precise anatomical location are extremely important to improve the chance of reaching a diagnosis (Fig 1.2).

In-house examination vs. submitting to an external laboratory

Unlike many diagnostic tests, cytology does not require especially expensive equipment. Aside from a decent microscope, all that is required are some needles, syringes, glass slides, staining dyes and a reasonably patient patient. Consequently, and because of its potential to give a rapid and accurate diagnosis, cytology lends itself to in-house examination.

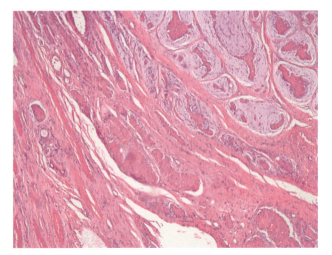

Fig 1.1 Histology specimen of collision tumour (perianal adenoma with invading soft tissue sarcoma) ×100

One purpose of this book is to illustrate how useful cytology can be in general practice. As already mentioned, however, cytology is a nuanced and occasionally bewildering subject. The second purpose of this book is to indicate to practitioners when they would be wise to refer their cases to an experienced cytologist. The text will show where the most common cytological traps occur, how to recognise them and how to avoid them, but there are many occasions where a practised eye can recognise patterns and avoid pitfalls (generally because they have fallen into those pitfalls themselves several times before – as Oscar Wilde once said, experience is simply the name we give our mistakes).

When starting out with cytology, it is useful to examine some slides in house and then submit the case to a pathologist for comparison. Many pathologists are happy to discuss the case in more detail, and to help to identify puzzling structures and cells in cases they have reported on. It is better not to stain every slide from the case with in-house stain, however – pathologists, mostly creatures of habit, are often much more used to their laboratory stains than stains used in practices (see staining, page 27, for the differences between in-house and laboratory) and whilst preparations can be restained, the appearance of the slides will be affected, which can make definitive identification challenging. The best approach is to stain some slides for in-house examination, leave some unstained, and submit all of them to the pathologist. Interesting or useful slides can then be returned to the practice if necessary.

More information on submitting cases to external laboratories is found in chapter 13, but one further point is worth making here – don't submit histopathology and cytology specimens together. Even limited exposure to formalin fumes has a significantly deleterious effect on the staining and preservation of cytological specimens and many perfectly cellular samples have been ruined by being packed next to a formalin-pickled specimen (Fig 1.3). Submit in separate packages to avoid this.

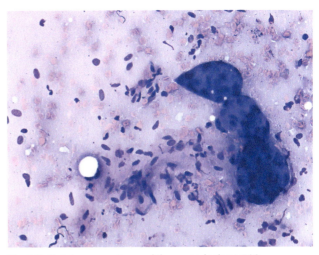

Fig 1.2 Cytology specimen of the same lesion ×500

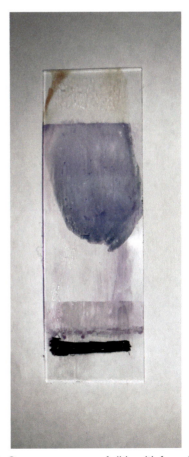

Fig 1.3 Gross appearance of slide with formalin fume damage; note the greenish tinge, especially at the edge of the smear

Pros and cons of cytology at a glance.

Pros
- Sampling relatively simple to perform and minimal discomfort to patient (similar to blood sampling).
- Equipment for sampling is cheap and easy to acquire.
- Equipment for in-house examination is also relatively cheap (microscope is the biggest cost).
- Rapid results (more or less immediate for in-house examination and within a few days for external lab submissions).
- A lot of information can be gained from samples – best at screening for neoplasia/infectious disease but potentially diagnostic.

Cons
- Less information gained than histopathology specimens, and higher chance of non-diagnostic samples.
- Some slight risks involved (such as seeding of neoplasia; see page 15 for more information).
- Some specimens can be misleading (when structures are complex – such as mammary tissue, or for inexperienced cytologists).

Many of the 'cons' above can be ameliorated with proper sampling and preparation technique – overall, cytology is a minimally invasive, safe, simple and cheap technique to perform with the potential for very rapid diagnosis.

Equipment for cytology
Microscopes (FIG 1.4)

The microscope is the single most expensive piece of equipment required for in-house cytology, but it need not be highly expensive. Prices and models vary widely, from simple monocular microscopes suitable for in-house parasitology to highly specialist powerful microscopes used in research laboratories. Although the quality of the images produced differs greatly, relatively

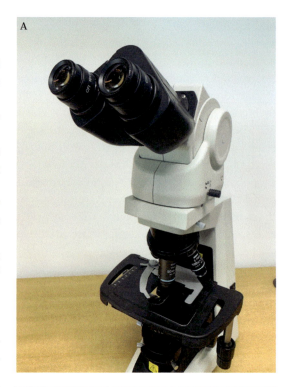
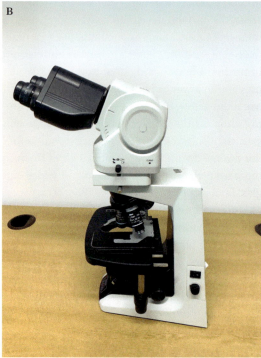

Fig. 1.4 Binocular microscope

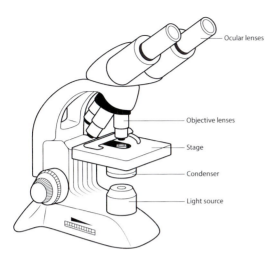

Fig 1.5 Anatomy of a microscope

low-end microscopes can still be used effectively for in-house cytological examination.

As with many areas of life, much can be achieved by getting used to the tools at your disposal. A clean and well-maintained basic microscope is likely to be more useful than an expensive but rarely cleaned and poorly maintained one.

There follows a brief examination of the most important components of microscopes (Fig 1.5), as well the author's preferences for microscope work.

Ocular lens (FIG 1.6)

For many microscopists, the first question they must ask themselves is this: 'Should I wear my glasses or not?' The simple answer is that it's up to you – the focus can be adjusted to suit your preferences either way – and there is no wrong way to do this. The author prefers to wear their glasses during cytology, mostly to avoid the constant removal and replacement of spectacles throughout the day, and also because it acts as a very visual reminder of when it is time to clean their spectacles.

The next question is whether to use monocular lenses or binocular. Here, the author's strong preference is for binocular lenses – monocular

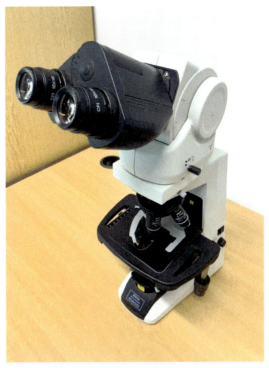

Fig 1.6a Ocular lenses in place on microscope

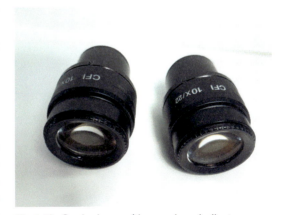

Fig 1.6b Ocular lenses (the numbers indicate the magnification – 10× – and the diameter of the diaphragm in the eyepiece – 22mm)

lenses become tiring to use after all but the very briefest of sessions at the microscope, and binocular lenses can be adjusted (usually by rotating the top of the lens, closest to the microscopist) to correct for variations in visual acuity from one eye to the other.

8 Part one | Cytological basics

> Ocular lenses have their own magnification factor, which is then multiplied by the lower objective lens. For most ocular lenses, this factor is ten times (×10), so images labelled '×100 magnification' have been acquired using the ×10 objective lens and the ×10 ocular lens, and so on.

Objective lens (FIG 1.7)

These are located within the rotating barrels just above the microscope stage and are used to adjust the magnification during examination. The microscopist should give some consideration to which objective lenses to use, and what quality. The cheapest objectives (*achromat*) contain only minimal correction for the curvature of the lenses and the differing wavelengths of light, whereas more expensive lenses (*fluorite/semi-apochromat* and the highly expensive *apochromat*) correct for all these factors.

The practical upshot of this is that cheaper objectives will produce blurrier or fuzzier images, especially at the periphery. '*plan*' lenses also correct for the curvature of the field of view. Therefore, in theory, '*plan apochromat*' objectives produce the sharpest image. In the author's experience, however, much can be achieved even with relatively cheap modern objectives such as '*plan achromat*'.

The most commonly used objective magnifications are ×4, ×10, ×20, ×40, ×50 and ×100 – for lenses with magnification over ×40, immersion oil is used (see below). Microscopes vary between the number of objectives that can be attached to them (usually three or four), and microscopists

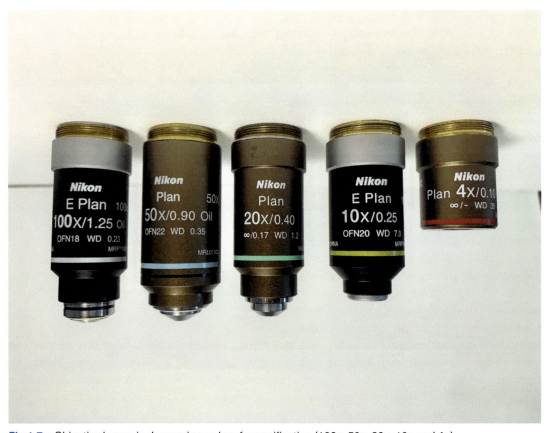

Fig 1.7a Objective lenses in decreasing order of magnification (100×, 50×, 20×, 10× and 4×)

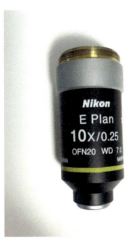

Fig 1.7b Objective lens; the inscriptions indicate (top to bottom): the make of the lens, the type of lens ('E plan' indicates a *plan* objective that fits a model 'E' microscope), the magnification (10×) and numerical aperture, the field number (the diameter in mm of the eyepiece field) and the working distance (the ideal distance in mm between the bottom of the objective lens and the top of the specimen)

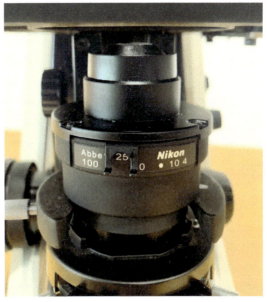

Fig 1.8 Condenser with adjustable diaphragm (partially open)

also vary with their preferences, although as a minimum the microscope should have a ×10 objective for low power examination and ×100 for detailed examination of individual cells.

Beyond this, the author's preference is to also use the ×4 objective for rapid scanning of slides, and ×50 for close examination but with a wider field of view. Many microscopists use ×20 objectives for more detailed low-power examination, or ×40 objectives for close examination without the need for immersion oil, but they have a few drawbacks: they are usually designed to be used with cover slips, and the image can be blurry without them, and these objectives are physically the same length as the ×50 and ×100 objectives, making it easy to absent-mindedly cover the objective lens with immersion oil, obscuring the view.

> **Key points**
>
> - Modern 'Plan achromat' objectives suitable for many purposes outside research laboratories
> - Minimum objectives: ×10, ×100, author's preference: ×4, ×10, ×50, ×100

Condenser stage (FIG 1.8)

The condenser is a lens on a (usually) adjustable substage below the main stage – the purpose is to gather the light emitted from the light source below and focus it into a cone to illuminate the sample directly above. The condenser can be adjusted for each objective, but in practice the author finds it usually sufficient for most purposes to have the condenser adjusted almost as high as possible, lowered slightly so that the image in the ocular lens is not focused on the lens of the condenser itself.

Many condensers have an adjustable diaphragm. Closing the diaphragm increases the contrast of the image but also increases artefacts on the image. For most purposes, the author works with the condenser diaphragm completely open.

Light source
Modern microscopes often have LED light sources. These are useful as they generally emit brighter and more reliable light than older bulb microscopes, but they are not essential for detailed microscopic examination.

Immersion oil (FIG 1.9)
As magnification increases, the refractive index of air becomes insufficient for detailed images to be produced – for magnifications above ×400, immersion oil is required to increase the refractive index and to produce clear images (×40 objectives can be either 'dry' or 'wet').

Immersion oil is used by rotating the objective slightly to one side, applying a drop of oil to the sample, and rotating the objective into the drop of oil. Many microscopists prefer to wear gloves whilst working to avoid becoming immersed in oil themselves.

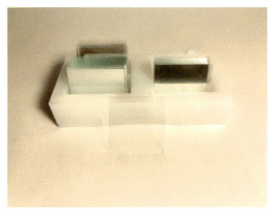

Fig 1.10 Cover slips

Cover slips (FIG 1.10)
Cover slips are rarely useful for cytological examination as they are not required to improve the quality of images (in fact they often obscure it) and are not required to preserve the material for the short periods of time between sampling and examination – even when submitting to an external laboratory.

Cover slips are sometimes required when using ×40 'wet' objectives. For this reason, the author prefers ×50 objectives.

Needles
The width of the needle required for fine needle aspirate biopsy somewhat depends on the lesion sampled. As narrow a needle as possible is recommended, because wider needles increase the risk of blood contamination, making sample assessment much harder. For the majority of lesions, 22 or 23 gauge needles will be sufficient. However, firm-feeling lesions may not exfoliate as well, and here 20 or 21 gauges may be used. Needles wider than this run the risk of aspirating a small tissue core rather than smaller sheets and clusters of cells. For very firm lesions such as bone masses, even larger needles may be required, although trying smaller needles first is still recommended.

The needle length does not affect the sampling except that shorter needles are easier to

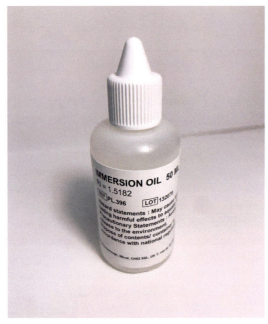

Fig 1.9 Immersion oil

manoeuvre; use the shortest needle required to reach the area aspirated.

Syringes

Many lesions can be sampled without applying negative pressure to the needle during aspiration (see page 16 re sampling). In these cases, the syringe is only used to expel the sample onto the slide. Pressure may need to be applied for firmer lesions, although the amount required varies. For most lesions, a 5ml syringe will be sufficient to acquire a suitable sample.

> **Key points**
>
> - Use as small a needle as possible to reduce blood contamination
> - 22–23 gauge needles are suitable for most lesions, possibly wider for firm lesions
> - If suction is required, 5ml syringes are usually suitable

Slides (FIG 1.11)

The main choice here is between completely clear glass slides and those with a frosted or coloured area at one end. The author recommends frosted slides, which can be written on with pencil. This is hard to erase (unlike labels with pen written on them), cheap and easy to perform. Even for in-house examination, labelling is extremely important to avoid misdiagnoses. For similar reasons, slides should never be reused between cases, including 'spreader' slides. Using a fresh set of slides for each case is not expensive and reusing them is not worth the risk of cross-contamination and misdiagnosis.

> **Key points**
>
> - Use frosted slides which can be easily labelled with pencil
> - NEVER reuse slides between cases (including 'spreader' slides)

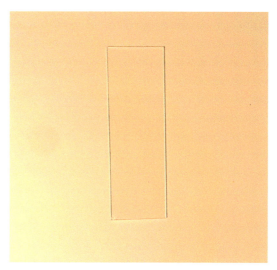

Fig 1.11 Frosted glass microscope slide

Stains (FIG 1.12)

Many commercial laboratories use automated stainers, but these are unlikely to be practical in practice – they are expensive and designed to deal with heavy caseloads, and hard to justify in general practice or even referral hospitals. However, as digital cytology improves and more cases are submitted online, automated stainers may become more useful. Their main advantage, other than speed and ease, is the uniformity of the stain applied – this is hard to reproduce with manual staining.

Most in-practice cytology, however, will be performed using manual stains. These stains have different appearances, however – this is mentioned at the beginning of the book but is worth repeating here: most laboratory stains use a type of methanol Romanowsky stain (MR) (such as Wright-Giemsa), whereas many in-practice stains (such as *Diff-Quik*) are aqueous Romanowsky stains (AR). Although the stains are very similar, there are some notable differences which are useful to bear in mind when examining the images. Firstly, AR stains often accentuate nuclear features, increasing the contrast within the nucleus – principally nucleoli often more prominent that displayed in

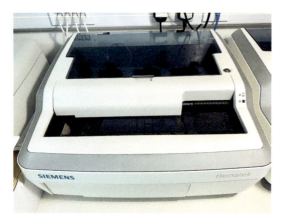

Fig 1.12a Siemens Hematek automated stainer

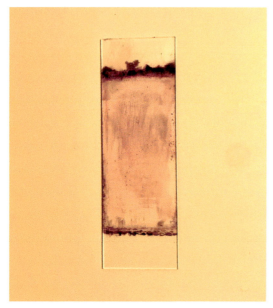

Fig 1.12b Areas of a slide stained by typical automatic stainer (notice the ends of the slide are not stained)

the pictures here, and care must be taken not to over interpret this finding as atypical.

Secondly, AR stains do not reliably stain many cytoplasmic granules, most notably mast cell granules, but also granules within basophils and lymphocytes, and this should again be considered when examining samples in house. Another effect of the poor staining of cytoplasmic granules is to make the cytoplasm of neutrophils appear paler on AR preparations than the images here (it appears as clear white rather than pale grey).

Manual stains (and automated stainers) need to be cleaned and changed regularly to avoid build of debris/stain precipitate, which obscures cytology specimens, and to reduce the risk of contamination of specimens (e.g. from bacteria growing in the stain). Some practices use separate 'clean' (e.g. masses not suspected to be infected) and 'dirty' (e.g. ear swabs, aspirates from suspected abscesses) stains to further minimise the risk.

> ### Key points
>
> - Stains need changing regularly to reduce contamination of specimens
> - Manual stains (AR) key differences from most laboratory stains (MR):
>   - Accentuated staining of nuclear features with AR (cells can appear more atypical)
>   - Unreliable staining of granules with AR (especially mast cells, lymphocytes)

Additional equipment (FIG 1.13)

Further equipment is unlikely to be required except in more specific situations, which will be covered in later chapters. For reference, these include: microhaematocrit tubes for blood films (covered in Chapter 13), a cytocentrifuge for poorly cellular fluid (covered in Chapter 12), a microhaematocrit reader (for manual PCV calculation), serum-coated slides, to aid preservation and a digital scanner, for uploading cytology for remote assessment.

Cytology explained | Chapter 1 13

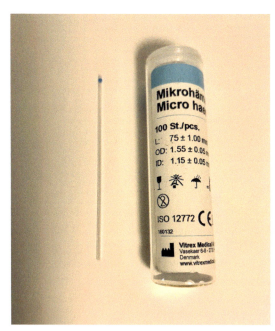

Fig 1.13a Microhaematocrit tubes

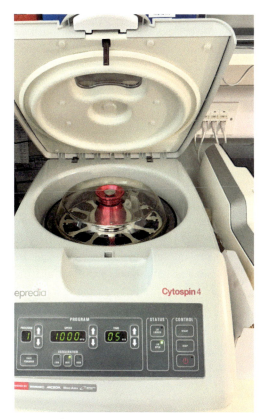

Fig 1.13b Cytocentrifuge

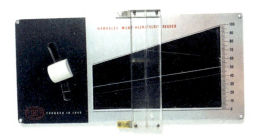

Fig 1.13c Microhaematocrit reader

Chapter 1 – take home messages

- Cytology and histology are separate (but related) disciplines, performed by different types of pathologists (clinical and anatomical, respectively).
- Microscopes do not need to be very expensive for cytology; a relatively cheap but well-maintained microscope that the clinician is familiar with is more useful than an expensive but rarely-used one.
- ×10 and ×100 objectives are the most useful for cytology; ×4 and ×50 are also useful if available.
- Cover slips are rarely required for cytological specimens.
- In-house stains must be changed regularly to prevent contamination (separate stains for 'clean' and 'dirty' specimens can help to reduce this).

Chapter 2

Sampling and preparation

Choice of sampling technique

Common sampling sites

Solid tissues and cysts
The most commonly harvested superficial specimens are from lesions within the skin, subcutaneous tissues and lymph nodes; the liver and spleen are the most commonly harvested internal viscera, but decent and often diagnostic samples can usually be safely taken from many others, including lung, thyroid, kidney, intestine, bladder, and the reproductive organs. If a lesion is visible on imaging, it can usually be successfully aspirated with at least some chance of a quick definitive diagnosis.

Whilst valuable diagnostic information can be gleaned from cytological examination of most masses, common exceptions include mammary lesions and fluid-filled cystic masses. Mammary masses often have a highly heterogeneous complex three-dimensional structure, and aspirates from there are often similarly mixed and confusing – the cytological appearance of mammary masses can correlate poorly with their behaviour. Whilst cytological examination of masses in mammary regions can be helpful to differentiate mammary masses from, say, mast cell tumours or lymph nodes, it is sometimes unhelpful in prognosticating about mammary neoplasia.

Examination of cystic masses is often unhelpful for a different reason – although many lesions can contain cystic areas, the cytological appearance of cystic fluid is similar regardless of the lesion in which they occur. Although cytology is sometimes valuable in reaching a diagnosis, histopathological examination of the wall of these structures is usually required for definitive assessment.

Fluids
The most frequently examined fluids are blood and pleural or abdominal effusions, but other fluid specimens which can be usefully assessed include urine, joint fluid, cerebrospinal fluid, and washes from a variety of locations (nasal, BAL, prostatic).

Impression Smears
Impression smears from ulcerated or inflamed cutaneous lesions often harvest predominantly surface inflammation only; only rarely do they provide helpful clues to underlying disease processes (such as acantholytic cells and non-degenerate neutrophils, raising suspicion for immune-mediated disease). Impression smears of swabs taken from the external ear canals, conjunctiva/cornea, sinus tracts, as well as smears of surgical biopsies, can provide limited information on infections and neoplastic processes more quickly than microbiological or histopathological examinations.

Sampling method by area

The diagnostic reward from these samples depends on the quality and preservation of the preparations – selecting the most appropriate sampling method greatly improves the chance of producing a diagnostic sample. Table 2.1 summarises the most appropriate sampling and preparation method for a variety of different tissues, based upon the author's and others' experience – although note that in most cases, using variety of sampling methods where possible (e.g. both suction and non-suction preparations for most solid lesions, direct, concentrated (or squash) and cytocentrifuged preparations for fluid) will improve preservation and therefore diagnostic chances.

For discussion of the techniques for these sampling methods, see Table 2.1.

Safety of cytological techniques and recommended precautions

Cytological sampling is minimally invasive and, in the majority of cases, can be performed without sedation. The risk associated with aspirating lesions is negligible in the majority of cases. Situations with slight risk of complications include the following.

- Aspiration of haemorrhagic lesions (such as thyroid masses, vascular neoplasms such as haemangiosarcoma).
- Aspiration of vascular organs (such as the liver or spleen) in patients with impaired coagulation ability.

Table 2.1 Recommended sampling and preparation techniques for different lesions

Lesion or specimen	Sampling method	Preparation technique
Hard masses, bone lesions	FNAB – suction (wider needle may be needed)	'Squash', 'blood smear'*
Soft masses, lymph nodes, vascular lesions/organs	FNAB – non-suction (smaller needles may be used to reduce blood contamination)	'Squash', 'blood smear'*
Effusions (bloody)	Fluid collection	Direct or buffy coat
Effusions (turbid), abscesses	Fluid collection	Direct or concentrated**
Effusions (clear), CSF, urine, other poorly-cellular fluids	Fluid collection	Cytocentrifuged preparation
Viscous fluid (e.g. synovial)	Fluid collection	Direct or squash
Surgical biopsy, ulcerated lesions	Impression smear	Imprint
Conjunctiva/cornea, very firm cutaneous lesions, plaque-like lesions	Scraping	Imprint or roll
Mucosae, ear canals, sinus tracts	Rolled swab	Roll
Respiratory tract	Tracheal wash or broncho-alveolar lavage	Direct, concentrated or cytocentrifuged**
Nasal masses, prostate***	Direct aspirate where possible, wash where not	'Squash', 'blood smear'* for direct aspirate, direct or concentrated** for washes
Bladder masses***	Direct aspirate where possible, traumatic catheterisation where not	'Squash', 'blood smear'* for direct aspirate, direct or concentrated** for washes

*where sufficient fluid/blood is present
**depending on cellularity
***although prostatic and bladder washes eliminate the risk of needle-tract metastasis from neoplasia, in the author's experience the diagnostic quality is generally inferior to direct prostatic aspirates

- Aspiration of mast cell tumours leading to histamine release.
- Aspiration of lesions in highly excitable patients.
- Aspiration of internal distended sites under pressure (e.g. abdominal abscess, distended gall bladder – risk of rupture/leakage).
- Failure of sterility (risk of implantation of infection).
- Aspiration of intra-thoracic lesions (slight risk of pneumothorax).
- Aspiration of adrenal masses with suspected phaeochromocytoma (hypertension followed by paradoxical hypotension has been reported).
- Aspiration of neoplastic lesions which may seed along the needle tract*.

Recommended precautions in these cases are as follows.

- When aspirating lesions suspected to be haemorrhagic, or from patients with impaired coagulation ability, then close monitoring of the patient for half an hour to an hour following sampling to assess for bleeding is recommended.
- Pre-sampling treatment of patients with suspected mast cell disease with antihistamines may be prudent, and having equipment and medication for anaphylaxis treatment close to hand is recommended.
- Highly excitable, stressed or aggressive patients may be sedated prior to sampling.
- Distended sites that may be under pressure should be sampled with care, especially if internal where rupture or leakage from the site may lead to surgical intervention.
- High standards of sterility should be maintained as much as possible during sampling.
- Pneumothorax is extremely rare following sampling of intrathoracic masses but appropriate equipment should be nearby to deal with the complication if it arises.
- Similarly, the risk of hypotension following aspiration of suspected phaeochromocytomas appears to be very rare, but caution, as above, is advised when attempting aspiration of these lesions.

*Needle-tract metastasis has been reported in urothelial (transitional cell) carcinoma, renal carcinoma, pulmonary adenocarcinoma, pancreatic carcinoma and osteosarcoma, but it is extremely rare, and implantation is most commonly associated with surgical procedures rather than needle aspirates. The relatively low risk of needle-tract implantation neoplasia must be weighed against the value of rapid diagnosis and the limited treatment options available for these neoplasms.

Sampling techniques
Fine needle aspirate biopsy (FNAB)

The preparation required for FNAB is similar or less than that required for blood sampling – clipping of the hair over the sampling area is often unnecessary but may be warranted where it will aid visualisation of the lesion, or where internal organs or body cavities are to be entered and where sterility or contamination is more of a concern. An alcohol swab is recommended for most lesions to clean the area and reduce the risk of contamination with surface commensal organisms where infection is suspected.

If ultrasound contact gel or anaesthetic cream is used, then as little as possible should be applied and excess gel/cream should be wiped away before sampling as it can have a significant effect on the diagnostic quality of samples (sterile water or surgical spirit can be used as alternative coupling media). (Fig 2.1)

Suction Vs non-suction

The simple answer to whether lesions should be biopsied with suction applied or without is usually 'both', as each technique has advantages or disadvantages. Unfortunately, limitations of

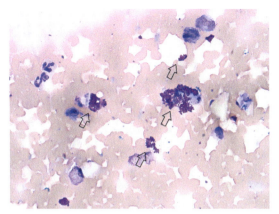

Fig 2.1 Gel contamination (open arrows; cytologically appears as irregular purple granules obscuring cells and other features)

FNAB without suction (fenestration technique) (FIG 2.2)

- Set aside a 5ml or 10ml syringe containing 4–6mls of air.
- Select a needle – 23–25 gauge is recommended (the softer or more vascular the lesion, the smaller the needle required).
- Introduce the tip of the needle into the lesion, holding the lesion firmly with the non-dominant hand.
- Gently rotate and the needle within the lesion to collect a core of cells within the needle hub; repeatedly move the needle back and forth within the same needle tract (this creates a slurry of cells and tissue fluid which move into the needle via capillary action).

time and the patient's patience often mean that one or the other must be chosen.

The non-suction technique (also known as fenestration) is slightly easier to perform, tends to reduce blood contamination and improve the preservation of fragile cells (such as lymphocytes). Cellular yield may be increased or decreased compared to suction techniques, depending on the type of lesion sampled.

The suction technique is most useful for lesions that do not exfoliate well and may be easier (or at least kinder) to perform in more sensitive areas, as adequate samples can often be obtained with a single needle penetration of the skin.

The choice of technique depends to some extent on experience and personal preference – as a general rule, the firmer the lesion is on palpation, the more likely it is to exfoliate poorly. Vascular lesions will usually produce haemodiluted samples when aspirated. Overall, soft lesions and vascular lesions will generally produce better samples without aspiration, whereas firmer lesions may require suction to be applied, although it should be noted that many firm lesions will exfoliate well enough with the non-aspiration technique to produce diagnostic samples.

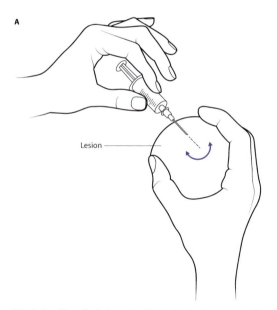

Fig 2.2a Needle is inserted into the lesion, rotated and moved back and forth

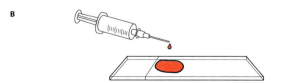

Fig 2.2b The syringe is attached and the sample is expressed onto a slide

- Withdraw the needle, attach the pre-prepared syringe, and express the sample onto a slide (see below for spreading).

Repeating this procedure in several different areas of the lesion will improve diagnostic accuracy.

FNAB with suction (aspiration technique)
(FIG 2.3)
- Select a 5 or 10ml syringe.
- Select a needle – 21–23 gauge is recommended (the softer or more vascular the lesion, the smaller the needle required) and attach to the syringe.
- Introduce the tip of the needle into the lesion, holding the lesion firmly with the non-dominant hand.
- Apply a small amount of negative pressure and release one to three times (redirecting the needle slightly each time may increase cellular yield, although avoid repositioning within the lesion when sampling within a body cavity (lateral movement of the syringe can occasionally damage blood vessels)). Instead, withdraw the needle slightly, reposition and reintroduce the needle. The appearance of material within the hub of the needle is a good indicator of successful sampling but is not necessary.
- Release pressure on the syringe and withdraw the needle from the lesion.
- Remove the syringe from the lesion, withdraw 4–6mls of air, then reattach the needle and express the sample onto a slide (see below for spreading).

General tips for FNAB
- If blood is noted in the syringe hub at any point, stop the current sample and prepare the slide – further sampling is only likely to increase the degree of blood contamination.
- If repositioning the needle during sampling with internal organs such as the liver, do not reposition *within* the lesion – lateral movement of the needle can act like a blade;

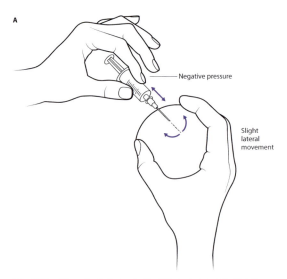

Fig 2.3a Needle is inserted with syringe attached and negative pressure applied

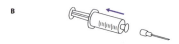

Fig.2.3b Syringe is detached, filled with 4–6mls of air and reattached ready to express the sample

instead, withdraw the needle from the lesion/organ, reposition and then reintroduce the needle.
- If fluid is aspirated, place in an EDTA tube (for better preservation) and a plain tube (if culture may be required – EDTA has mild antibacterial properties) then repeat aspiration to attempt to retrieve soft tissue.
- The core of larger lesions may be necrotic – sampling the periphery of these lesions is more likely to be useful; bony lesions, however, are often surrounded by peripheral osteomyelitis – sampling the centre of these lesions is more likely to be rewarding; sampling from multiple sites of larger lesions (centre, periphery, different anatomic locations) may be useful.
- Mammary lesions in particular often have complex and mixed pathology and can be challenging to interpret cytologically; histopathological examination is usually more

useful for mammary masses (especially in dogs).
- The use of smaller gauge needles, where possible, will reduce blood contamination and minimise pain/discomfort associated with the procedure.

Slide preparation techniques for FNAB

Expel a small drop of sample, roughly the same amount as that required for the production of a blood smear, onto a clean slide. Again, similar to a blood smear, the sample should be placed approximately a third of the way along the slide, rather than directly in the centre (fig 2.4).

The sample now needs to be spread so that the cells within it can be examined. Ideally spreading creates many areas of monolayer – that is, areas on the slide where cells are in a single layer, so that they can be easily assessed – without rupturing the cells.

There are several techniques described to obtain this ideal outcome; the author's preferred methods are summarised below, along with several techniques which generally produce poor samples.

'Squash' preparation (slide over slide)
(FIG 2.5)
- Place sample on a clean slide, as above.
- Take a second clean slide (the 'spreader').
- With the spreader at right angles to the sample slide, lay the spreader on top of the sample material on the sample slide. Do not press the slides together as this may lead to cell rupture*.

- Lightly move the spreader slide across the length of the sample slide – again with no downward pressure*.
- Both the sample slide and the spreader slide can now be stained for examination.

*Very thick or viscous samples may require slight downward pressure to help spread them, however this must be kept to a minimum to reduce cell rupture.

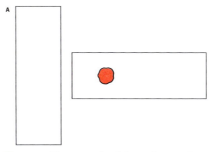

Fig 2.5a The sample slide and spreader at right angles to each other are gently moved together (avoid squeezing together)

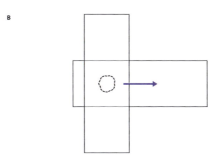

Fig 2.5b The spreader is moved lightly across the sample slide and removed at the end

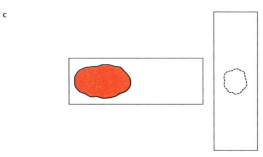

Fig 2.5c Both spreader and sample slide should now have well-spread cells and material

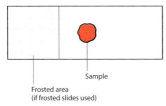

Fig 2.4 Ideal positioning of sample on slide

'Blood smear' preparation (FIG 2.6)

This technique is suitable for more fluid samples and is often very useful for lymph node aspirates.

- Place sample on a clean slide, as above.
- Take a second clean slide (the 'spreader').
- Incline the spreader to 45 degrees and place on the sample slide in front of the specimen.
- 'Reverse' the spreader gently onto the specimen so the material spreads along the edge of the spreader slide.
- In a single smooth motion, slide the spreader forward across the sample slide.
- The sample slide is now ready to be stained.

> Note: for fluid samples with low cellularity, the 'line smear' variant is useful; instead of spreading the fluid all the way across the slide, the movement is stopped abruptly to concentrate the cells in a thin line.

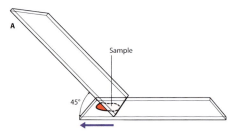

Fig 2.6a The spreader slide is held at 45 degrees in front of the sample

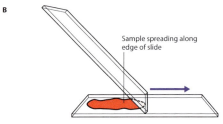

Fig 2.6b The spreader is reversed onto the sample

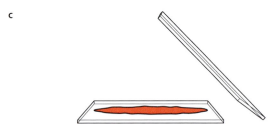

Fig 2.6c The spreader is moved in a single motion across the length of the sample slide

General tips for slide preparation

Avoid placing or spreading the specimen to the very end of the slide – the edges of samples are often the best areas of monolayer and may be lost if they fall off the edge of the slide; also, many automated stainers (used in most commercial labs) do not stain 1–2cm at either end of the slide.

Not recommended – 'Shotgun' preparation and 'Starfish' preparation

Despite their more exciting names, these techniques are not recommended unless other techniques are not possible as they usually produce thick, dense areas of material with only small areas of monolayer at the periphery of the specimens. (Fig 2.7)

The 'shotgun' technique involves blasting the specimen in multiple small droplets across the preparation without further spreading. Although it is sometimes necessary due to limitations of time or the specimen sampled, it is to be avoided where possible.

The 'starfish' technique is a method of spreading material across the slide using the tip of a needle. Although cell preservation is often better than may be expected, the technique does a poor job of spreading the material.

Fluid and wash preparations

Fluid collection is straightforward for most samples, although specialist techniques and great attention to sterility are required for some samples (see below).

Preparation of fluid samples is dependent on the amount of material aspirated. With an

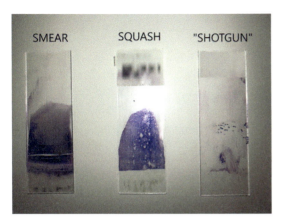

Fig 2.7 Well-prepared stained smear and squash techniques, and an example of 'shotgun' preparation

a broad assessment of appearance and overall cellularity.

Concentrated preparations are useful for less cellular fluids – the 'line smear' variant of the blood smear technique (see below) is useful for this. Alternatively, a clean wooden, plastic or glass stick can be drawn through concentrated droplets of fluid to spread them across the slide. (Fig 2.8)

Cytocentrifuges are used in commercial labs to concentrate fluid with very low cellularity (such as CSF, urine or BAL samples). Although cytocentrifuges are expensive and impractical to use in general practice, several papers have described using kitchen salad spinners instead

ample harvest, and where fluid is to be submitted to an external laboratory, the sample should be divided between EDTA and plain tubes. EDTA is most suitable for cytology and cell counts as it preserves cells, but it has a mild antibacterial effect (due to prevention of biofilm formation) – sterile plain tubes are more useful if culture is to be performed, and if biochemistry is required on the submitted fluid.

The author recommends not routinely adding formalin if preparations are to be examined immediately – formalin condenses cells and makes them harder to identify. If sending to an external laboratory, check with them first to see whether they would prefer formalinised or non-formalinised samples.

Fresh fluid preparations will be needed for in-house examination, and they will also be valuable when submitting to an external laboratory, where sample permits. Even if the sample is not going to be examined immediately, fresh fluid preparations should always be made as soon as possible (to avoid deterioration of cells, and therefore to improve sample preservation). Direct smears of fluid (prepared in an identical fashion to the 'blood film' technique above) are most useful for cellular smears and fluids where cellularity is unknown, although they should be performed on all fluids to give

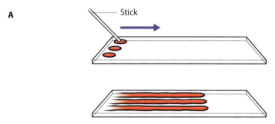

Fig 2.8a 'Stick' preparations – the fluid is concentrated (via sedimentation or low-speed centrifugation) and a stick is drawn through droplets of concentrated fluid

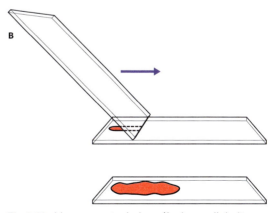

Fig 2.8b Line smear technique (for low-cellularity fluids): The procedure is identical to making a blood smear except that the movement of the slide is abruptly halted to concentrate the cells in a line at the end of the smear

to similarly concentrate samples with encouraging results (see Bibliography). As an alternative, using centrifuges at low-levels (roughly 1,500 rpm) for ten minutes should help to concentrate samples without excessive cell lysis.

For highly blood-contaminated samples, a buffy coat preparation can be made: the sample is placed in a microhaematocrit tube and centrifuged at high speed. The tube is then cut at the thick buffy coat, containing the concentrated cells, and this material is placed upon a slide and prepared as for other specimens. (Fig 2.9)

Synovial fluid

The approach to sampling synovial fluid depends upon the joint sampled – the simplest joints to sample are usually the stifles, whereas the carpus and tarsus are the most difficult (largely due to the volume of fluid within these spaces, as well as the anatomical challenge of introducing the needle). A detailed description for sampling each joint is beyond the scope of this book, but the following general points are consistent for synovial fluid aspirates.

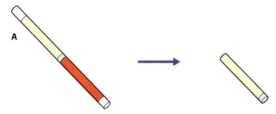

Fig 2.9a The microhaematocrit tube is cut at the level of the buffy coat

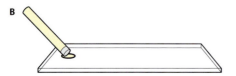

Fig 2.9b The material at the cut is expressed onto the slide and spread as with other techniques (most typically as a blood smear)

- Full aseptic technique must be followed for synovial samples, as normal joint spaces are sterile.
- Synovial fluid is viscous and therefore suction is likely to be required, especially for joints with minimal or no effusion.
- Needle sizes of 21–23g will be suitable, although for smaller patients (and smaller joint spaces), 25g may be used.

Procedure

- Select a 21–25g needle (see above) and attach to a 2.5ml syringe.
- The patient is suitably restrained and (usually) placed in lateral recumbency, with joint to be sampled (aseptically prepared) uppermost.
- Flexion or hyperextension of the joint, where possible, should aid identification of the joint capsule.
- Carefully advance the needle through the joint capsule into the joint space (gentle movements to avoid damaging the articular surfaces are recommended).
- Apply gentle suction to the needle to aspirate joint fluid (the amount produced will vary due to the joint sampled and the underlying condition).
- Release suction before withdrawing the needle from the joint space (to reduce the risk of blood contamination).
- Prepare fresh smears using the 'blood smear' technique described above and divide sample into an EDTA tube (for improved preservation) and plain tube (for culture), as above, although there is likely to be limited sample – prioritise based upon the most pressing clinical requirement.

Tracheal wash/broncho-alveolar lavage

These are both techniques for sampling the respiratory tract, most useful for assessment of patterns of inflammation. Neoplasia within the respiratory tract only rarely exfoliates into fluid samples; where this is suspected, direct aspiration of suspected lung lesions is more likely to produce a diagnosis.

Trans-tracheal washing (TTW) is a technique whereby a catheter is inserted into the trachea via a cutaneous incision in the neck, or intra-orally alongside an endoscope. Although it can be used in small animals (particularly those deemed too much of an anaesthetic risk for broncho-alveolar lavage), it is most commonly used for larger patients (mostly horses). Samples from tracheal washes, perhaps unsurprisingly, are more likely to reflect inflammation and pathology within the wider airways such as the trachea and bronchi.

Bronco-alveolar lavage (BAL) is more likely to be familiar to small animal practitioners. Samples using this technique are more likely to reflect deeper respiratory inflammation and pathology within smaller airways. Although this theoretically allows for localisation of washes to specific areas of pathology, in the author's experience samples taken from different areas of the deep respiratory tract of the sample patient seldom produce significantly different samples. BAL is most usefully performed using a bronchoscope, but the technique can be carried out very effectively without ('blind BAL'); a brief summary of this procedure follows. (Fig 2.10).

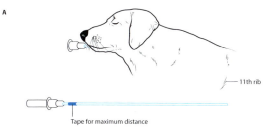

Fig 2.10a The catheter is measured against the patient from the nose to the 11th rib and this distance (which represents the maximum distance the catheter can be inserted) is marked with tape

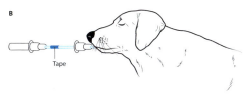

Fig 2.10b The marked catheter is inserted into the ET tube to somewhere between the 4th and 11th rib

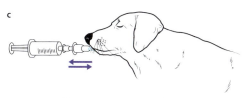

Fig 2.10c Warmed saline and air is injected into the catheter and immediately withdrawn (up to three times)

- The patient is anaesthetised and placed in sternal recumbency or lateral recumbency (with the most severely affected lung on the table). Pre-oxygenation is recommended.
- Select a small sterile urinary catheter (5-Fr is usually suitable) and mark the distance (with surgical tape or similar marker) from the nose of the patient to the level of the 11th rib (this is the **maximum** distance the catheter should be inserted).
- Thread the catheter through the endotracheal tube, taking care to avoid the oropharynx (oropharyngeal contamination makes assessment of the sample much more challenging) gently until resistance is felt, then slightly withdraw the catheter (this should be somewhere between the 4th and 11th rib spaces for suitable sampling).
- Attach a syringe containing warmed sterile saline to the catheter (volume required: 5ml/Kg for cats, 2–5ml/Kg for dogs) and a further 5ml of air (to ensure the whole amount of fluid is introduced.
- Introduce the fluid/air rapidly into the catheter then immediately withdraw until no more fluid is obtained.
- Repeat aliquots of fluid may be introduced to ensure sufficient sample is retrieved but no more than three aliquots should be used.
- Prepare fresh, concentrated and (where possible) centrifuged smears as described above

(BAL preparations are usually very poorly cellular); where fluid is to be submitted to an external laboratory, use EDTA tubes for preservation and plain tubes for culture (where possible).

Nasal flushes

Nasal flushes are often unrewarding for clinicians, cytologists and patients. They can be performed retrograde or anterograde; results are generally similar. There follows a brief description of a technique for sampling anterograde (Fig 2.11).

Advance a small gauge catheter into the external nares, flushing and aspirating small volumes (5–10ml) of warmed saline whilst advancing and retracting the catheter. The sample yield can be improved by making a small nick in the side of the catheter, providing a rough surface that can help dislodge tissue. The patient should be anaesthetised with an inflated ET tube or a packed nasopharnyx to prevent aspiration.

Traumatic catheterisation (bladder samples)

Lesions within the wall of the bladder can exfoliate into urine, but this is unpredictable and uncommon. Direct aspiration of bladder wall lesions is most likely to yield a diagnostic sample, but where there are significant concerns about using this technique (such as needle-tract implantation of neoplasia, discussed on page 15), traumatic catheterisation can be a useful technique for sampling (Fig 2.12).

- Perform under anaesthesia or heavy sedation.
- Select a suitable urinary catheter size for the patient, as well as a 10ml (small patients) or 20ml (large patients) syringe.
- Introduce the urinary catheter into the urethra (the author is aware this is easier to write here than to perform in female patients) and empty the bladder.
- Locate the mass via rectal palpation or ultrasound (many suspect masses will be located

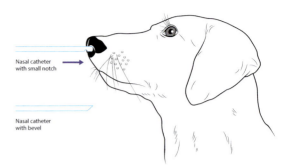

Fig 2.11 The nasal catheter can have a small nick or bevelled edge to provide a rough surface to aid tissue sampling

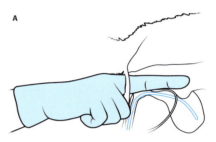

Fig 2.12a The catheter is localised over the mass, confirmed by rectal palpation

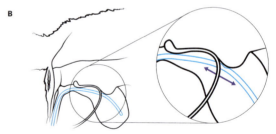

Fig 2.12b The catheter is moved back and forth over the mass whilst negative suction is applied to the syringe attached to the catheter

in the trigone (i.e. the caudal dorsal bladder) and place the catheter adjacent to it.
- Apply negative pressure to the syringe whilst moving the catheter back and forth over the mass.
- Prepare direct and concentrated preparations of the aspirated material, as above (if small sections of the mass exfoliate, prepare squash preparations of these, as above).

Prostatic wash

As discussed above, the risk of needle-tract implantation of neoplasia is relatively small, and in the majority of cases where prostatic lesions are to be sampled, direct aspiration is much more likely to produce a diagnostic sample. Techniques for prostatic wash have been described, but in the author's experience this sampling method often only samples the urethra as it passes through the prostate, rather than the prostate itself. Additionally, the sample quality is often very poor.

These factors combine to give a high risk of false negative samples where prostatic neoplasia is concerned, and for this reason prostatic washes should only be performed where there is significant concern about the risk of direct aspiration.

Impression smear

Impression smears of ulcerated lesions are frequently unrewarding, as they often only exfoliate surface inflammation and infection, rather than material from deeper lesions, but they can occasionally be helpful in identification of infectious agents.

Impression smears from surgical biopsies, in contrast, can provide rapid valuable and often diagnostic information while awaiting histopathology results (Figs 2.13 and 2.14). The recommended procedure is as follows.

- Cut the surface of the excised tissue and blot with paper towel or filter paper to clear excess blood and fluid.
- Press the cut surface of the tissue firmly onto a clean slide in several places (often the yield increases with each press – the final preparation is often the best.
- For very fibrous tissues, scarifying the surface of the sample with a scalpel blade will help to improve yield.
- No further spreading is required.

Scraping

This technique is used for very firm lesions, as well as surfaces that can't readily be aspirated (such as the cornea) (Fig 2.15).

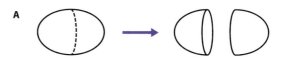

Fig 2.13a The excised sample is sectioned and blotted with filter paper to reduce blood contamination

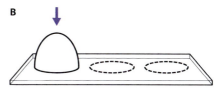

Fig 2.13b The sectioned sample is pressed onto a clean slide

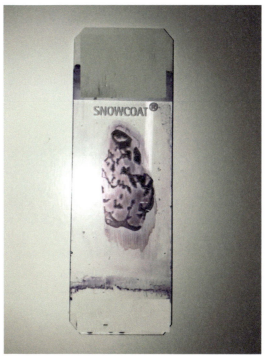

Fig 2.14 Gross appearance of surgical impression smear from a testicular neoplasm (already stained)

- Clean the surface of the lesion with a cotton swab or by flushing with saline to remove surface inflammation (which is often secondary).
- Using a sterile spatula (such as a Kimura spatula) or the blunt edge of a sterile scalpel blade, gently scrape the surface of the lesion, ideally along the margin, in one direction, until a small drop of the specimen appears.
- Transfer to a slide and smear as above.

Rolled swabs

Used for difficult-to-reach areas and lesions where the superficial inflammatory pattern or microorganism is of prime interest (e.g. ears, mucosae) Fig 2.16.

- A plain cotton swab is suitable for most lesions.
- For dry areas, moisten the swab prior to sampling (to improve adhesion to the swab).
- Gently swab the lesion and roll over the centre of a slide (rolling, rather than dragging, to reduce cell rupture) in one direction (do not roll back and forth over the same area).

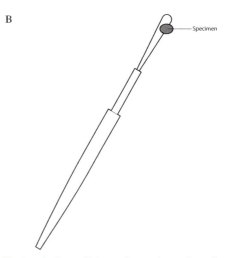

Fig 2.15b A small drop of sample on the edge of the spatula/scalpel

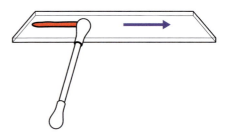

Fig 2.16 The swab is rolled over the slide in a single direction

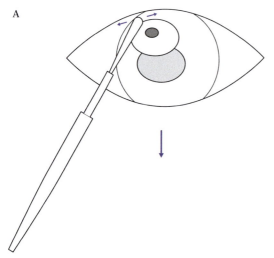

Fig 2.15a The spatula/scalpel is scraped along the margin of a lesion

Drying

Samples must be completely dry prior to staining or placing in slide containers (to avoid drying artefact and poor preservation) – air drying is suitable for preserving most cytological specimens and, once dried, the slides will remain usable for many months. The majority of specimens will dry very quickly in air, but for some samples (such as synovial fluid), a hair dryer set to cold or a fan can speed up the process.

Avoid blowing on the slides as this can lead to droplets of saliva contaminating the sample, as well as allowing the cytologist to judge the sampler's oral hygiene regimen.

Key points

Tips to improve preservation

- Use the non-aspirate (fenestration) technique wherever possible, especially lymph nodes, as it will reduce cell rupture
- Always be gentle when smearing samples; in particular, avoid downward pressure when using the 'squash' technique except in firm or gritty samples (Fig 2.5)
- Clear excess ultrasound/anaesthetic gel prior to sampling
- Sample the margins of larger lesions which may be necrotic rather than the centre (exception: bone lesions)
- Avoid talking over or blowing on specimens to reduce saliva contamination
- Ensure specimens are completely dry prior to staining/placing in slide boxes
- Never place histopathological and cytological specimens in the same package – formalin fumes ruin cytological samples!

Staining

Most standard cytological examinations use Romanowsky stains, with which material on the slide takes up different stains depending largely on the pH – acids take up red (eosinophilic) stain, whereas bases take up blue-purple (basophilic) stain.

Most commercial labs use methanol Romanowsky (MR) stains such as Wright or Wright-Giemsa, but in practice the use of aqueous Romanowsky (AR) stains such as *Diff-Quik* is more common. Both stains involve methanol fixation, although in MR stains, the dyes are dissolved in methanol, whereas in AR stains the dyes are dissolved in water and the methanol fixation is a separate step (the first 'dip').

There are some differences between MR and AR; principally, AR stains do not reliably stain cytoplasmic granules such as mast cell granules, basophil granules and lymphocyte granules, and this should be borne in mind when examining specimens.

The actual technique of staining the specimens varies depending on the stain used; the manufacturer's instructions should be followed in each case. Stains should not be left idle for too long – contaminants can build up in old stains and bacteria can eventually begin to grow, causing confusion or misdiagnosis of infection on the stained samples.

Labelling

Even for samples that are to be evaluated in-house, accurate labelling is important to prevent mix-ups and misdiagnoses. Minimum labelling should include the patient's surname and date of sampling. Ideally, if time permits, it will include the patient's full name and location of sampling too.

There are a variety of methods of labelling samples, from sticky labels to etching the slide. The author recommends using a frosted slide and writing on in pencil – this is hard to erase and simple to perform. Dedicated or aesthetically sensitive readers may consider using different coloured slides for ease of recognition and retrieval, but this is seldom necessary in practice. Label the slides themselves, rather than the

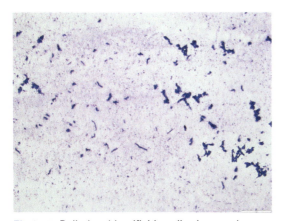

Fig 2.17 Rolled, unidentifiable cells, damaged during spreading (×100)

slide boxes they are stored in – this avoids mixing the slides up later.

For slides to be submitted for external evaluation, accurate labelling is essential (see chapter 13).

Storage

Once dried, either before or after staining, slides from cytological specimens can be safely stored for many weeks or months without significant sample deterioration. Refrigeration is not required – in fact it is not recommended as it can lead to condensation, adversely affecting preservation.

As mentioned in chapter 1, cover slips are not required for the relatively short period of time (weeks-months) that cytological slides are stored, although they may reduce deterioration in the longer term.

Chapter 2 – take home messages

- Mammary lesions and cystic structures are exceptions to the general rule of the high diagnostic utility of cytology; consider histopathology instead for these masses.
- Generally, the softer the lesion is, the smaller the needle required, and many cytological samples can be retrieved without suction; small needles and minimal aspiration reduce the risk of blood contamination.
- Wipe the area to be sampled clear of anaesthetic gel or ultrasound gel prior to sampling; gel contamination ruins cytological samples!
- Spread samples using the 'smear' or 'squash' techniques – avoid 'starfish' and 'shotgun'.
- When submitting externally, package histological and cytological specimens separately – formalin fumes also ruin cytological samples!
- Impression smears from ulcerated lesions are rarely as diagnostically valuable as aspirates from the same lesion.

Chapter 3

The basics of cytology

The sample has been taken. The patient, relieved, has escaped the consulting room, and the slide is labelled and prepared. Now for the difficult bit: *What do all the blobs mean?*

This chapter covers the very basics of cytology and is aimed at people who haven't looked down a microscope since long-ago student days, or for those completely new to the subject. It covers the very basics of microscopy and is intended to smooth the transition from beginners to cytologists. If you find that this material veers towards patronising, then you can probably safely skip to Chapter 4, where a more detailed discussion of cytological features begins.

What is all this stuff? (FIG 3.1)

Even 'poor' cytological samples often contain a lot of things to examine. The glib answer to 'What can I safely ignore?' is nothing! This was a sample taken at some cost to the patient, the client and the clinician, and it behoves the cytologist to interrogate the material.

Except... that's not really true. A great deal of material on that hard-won sample is likely to be irrelevant: ruptured cells, blood and its associated leukocytes, fingerprints and other keratin, debris from the slide or the stain, saliva from clinicians, bacterial commensals and contaminants, and so on. Diligently describing everything that is visible on a preparation in detail will produce a report that even Leo Tolstoy would think was 'a bit wordy'; the actual clinically relevant details will be lost in the forest of words.

Learning what is relevant and what isn't is an important cytological skill. It comes with patience, time and experience. The rest of this chapter is devoted to helping those new to the microscope to develop it.

What am I actually looking at?

The amount of material harvested from the patient varies greatly depending on the lesion. This is covered in more detail in Chapter 4 (see page 56), but lesions that have yielded a good cellular harvest are said to have *exfoliated* well, those that haven't have exfoliated poorly. (Figs 3.2 and 3.3)

The material will probably comprise a mixture of acellular debris, other acellular material, red blood cells and nucleated cells, in varying amounts. For most cytological cases, we are interested in examining nucleated cells, so let's start with a discussion of the nucleus, the cytoplasm, and the important things to note when examining them. After this, there will be a brief discussion of cytological artefacts and irrelevant material that can find its way onto cytological slides.

Nucleated cells (FIG 3.4)

By definition, these cells comprise a nucleus, and the surrounding supportive watery jelly-like material – cytoplasm. The size of the nucleus and the amount of cytoplasm vary greatly depending on the function of the cell and the stage of development, but the key point is that

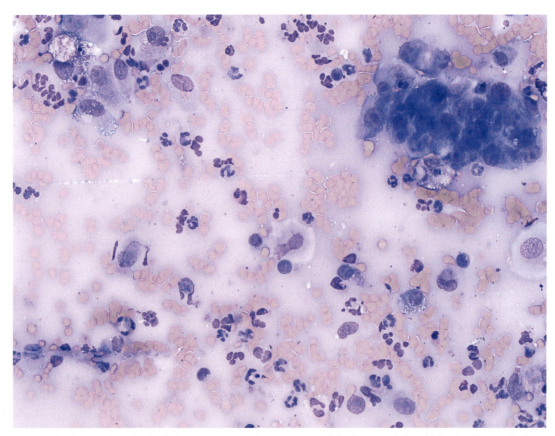

Fig 3.1 A mixture of cytological elements: macrophages, neutrophils, bare nuclei, red blood cells, atypical epithelial cells and lymphocytes

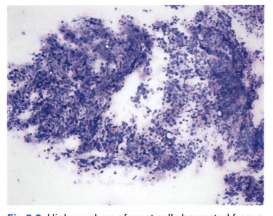

Fig 3.2 High numbers of mast cells harvested from a mast cell tumour – good exfoliation (×100)

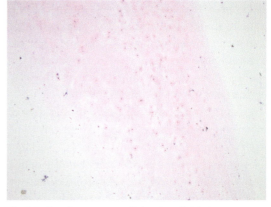

Fig 3.3 Small amounts of blood and debris harvested from a skin thickening – poor exfoliation (×100)

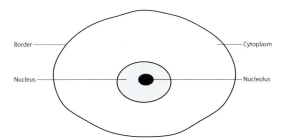

Fig 3.4 Diagram of an intact cell with nucleus, a single nucleolus and moderate amounts of cytoplasm

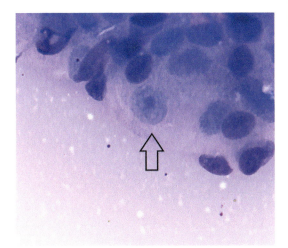

Fig 3.5a Cell with a single prominent nucleolus (open arrow) in a cluster of hepatoid epithelium from a perianal adenoma (×1000)

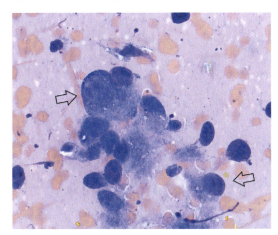

Fig 3.5b Cells with prominent multiple nucleoli (open arrows) from a malignant cutaneous neoplasm; small yellowish-brown haematoidin crystals are also present (×1000)

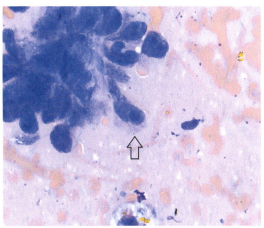

Fig 3.5c Cell with a prominent macronucleolus (open arrow) – note its size compared to the adjacent red blood cell – from the same neoplasm as 3.5b (×1000)

both the nucleus and cytoplasm should be visible through the microscope if a cell is intact. A common early mistake is attempting to interpret ruptured cells or bare nuclei.

Nuclei, nucleoli, bare nuclei and basket cells

The nucleus of a cell is packed with genetic material and its supporting apparatus, collectively termed *chromatin*. This chromatin is surrounded by a membrane, and the visible texture of the chromatin varies between cell types – this is the *chromatin pattern*, more on which later.

Nuclei are not featureless – they often contain *nucleoli*. These represent areas of activity (usually representing ribosome synthesis, a precursor to most cellular functions, particularly protein synthesis). As a general rule, the more nucleoli present, the more biologically active a cell is (Fig 3.5). Microscopically, nucleoli are usually visible as round dark patches against the paler chromatin, although some nucleoli appear paler than the surrounding chromatin (usually in cells with already dense dark chromatin, such as lymphocytes). Some nucleoli are linear, rather than round, particularly in neoplastic cells. Very large nucleoli (larger than a red blood cell) are termed *macronucleoli*, a finding strongly associated with malignant neoplasia.

Bare nuclei are often present to some degree in any reasonably cellular sample. These are cells that have ruptured during sampling and have had their cytoplasm stripped away from them. They can be confusing when first starting cytology because they can be confused for intact nucleated cells. They are quite easy to distinguish when no nucleoli are present, as they appear as irregular circles or ovals with no other circles within them.

Where nucleoli are present, they can be mistaken for cell nuclei, and the nucleus as a whole can be mistaken for cytoplasm. In general, bare nuclei are large, irregular and often have a moth-eaten appearance to the chromatin, frequently with irregular edges where the nuclear membrane has ruptured. Bare nuclei are sometimes termed 'basket cells', because of their very slight resemblance to the texture of a wicker basket, although the term is generally best avoided as they are not complete cells. (Fig 3.6)

For the most part, bare nuclei should be ignored and not interpreted, although the presence of high numbers of bare nuclei is worth noting, as they are found more commonly in very fragile neoplasms (such as lymphoma or neuroendocrine tumours – see pages 86 and 76, respectively).

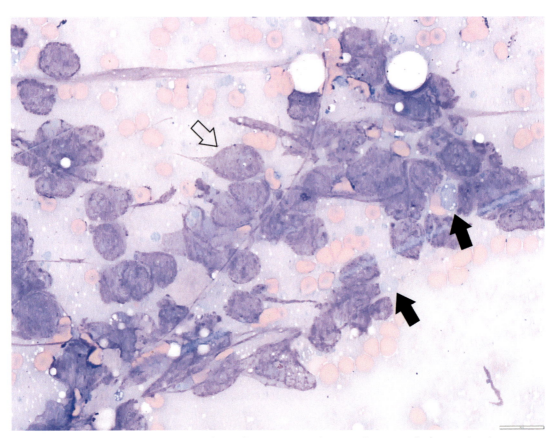

Fig 3.6 Bare nuclei aspirated from a lymphoma (open arrow and many other examples); note also the presence of cytoplasmic fragments, stripped away from their nuclei (closed arrows and other examples) – these are commonly found with ruptured lymphocytes and are sometimes termed 'lymphoglandular bodies' (×1000)

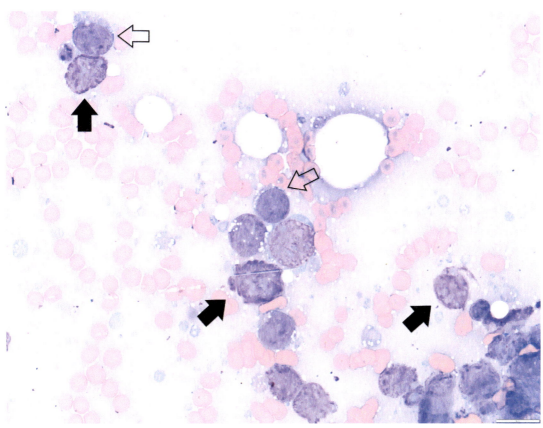

Fig 3.7 A mixture of intact and ruptured lymphocytes: intact cells (open arrows) have a thin rim of pale blue cytoplasm just visible, with rounder and denser nuclei; ruptured cells (closed arrows) have irregular nuclear borders, less dense nuclei and no visible cytoplasm. Cytoplasmic fragments are also present (×1000)

One challenge for novice cytologists is distinguishing between small lymphocytes and bare nuclei. Small lymphocytes are about as small as it is possible for a nucleated cell to be – they have small dense nuclei (about the size of a red blood cell, or very slightly larger) with a very small amount of cytoplasm. This tiny amount of cytoplasm can be difficult to spot, and often just appears as a thin pale blue rim around the edge of the cell. Close examination is often required to find this rim. If it is present, the cell is a small lymphocyte, if not then it is a bare nucleus. As the author will never tire of saying in this textbook, context is important – if the cells are surrounded by many other small lymphocytes, then they are likely to also be small lymphocytes. Similarly, bare nuclei are more likely to be surrounded by other bare nuclei. (Fig 3.7)

Streaming chromatin

Sometimes, not only the cell ruptures, but the nucleus does too. In these cases, the chromatin streams across the preparations, appearing as wispy purple ribbons, the same colour as chromatin (Fig 3.8). When this occurs, any hope of identifying the cell is lost, although it seems to occur most commonly with neutrophils. On preparations with large amounts of streaming chromatin, it may be helpful to search amongst the ribbons for intact neutrophils or bacterial organisms.

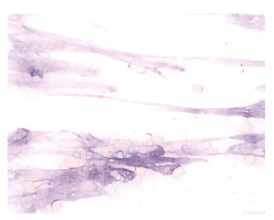

Fig 3.8 Ribbons or 'streams' of chromatin from ruptured neutrophils (×1000)

Rolled cells

Similar to streaming chromatin, rolled cells are the burst and rolled up nuclei of cells. Rather than wide ribbons of material, rolled cells appear as discrete basophilic linear structures, somewhat resembling (with a little imagination) an irregular roll of paper (Fig 3.9). Once again, whatever the cells once were, they are now impossible to identify, although this seems to occur more commonly to round cell tumours. When cells appear rolled, it appears to affect most of the cells present; that is, it is rare to find any intact cells accompanying them.

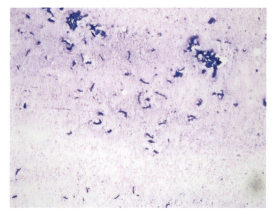

Fig 3.9 Rolled and identifiable cells from a cutaneous lesion (×100)

> **Key points**
>
> **Bare and intact nuclei**
> - Intact cells should have both a nucleus and cytoplasm visible
> - Macronucleoli (nucleoli larger than a red blood cell) are a strong feature of malignancy
> - To distinguish between bare nuclei and intact cells: bare nuclei are large, irregular and often have a moth-eaten appearance to the chromatin, frequently with irregular edges where the nuclear membrane has ruptured
> - In most cases, ignore bare nuclei and do not interpret

Examining and describing nuclei

The nucleus of a cell can reveal a great deal about it – the features below can all help to identify what type of cell is being examined:

Size

The size of the nucleus is most easily estimated by comparison to easily available structures of known sizes – neutrophils and red blood cells. Whilst both of them can vary in size somewhat, they are the closest available structure that a cytologist has to a standard reference size (Table 3.1). The size of the nucleus can then be estimated directly (by checking the size of neutrophils and erythrocytes in μm (see below) and then extrapolating the size of the nucleus, but in general it's easier to simply compare the nucleus with the chosen reference cell (e.g. the nucleus is 2–2.5 erythrocytes in diameter). The amount of variation in size (*anisokaryosis*) should also be assessed (Fig 3.10).

Table 3.1 Size of erythrocytes and neutrophils in dogs and cats (μm)

Average size (in μm)	Cat	Dog
Erythrocyte	5–6	7
Mature neutrophil	12–15	12–15

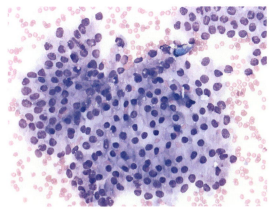

Fig 3.10a A cluster of prostatic epithelium; the cells display minimal anisocytosis and anisokaryosis (minimal variation in cell size and nuclear size) (×1000)

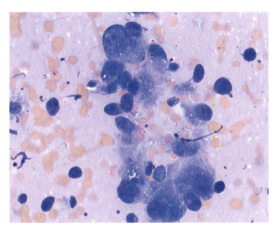

Fig 3.10b A cluster of atypical epithelium from a malignant cutaneous lesion; the cells display marked anisocytosis and anisokaryosis (marked variation in cell size and nuclear size); small yellowish-brown haematoidin crystals are also present (×1000)

Shape

Nuclei tend to be round or oval in shape – round nuclei are more often found in epithelial cells and round cells (see page 82), whereas oval nuclei are found in mesenchymal cells, although there is significant overlap, especially when cells are atypical (i.e. dysplastic or neoplastic). Some cells have 'indented' nuclei, others have 'floriform' or 'cerebreform' nuclei – this means the nuclei have multiple irregular indentations and so resemble a flower or a cerebrum (with a little imagination). (Fig 3.11)

Position

Briefly: central, eccentric (i.e. touching the cell membrane on one side) or paracentral/paracentric (slightly eccentrically positioned but not right at the edge of the cell) (Fig 3.12). There will be variation in this due to the way cells are spread out onto a slide; the important thing to decide is the most common position of the nucleus (for instance, histiocytes usually have central nuclei, whereas plasma cells have mostly eccentric nuclei – this is valuable when trying to distinguish between a histiocytoma and a plasma cell tumour).

Chromatin Pattern

The 'pattern' of chromatin refers to the density of the nucleus, and this is useful to assess because it often gives an indication to the activity of the cell – inactive cells usually have densely packed chromatin, and as activity increases, more DNA is unpacked for protein synthesis.

Cytologically, this broadly means that the darker and denser the chromatin appears, the less active the cell is. As cells become more active, chromatin 'opens' – it appears paler, less dense, and more nucleoli (see page 31) start to appear.

The 'texture' of chromatin (i.e. how open it appears) is hard to express linguistically. Some suggested terms are listed below (from broadly less active to more active cells, and from denser to less dense chromatin), but there is considerable variation in the way that the appearance of chromatin is reported. (Table 3.2 and Fig 3.13)

There are many exceptions to these general rules, and many cells have distinctive textures – mast cells, for instance, have 'smooth' or 'smudged' chromatin (where it is visible at all, it is often obscured by granules), as if someone has smeared the chromatin with their thumb. The 'cracked' chromatin in the table above, in plasma cells and nucleated red cells, is also

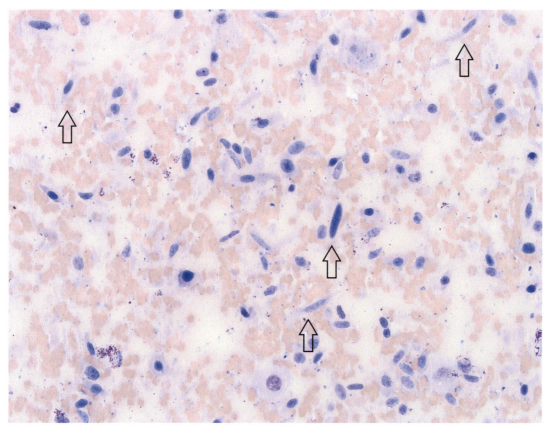

Fig 3.11a Oval nuclei (open arrows) aspirated from a fibroma; some cells are ruptured; others have small amounts of cytoplasm (×500)

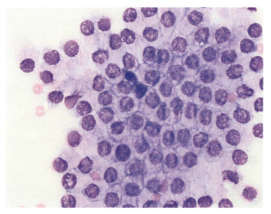

Fig 3.11b Round nuclei in prostatic epithelial cells (×1000)

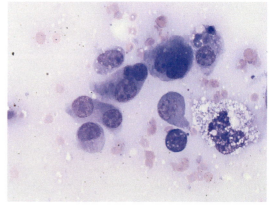

Fig 3.11c 'Polygonal' (rounded but variably-shaped) nuclei from a malignant neoplasm (×1000)

The basics of cytology | Chapter 3 37

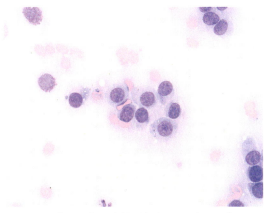

Fig 3.12a Central nuclei in histiocytes (×1000)

Table 3.2 Chromatin pattern descriptions

Description	Example cell type
Dense, hyperchromatic	Small lymphocyte, basal epithelium
Clumped, cracked	Plasma cell, nucleated erythrocyte
Coarse	Hepatocyte
Coarsely stippled	Histiocytes, macrophages
Stippled	Uncommon; sometimes malignant cells
Lacy, reticular	Germ cells (testicular, ovarian)

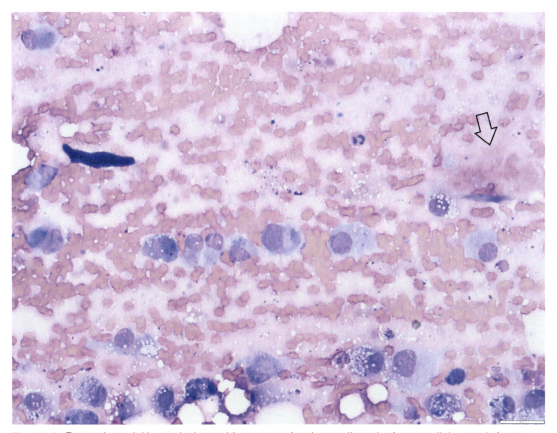

Fig 3.12b Eccentric nuclei in atypical osteoblasts; note also the small patch of extra-cellular matrix (open arrow) (×500)

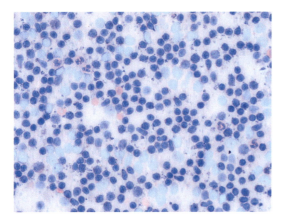

Fig 3.13a Dense chromatin in lymphocytes (×1000)

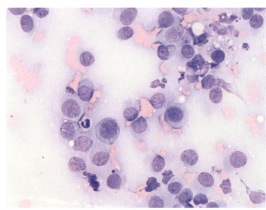

Fig 3.13d Coarsely stippled chromatin in histiocytes (×1000)

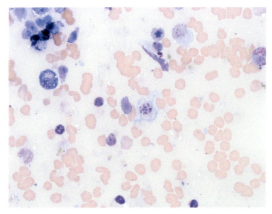

Fig 3.13b Clumped or 'cracked' chromatin in plasma cells (×1000)

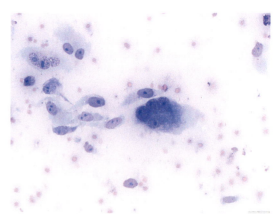

Fig 3.13e Stippled chromatin in a malignant mesenchymal neoplasm (×1000)

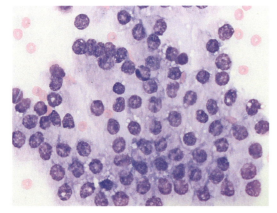

Fig 3.13c Coarse chromatin in prostatic epithelium (×1000)

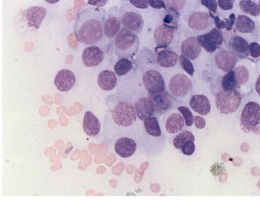

Fig 3.13f Lacy chromatin in a germ cell neoplasm (×1000)

distinctive, appearing something like a dried-up river bed. (Fig 3.14)

Describing chromatin patterns is challenging and different pathologists often disagree on which term to use in a particular cell, but broad general rule of 'more open = more active' is a useful one to keep in mind when examining cells.

> **Key points**
>
> **NUCLEI**
> - Size estimate by comparison to neutrophils or red blood cells
> - Epithelial cells – usually round nuclei; mesenchymal cells – usually oval nuclei
> - Dark dense chromatin usually indicates less biologically active cell; 'open' chromatin indicates more active cell

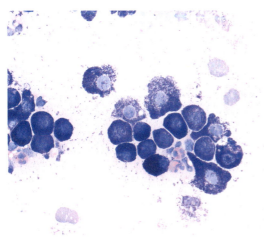

Fig 3.14a Smooth chromatin in mast cells (×1000)

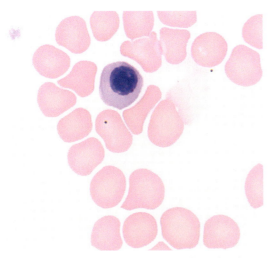

Fig 3.14b Cracked chromatin in a nucleated red blood cell (metarubricyte) (×1000)

Cytoplasm

The jelly-like cytoplasm, surrounding the nucleus and containing the cellular organelles, appears as a variably-coloured clear substance. Many cells have pale pinkish red or pale blue cytoplasm. RNA bound to protein (ribonuclear protein) stains blue with Romanowsky stains, and therefore, as a general rule, the more deeply blue the cytoplasm of a cell, the more metabolically active it is (see, for instance, plasma cells – page 68). (Fig 3.15)

Cytoplasmic fragments (lymphoglandular bodies)

Some preparations contain small grey fragments, slightly resembling platelets but with no obvious material inside, although they occasionally contain small punctuate (meaning 'tiny holes or dots') vacuoles. These are fragments of cytoplasm that have been stripped from the cells during sampling. They are sometimes called 'lymphoglandular bodies', as they were originally thought to be specific for malignant lymphoid neoplasia. They can actually appear with other cells than lymphocytes, although in practice if a preparation contains high numbers of cytoplasmic fragments, it is very likely that lymphoid tissue has been sampled.

They are not specific for malignancy, however. Neoplastic lymphocytes are often more fragile than reactive lymphocytes, and so cytoplasmic fragment numbers may be higher with

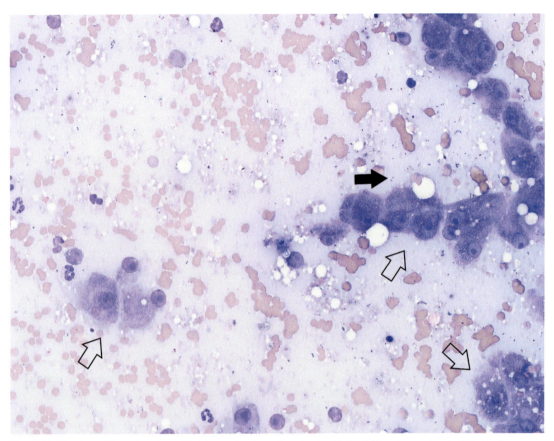

Fig 3.15 Clusters of hepatocytes with bluer cytoplasm than typical (×500) (due to presence of bacterial infection – scattered bacteria are present in the background, some indicated with solid arrow) (×1000)

neoplasia, but the presence of cytoplasmic fragments alone is not sufficient to diagnose lymphoid neoplasia. (Fig 3.16)

Granules and vacuoles

Cytoplasm is not featureless – it often contains vacuoles (clear, usually round, droplets) or granules (coloured, variably shaped and sized), which often helps to identify the origin of the cells.

Commonly encountered cells with vacuoles include sebaceous epithelium (see page 132), macrophages (see page 62) and hepatocytes (often with more diffuse vacuolation (i.e. vacuoles with indistinct borders; the overall effect is patchy paler cytoplasm – see page 188). (Fig 3.17)

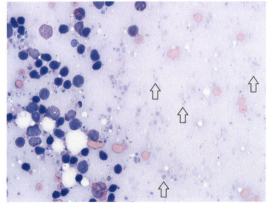

Fig 3.16 Cytoplasmic fragments in an inflamed lymph node (open arrows and many other examples) (×1000)

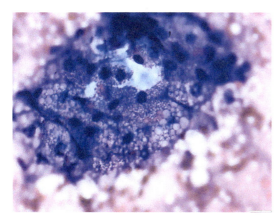

Fig 3.17a A cluster of well-differentiated sebaceous epithelium (×1000)

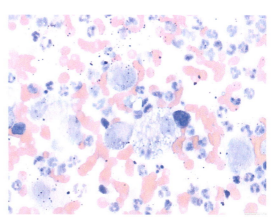

Fig 3.17b Large vacuolated activated macrophages (accompanied by neutrophils) (×1000)

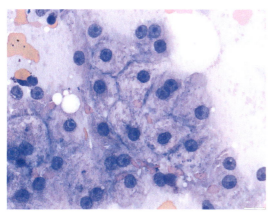

Fig 3.17c 'Indiscrete' vacuolation in hepatocytes – cytoplasm appears paler but obvious vacuoles are not evident; this is a common and quite non-specific finding (×1000)

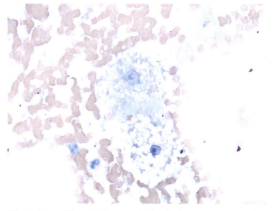

Fig 3.17d 'Discrete' vacuolation in hepatocytes – the vacuoles are more clearly defined; this is usually associated with increased lipid deposition within the cells (×1000)

Commonly encountered cells with granules include mast cells (dense purple granules), eosinophils (large red granules, round in dogs and oval in cats), lymphocytes (scattered small magenta granules, indicating the cell is either a T lymphocyte or a natural killer (NK) cell) and hepatocytes (small granules giving the cytoplasm a rough pinkish appearance similar to sandpaper). (Fig 3.18)

Remember that some granules, particularly mast cell granules, stain very poorly with aqueous Romanowsky stain (see page 27).

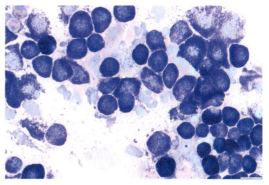

Fig 3.18a Heavily-granular mast cells in a mast cell tumour; granules from ruptured mast cells are also present in the background (×1000)

42 Part one | Cytological basics

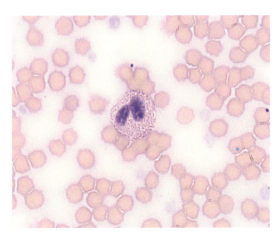

Fig 3.18b Feline eosinophil (centre of image) in a blood film; note the rod-shaped granules (canine eosinophils have round granules) (×1000)

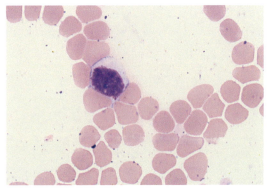

Fig 3.18c Granular lymphocyte in a blood film – very low numbers of faint reddish-purple granules are just visible in the pale blue cytoplasm (×1000)

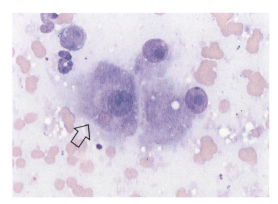

Fig 3.18d An intact hepatocyte with finely granular cytoplasm (open arrow); two ruptured hepatocytes are adjacent with similar cytoplasm (×1000)

> **Key points**
>
> **Cytoplasm**
> - More basophilic (bluer) cytoplasm typically indicates a more active cell
> - Cytoplasmic fragments often (but not always) indicate the presence of lymphocytes

Intact cells – examination and description

So far, we've discussed examining the nucleus and the cytoplasm as separate entities, but assessing the cell as a whole is critical to identifying them. The following section contains a guide to the important overall features to recognise and assess, as well as a brief guide to which features are typical of which cells (this is discussed in more detail in Chapter 4).

Cell shape

Specific cell shapes (specific for each tissue type e.g. cuboidal, caudate) are discussed in Chapter 4, but the general shape of the cells should be assessed (Fig 3.19). The most commonly noted shapes are:

Round – round cells, lymphocytes, epithelial cells

Fusiform (spindle-shaped or oval) – mesenchymal cells

Polygonal (irregular, often broadly round but can be slightly oval, varies from cell to cell) – macrophages, fibroplasias, malignancies

Cell borders

Cell borders should be assessed for how clearly defined they are. (Fig 3.20)

Distinct borders (clear demarcation of the edge of the cell) – round cells, epithelial cells

Indistinct borders (the cells fade into the background; the border is unclear and often 'wispy') – mesenchymal cells, neuroendocrine cells

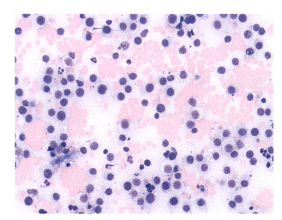

Fig 3.19a Round cells with round nuclei from a transmissible venereal tumour (×500)

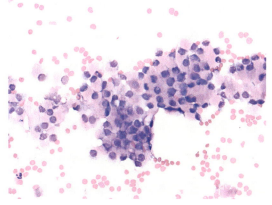

Fig 3.20a Distinct borders in prostatic epithelium (×500)

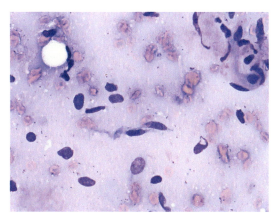

Fig 3.19b Fusiform (spindle-shaped) cells (centre of image) from a fibroma (×1000)

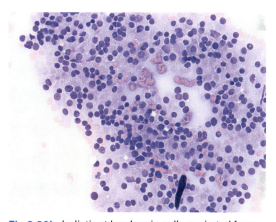

Fig 3.20b Indistinct borders in cells aspirated from an anal sac apocrine gland adenocarcinoma; note that the cells appear more like bare nuclei embedded in a pool of pale blue cytoplasm

Nuclear to cytoplasmic ratio (N:C)

Broadly, assess how much of the cell is taken up by the nucleus – cells with high N:C have very little cytoplasm surrounding their nucleus, and vice versa (Fig 3.21). With neoplasia, the N:C usually increases, and this is an important feature to help distinguish between malignant cells and other cells which mimic malignancy (such as activated macrophages – see page 323).

High N:C – lymphocytes, basal epithelium, neoplasia

Low N:C – macrophages, most other mesenchymal and epithelial cells

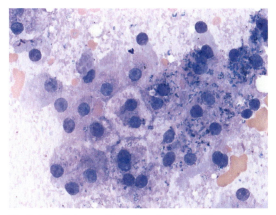

Fig 3.19c Polygonal hepatocytes (×1000)

44 | **Part one** | Cytological basics

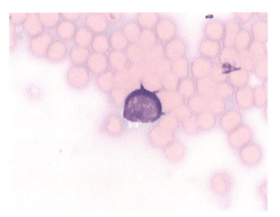

Fig 3.21a High nuclear: cytoplasmic ratio in a lymphocyte (centre of image) (×1000)

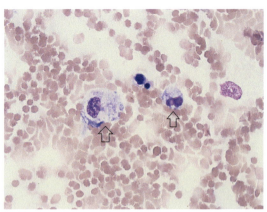

Fig 3.21b Low nuclear: cytoplasmic ratio in macrophages (open arrows) (×1000)

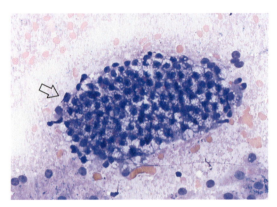

Fig 3.22a Minimal variation in nuclear and cell size and shape in a cluster of biliary epithelium (open arrow) (×1000)

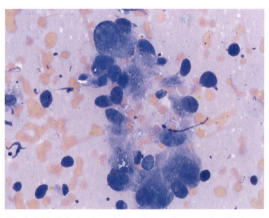

Fig 3.22b Marked variation in nuclear and cell size and shape in a cutaneous carcinoma (×1000)

Anisokaryosis, anisocytosis, and pleomorphism (FIG 3.22)

All of these have been discussed previously, but for clarity they are mentioned here as they are generally assessed together. They are all assessments of variation *between* cells (they are meaningless for an individual cell).

Anisokaryosis means variation in nuclear size between cells. *Anisocytosis* means variation in overall cell size. *Pleomorphism* indicates variation in cell shape.

As a general rule, the more variation in a cellular population, the more atypical (and potentially neoplastic) the cells are, but there are many cells that break this rule. For instance, activated macrophages can display marked pleomorphism and anisocytosis, although usually very little anisokaryosis; reactive mesothelial cells can display marked anisocytosis, anisokaryosis and pleomorphism. In contrast, lymphoma usually displays only mild anisocytosis, anisokaryosis and pleomorphism.

Cohesion

Cohesion is a measure of how tightly adhered to each other cells are and is very important to help identify they type of

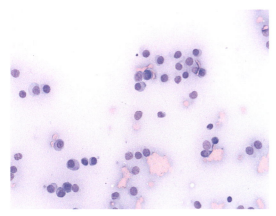

Fig 3.23a No cohesion amongst these cells from a plasmacytoma (×1000)

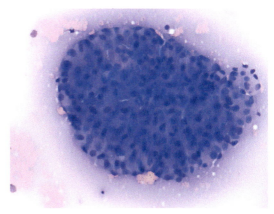

Fig 3.23c Tight cohesion in this cluster of hepatoid epithelial cells (×500)

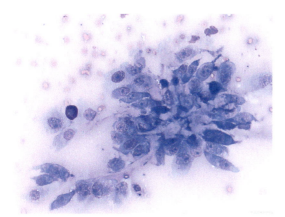

Fig 3.23b Loose cohesion in this aggregate of mesenchymal cells (×1000)

tissue being examined (discussed more in Chapter 4 – see page 72, Table 4.2). It is sometimes difficult to distinguish between high numbers of cells that are merely close to each other and cells that are actually stuck together. It is often more apparent on less cellular samples but with practice the distinction can often be made even on densely packed samples. (Fig 3.23)

- No cohesion (individual, discrete cells with no clear connection) – leukocytes, round cell tumours, poorly differentiated tumours.
- Loose cohesion (cells are sometimes found individually, sometimes in loose 'aggregates'); these aggregates often have frayed or irregular edges (see page 78) – mesenchymal cells.
- Tight cohesion (tight dense 'clusters' of cells, usually with rounded edges (see page 71); cells are rarely found individually) – epithelial cells, epithelioid macrophages (see page 65).

Nuclear moulding is a useful feature to notice when examining cohesion. It basically means that the nuclei of some cells are constrained by the cells (or nuclei) surrounding them, and so the shape of the nucleus takes on the contours of its surroundings. It can occur to nuclei within multinucleate cells (the nucleus conforms to the other nucleus or nuclei around it) or mononuclear cells (the nucleus conforms to the borders of the cells surrounding it); in either case, the presence of nuclear moulding is suggestive of malignant cells. (Fig 3.24)

The 3 (or 5) 'm's of description

When describing cytology for other clinicians, simpler terms are preferred to avoid confusion. As a description of scale, the author prefers to use 3 'm' adjectives, usually sufficient for most purposes, with a further two held in reserve for more extreme situations. They are not specific,

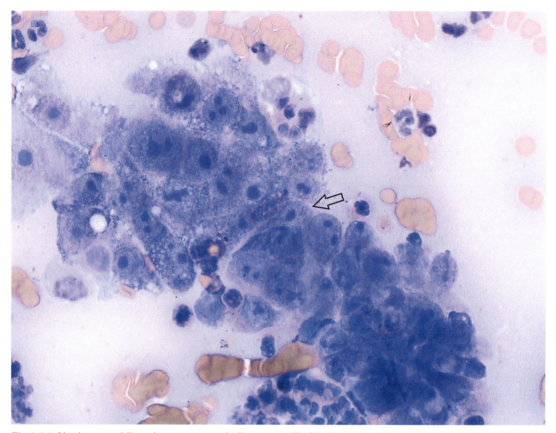

Fig 3.24 Nuclear moulding; the open arrow indicates a cell with a 'squashed' nucleus, conforming to the shape of its neighbouring nuclei; other examples are also visible (carcinoma) (×1000)

but are useful for comparison, and entirely appropriate for cytology, given the high degree of subjectivity. The adjectives are, in ascending order:

- (minimal)
- mild
- moderate
- marked
- (massive).

(Example: cellularity is minimal; the cells display moderate anisocytosis and anisokaryosis etc.)

> **Key points**
>
> **Examination and description of cells**
>
> *Nucleus*
> - Position
> - Size
> - Shape
> - Chromatin pattern
> - Nucleoli
>
> *Cytoplasm*
> - Colour
> - Vacuoles
> - Granules
>
> *Cell features*
> - Cell size
> - Cell shape

> **Key points**
>
> **Tips to improve preservation**
> - Borders (distinct/indistinct)
> - Nuclear to cytoplasmic ratio (N:C)
>
> **Tissue features (comparison of multiple cells)**
> - Anisocytosis, anisokaryosis, pleomorphism
> - Cohesion

Non-nucleated cells

Erythrocytes (FIG 3.25)

Red blood cells are present on almost every cytological preparation and are usually the smallest intact cells – even small lymphocytes are larger than erythrocytes. High numbers of them can make the assessment difficult, as they dilute the nucleated cells, which are usually of more interest, and make judging inflammation hard (see page 53, below).

Page 98 discusses how to distinguish between bleeding before sampling and haemorrhage during sampling (briefly: platelets are most suggestive of contamination during sampling, and macrophages containing red cells or red cell breakdown products indicate bleeding before sampling).

Red blood cells can also be a useful guide to preservation – erythrocytes have a standard appearance, and if they are poorly preserved then the appearance of the nucleated cells is not to be trusted (for instance, if they are markedly pleomorphic or varying in size, this may be due to preservation rather than representing true atypical cells).

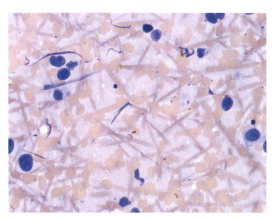

Fig 3.26 Haemoglobin crystals (the long linear needle-like structures, the same colour as red blood cells); bare nuclei, haematoidin crystals and streaming chromatin are also visible (×1000)

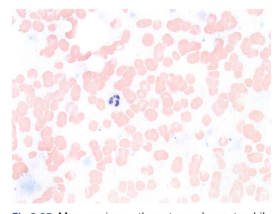

Fig 3.25 Many canine erythrocytes and a neutrophil (note that the neutrophil in this case contains faint reddish granules; this can make such cells difficult to distinguish from eosinophils, but eosinophils typically have many more and much larger granules) ×1000

Haemoglobin crystals

Very poorly preserved red blood cells are often found cytologically as haemoglobin crystals – linear crystals the same colour as erythrocytes (Fig 3.26). Their presence indicates drying artefact (i.e. the specimen was not properly dried before being placed into a slide holder) and, as above, suggests the preservation of nucleated cells is also likely to be suboptimal.

Common Cytological Artefacts (Or… what can I safely ignore?)

Cytological specimens are often messy, busy and chaotic. To apply some order to the slide, it is useful to be able to recognise common artefacts from the environment, not the patient.

Acellular debris

Scattered in amongst the red cells, leukocytes and other nucleated cells, there is likely to be at least some, and often a lot, of debris – small flecks of non-cellular material. Keratin is the most common component of this – see below. Other debris includes hair, crystalline fragments, glass fragments and contaminants from the stainer. Most of this material can be safely ignored, although large amounts of debris should be noted, if only because it makes the rest of the examination difficult. (Fig 3.27)

Contact gel

This is often found in samples from internal organs, but dermal preparations such as local anaesthetic cream or steroid ointment appear similar cytologically. Contact gel and ointments are frustrating because they often obscure large portions of the sample and render otherwise perfectly good samples non-diagnostic.

Cytologically, gels, creams and ointments appear as clumps of irregular purple granular material. (Fig 3.28)

Stain precipitate

This material is formed within the dyes used to stain cytological specimens. Over time, the dyes precipitate out into small round clumps, which if present in large numbers can obscure specimens, as with contact gel above. Stain precipitate can be particularly frustrating on blood films, as the small dark blue structures can strongly resemble Mycoplasma organisms. Regular changing of dyes, or at least changing when significant precipitate is noted on specimens, reduces the incidence of this problem. (Fig 3.29)

Fingerprints (keratin)

Everywhere we touch, we shed small amounts of the anucleate keratinised cells from the surface of our skin. If we touch a slide, we'll smear keratin bars (scrolls of keratin which appear as dense deep blue straight bars with angular ends) onto it, which can lead to the inaccurate interpretation that the structure aspirated is an epidermal inclusion cyst.

Additionally, squames and keratin bars are often floating in the air in the form of dust, and often find their way onto cytological specimens. It is a rare cytology slide which does not contain at least a small amount of keratin. Distinguishing contamination from true aspiration of keratin can be challenging, but in lesions which genuinely contain keratin, the material is most often aspirated in large irregular clumps and is often smeared across the slide during the spreading process, whereas contaminant keratin is usually

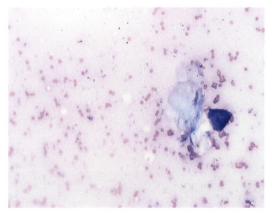

Fig 3.27a Keratinaceous debris (×500)

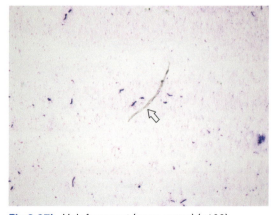

Fig 3.27b Hair fragment (open arrow) (×100)

The basics of cytology | Chapter 3 49

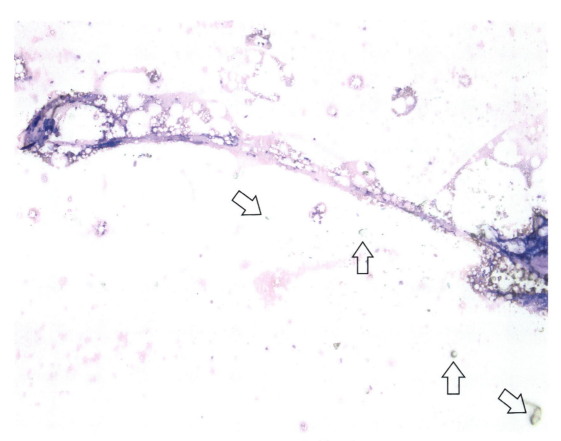

Fig 3.27c Crystalline debris (open arrows and other examples) (×100)

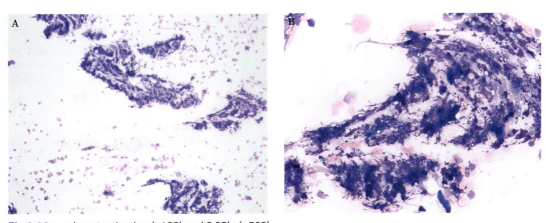

Fig 3.28a gel contamination (×100) and 3.28b: (×500)

found in small even amounts through the whole preparation (mostly where the slide was wet) or in shapes clearly visible as fingerprints. (Fig 3.30)

Haemodilution

There is some debate about the accuracy of this word – some pathologists argue that 'haemodilution' literally means 'dilution of blood with some

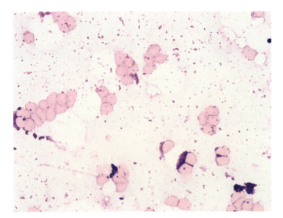

Fig 3.29 Stain precipitate with erythrocytes (×1000)

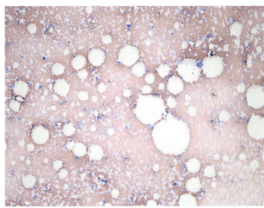

Fig 3.31 Marked haemodilution (×100)

Fig 3.30 Fingerprint contamination (×500)

other substance, rather than the more generally understood meaning of 'a specimen diluted with peripheral blood'). In this book, the author will use the term with the later, more commonly understood, definition, as it is the meaning most often encountered in pathological reports.

Haemodilution, as the name suggests, spreads out the cells of interests, and dilutes them with red cells, platelet clumps and blood-borne leukocytes. It is of particular frustration in samples of joint fluid and CSF, partially because it is hard to avoid during sampling, and partially because it makes the presence of neutrophils and other leukocytes difficult to interpret – is there genuine neutrophilic inflammation, or did they all come from the blood? (Fig 3.31)

Page 98 in Chapter 4 discusses how to distinguish between blood contamination and haemorrhage prior to sampling (but as a quick reminder: platelets usually indicate contamination, and haemosiderin/haematoidin pigments indicate bleeding before sampling). Estimating inflammation in the face of blood contamination is discussed on page 53.

Fibrinocellular aggregates

These are clumps of platelets, fibrin clots and leukocytes, mostly neutrophils, which can often be large (Fig 3.32). To the inexperienced cytologist, they can appear to be important, if poorly preserved, structures, sometimes mistaken for mesenchymal aggregates or epithelial clusters. They are, unsurprisingly, more common in significantly haemodiluted specimens.

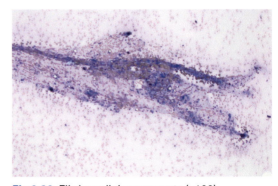

Fig 3.32 Fibrinocellular aggregate (×100)

Iatrogenic oral contamination

Whilst it may be dramatic to suggest that in a cytological sense, careless talk cost lives, it can certainly lead to a misdiagnosis. Chattering whilst sampling can lead to flecks of human spittle on the specimen which, when stained, appear as droplets of pale pink fluid. The fluid can sometimes contain oral squamous epithelial cells and, occasionally, even neutrophils and bacteria (Fig 3.33). Aside from the danger of over interpreting this material, observing it can make many cytologists feel rather queasy, and therefore minimising above-slide conversation is recommended.

Fungal spores, yeasts and bacteria

Fungal spores from moist or dusty environments, and commensal bacteria from the skin surface, the patient's (or clinician's) oral cavity

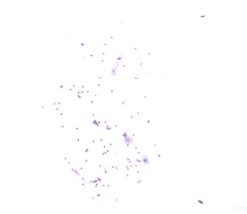

Fig 3.33 Human saliva contamination (×100)

or from external sites (such as contaminated dye) can make their way onto cytological specimens, and it can be challenging to distinguish them from pathogens (Fig 3.34). The most reliable clue that organisms represent contaminants

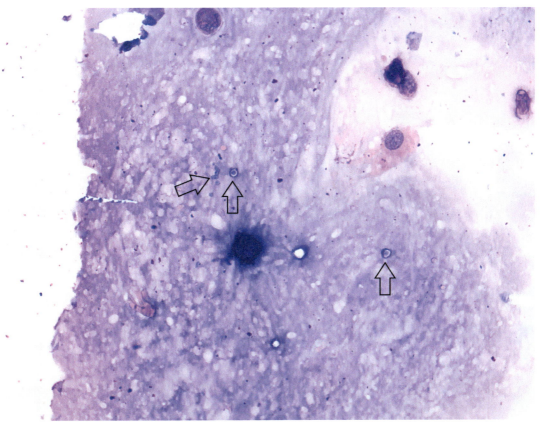

Fig 3.34 Fungal spores or yeasts contaminating a respiratory wash (note lack of inflammation) ×500

is a lack of inflammation, as opposed to the marked inflammation usually associated with pathogens. This is not a wholly reliable indicator, however – contamination can occur within specimens containing inflammation present for other reasons, and some pathogens can elicit surprisingly little inflammation.

See Chapter 5 for a discussion of how to distinguish these possibilities, but as a quick reminder: degenerate neutrophils are often associated with bacterial toxins, and organisms phagocytosed within leukocytes (usually neutrophils for bacteria and macrophages for fungal organisms) confirm the presence of infection.

Plant material, hairs and other objects

Contaminants from the environment and from the patient's coat are often seen on cytological specimens, and some plant structures can appear highly intriguing on cytology. As with infectious organisms above, a relatively simple rule of thumb applies to whether an observed peculiar unidentified structure is likely to be significant – is there inflammation associated with it? If not, then whilst it is useful to examine, describe, and document, it is likely to be unrelated to the reason for sampling. (Fig 3.35)

Relevant acellular material

Despite the minefield of contaminants and irrelevant material, some acellular material is useful or even essential for a diagnosis. Recognising this can be helpful even when no cells have been harvested. For a detailed discussion of the most relevant acellular material, see the last section of Chapter 4.

> **Key points**
>
> **Red cells and acellular material**
> - Haemoglobin crystals usually indicate poor preservation (often drying artefact)
> - Keratin is the most common acellular contaminant (often from fingerprints)
> - Some lesions such as chondrosarcoma or myxosarcoma predominantly comprise extracellular matrix

Other useful cytological concepts
Windrowing

The term 'windrowing' comes from agriculture, where it describes crops and vegetation that has been cut and laid out in long narrow rows; cytologically, it refers to cells doing the same thing: lining up in thin (usually single cell) narrow rows within the background (Fig 3.36). It usually occurs with erythrocytes (where it resembles rouleaux – see page 290) but can occasionally be observed with leukocytes and other non-cohesive cells.

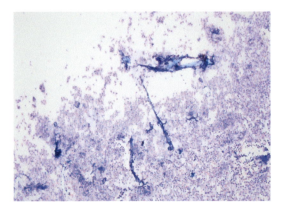

Fig 3.35 Large angular basophilic plant material contaminating a respiratory wash (×100)

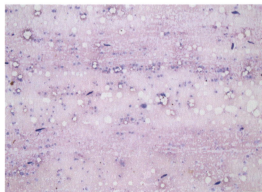

Fig 3.36 Windrowing at low power (myxosarcoma) (×100)

Windowing is a very useful cytological finding as it indicates increased viscosity in the sample structured; it is commonly seen in joint aspirates, as well as samples from salivary mucocoeles (see page 168), myxomas (see page 265) or other structures containing mucous or viscous material.

Estimating inflammation with blood contamination

One of the biggest problems of specimens containing large amounts of blood is estimation of inflammation; not only does the blood dilute the cells that were already present, it contains leukocytes. Additionally, leukocyte numbers within the blood vary depending on the state of health, stress or inflammation of the patient. Consequently, assessing the relevance of leukocytes (that is, whether or not inflammation is present), particularly neutrophils, is very difficult when blood contamination is present. Samples from many internal organs, particularly the liver and spleen, almost always contain large amounts of blood, making it always a challenge to estimate inflammation in these cases. (Fig 3.37)

There is no standard way of accounting for blood contamination. The author finds it helpful to imagine they are looking at a blood film, and asking themselves 'Would I consider this blood film to have an increased white blood cell count?' If so, then inflammation is possible (although, of course, the patient may *actually* have an increased white blood cell count). Additionally, with true inflammation, there is almost always

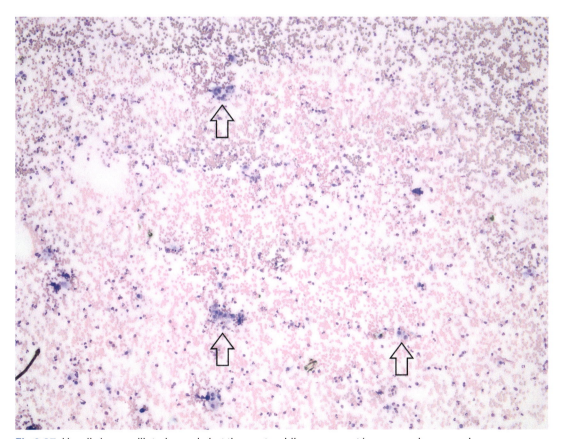

Fig 3.37 Heavily haemodiluted sample but the neutrophils are present in uneven clumps, and are accompanied by macrophages and mesenchymal cells (open arrows), consistent with inflammation (×100)

some other evidence that would not typically be found in blood alone (such as plasma cells, macrophages, mast cells or mesenchymal cells).

With very heavily haemodilution, the erythrocytes can pile up in multiple layers on the preparation, making it very hard to actually estimate how much blood is present, and consequently difficult to estimate how many of the leukocytes would be expected for blood contamination alone.

> **Chapter 3 – take home messages**
>
> - Avoid interpreting bare nuclei; intact cells should have nucleus and cytoplasm visible.
> - Round nuclei are more often found in epithelial cells and round cells; oval nuclei are found in mesenchymal cells.
> - Dark dense chromatin usually indicates less biologically active cell; 'open' chromatin indicates more active cell.
> - In general, the more variation in a cellular population, the more atypical (and potentially neoplastic) the cells are (although there are many exceptions including lymphoma, macrophages and mesothelial cells).
> - Some granules, particularly mast cell granules, stain very poorly with aqueous Romanowsky stain (i.e. *Diff-Quik*).
> - Haemoglobin crystals usually indicate poor preservation (often drying artefact).

Chapter 4

General principles of cytology

Stepwise approach to evaluating cytology smears

Cytological specimens are not standardised – they have great variation in the number of cells, their preservation, the material present in the background and the overall pattern. This variation leads to a near-infinite variety of appearances – even when the basics of cellular examination are understood (see Chapter 3), evaluating them can be overwhelming at first, particularly in samples with highly mixed cellularity. A stepwise, logical approach is recommended for each slide. Rational and repetitive examination applies order to the chaos and, with practice, allows a cytologist to rapidly and efficiently assess specimens.

With this in mind, there follows a suggested technique for evaluation of cytological specimens.

Initial examination and assessment of cellularity/preservation

On low power (4× or 10× objectives), scan the specimen whilst asking yourself the following questions.

- Does the sample have enough cells or other material (such as keratin) to draw a meaningful conclusion about its contents?
- Is the material on the sample likely to be representative of the lesion given the collection technique? (e.g. adipocytes present on a sample taken from a cutaneous mass are more likely to reflect inadvertent aspiration of subcutaneous fat than be a true representation of the lesion).
- Is the sample free of blood contamination (significant enough to hamper interpretation)?
- Is the cellular material adequately preserved? Are the cells present ruptured, rolled, or otherwise unidentifiable?
- Has the material on the preparations taken up adequate amounts of stain?
- Is the material evenly spread throughout the preparations? Are there suitable areas of monolayer for examination?
- Is the sample free of ultrasound gel, drying artefact, damage from formalin fumes or other contaminants (such as fingerprints/saliva) which are obscuring the detail of the preparations?

If the answer is 'no' to one or more of the above questions, it may be more useful to re-sample, where feasible.

Cellularity and preservation

Cytological examination is subjective. One cytologist's 'stippled' chromatin pattern may be another's 'lacy' (see page 37, Table 3.2 for more information on chromatin patterns). Nevertheless, cytologists find it helpful to label and describe what they're observing, partially so that other cytologists can understand what they have seen (although this will become less important with the rise of digital cytology and the ease of sharing images as well as descriptions – see Chapter 14), but also to help them order their thoughts and, ultimately, come to a decision upon their specimen.

One of the first things a cytologist is likely to do is describe the sample's cellularity (low, moderate, high) (Fig 4.1) and preservation (poor, moderate, good) (Fig 4.2). Deciding upon this at the beginning of the examination helps the cytologist decide how much information they are likely to get out of their sample. In general, of course, the more highly cellular and better preserved the material is, the more likely a diagnosis is to be reached, although the context of the sample is important; for instance, the mere presence of high numbers of cells within synovial fluid is likely to be relevant even if poor preservation makes their identification challenging.

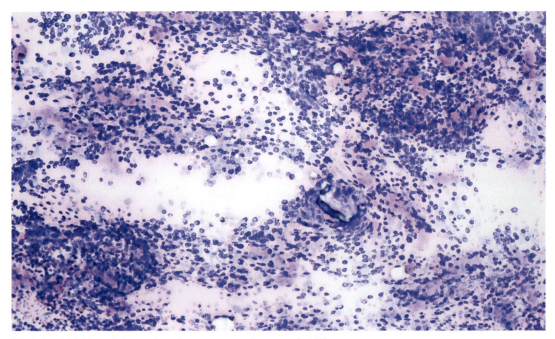

Fig 4.1a A highly cellular aspirate from a mast cell tumour (×100)

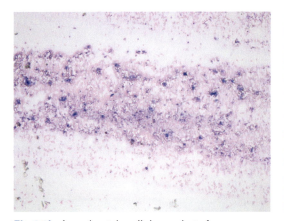

Fig 4.1b A moderately cellular aspirate from a malignant neoplasm (×100)

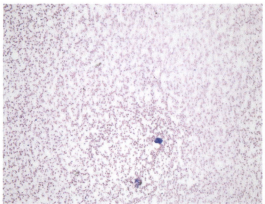

Fig 4.1c A poorly cellular aspirate from a cutaneous lesion (×100)

General principles of cytology | Chapter 4   57

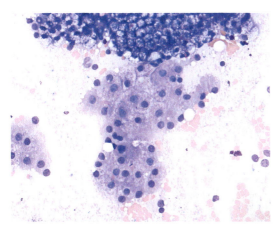

Fig 4.2a Well preserved hepatic and biliary epithelium (×500)

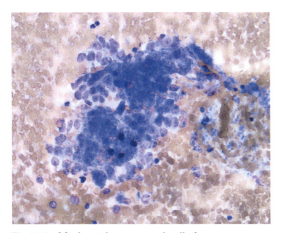

Fig 4.2b Moderately preserved cells from a malignant neoplasm (×500)

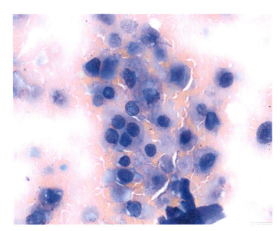

Fig 4.2c Poorly preserved cells from a cutaneous mass (×1000)

There is no definitively correct answer to how cellular or how well-preserved a sample is; judging this accurately comes with experience, and there is considerable variation between cytologists in these descriptions. The important point, however, is to make a judgement on cytology and preservation which is meaningful to yourself, and to do this early in the examination.

Assessing cell types

Once cellularity and preservation are assessed, a stepwise approach to assessing the material can begin. Again, scan the slide from low power to high power whilst asking yourself a series of logical questions. The author finds the following simple approach to be useful.

- Is this lesion predominantly inflammatory or neoplastic? (Or is it mixed? Or neither? (i.e. necrosis, mineralisation)).
- If inflammatory, what is the predominant leukocyte (neutrophils, macrophages, eosinophils, lymphocytes) or is this a mixed inflammatory pattern?
- If neoplastic, what is the predominant cell type present (epithelial, mesenchymal or round cells)?
- Is there any relevant acellular material present (keratin, extracellular matrix, crystals, fat droplets)?
- Are there any visible infectious agents?

The following flowchart in Table 4.1 summarises this process in more detail.

Backgrounds (FIG 4.3)

Some information about a specimen can be gleaned from the background to the material, especially with experience. Assessments should be made of the colour (eosinophilic (red), basophilic (blue-purple), amphophilic (a mixture of both colours)), intensity (faint, mid, deep/intense) and texture (smooth, lightly stippled, heavily stippled).

Table 4.1 Stepwise approach to cytological evaluation

```
┌─────────────────────────────────────┐
│ Evaluate cellularity, preservation, │
│ staining and contamination          │
└─────────────────────────────────────┘
                   │
                   ▼
┌─────────────────────────────────────┐
│      Is this lesion predominantly:  │
│                                     │
│   Inflammatory?         Neoplastic? │
└─────────────────────────────────────┘
         │                    │
         ▼                    ▼
```

Inflammatory	Neoplastic
Predominant leukocyte? Neutrophilic/ macrophagic/ eosinophilic/ lymphocytic/ plasmacytic/ mixed	**Predominant cell type?** Epithelial/ mesenchymal/ neuroendocrine/ round
Are the cells present degenerate or non-degenerate? Activated or inactive?	Do the cells appear benign or malignant? Are granules present?
Are infectious agents present? Are they phagocytosed or free in the background?	Is concurrent inflammation present? What type?
Is there any foreign material present?	Is there evidence of necrosis or apoptosis?

Is there any other relevant extracellular material? (Keratin, extracellular matrix, secretory material)

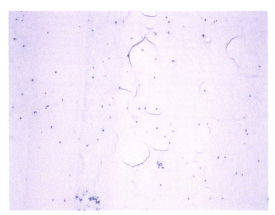
Fig 4.3a Proteinaceous background (seroma) (×40)

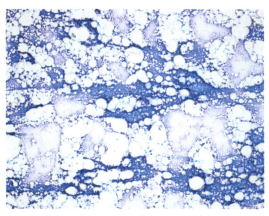
Fig 4.3b Fatty background (panniculitis) (×40)

Proteinaceous fluids, such as from a seroma, tend to have highly stippled eosinophilic to amphophilic backgrounds, often with small clefts. Aspirates from fatty areas are usually clear and smooth, with numerous fat spaces (fat is dissolved by methanol, and therefore is clear with Romanowsky stains). Haemodiluted samples often have a smooth eosinophilic background.

Knowledge of backgrounds can help judge whether a sample aspirated from near a joint contains synovial fluid or whether a sample containing mostly ruptured cells could be a histiocytoma. Some examples are found in Appendix C.

> **Key points**
>
> **Initial examination**
> - A stepwise, logical approach to cytological specimens is helpful to organise their variable appearance
> - If cellularity or preservation are poor, or there is significant contamination, resampling should be considered (where feasible)
> - The background to preparations can give valuable information (particularly where cellular details are not visible) – see Appendix C

Cytology of inflammation

When inflammation is present, the first question is – what type? Different patterns of inflammation have very different causes, which can give a useful insight into the underlying lesion. Almost all inflammatory patterns are mixed to some extent but, in most cases, there is a predominant cell type present, or increased numbers of less commonly-seen cells (such as eosinophils).

Although leukocytes have varied and distinctive morphologies, they often condense in high protein environments (such as joint fluid and exudates) or urine, appearing as small round dense nuclei with small amounts of pale eosinophilic cytoplasm. Distinguishing between leukocytes in such fluids can be difficult. Similar condensing of cells can occur with the addition of formalin to fluid specimens, which is not recommended for this reason.

Neutrophilic inflammation

Also known as 'suppurative' or 'purulent' inflammation, inflammation is defined as neutrophilic when 85% or more of the observed leukocytes are neutrophils (Fig 4.4). They are often accompanied by low numbers of macrophages. Neutrophils are the first responders and the

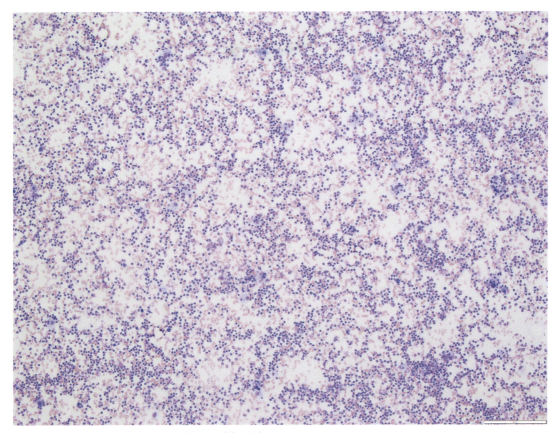

Fig 4.4 Neutrophilic inflammation (abscess) (×100)

foot soldiers of the immune system. They are rapidly mobilised in most causes of inflammation, honed by natural selection to phagocytose bacteria and release toxic substances to destroy invaders.

In samples taken from tissues with a relatively benign environment (most tissues except for bile, urine, and some other fluids), neutrophils are usually *non-degenerate* – non-degenerate neutrophils have sharply-defined nuclear borders with dark, dense nuclear chromatin and well-segmented nuclei. Their overall appearance is similar to mature neutrophils in peripheral blood (Fig 4.5).

In more toxic environments, particularly those created by bacterial toxins, neutrophils undergo hydropic change, as the cells begin to lose their membrane integrity and swell up.

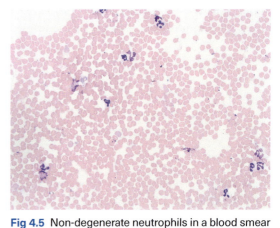

Fig 4.5 Non-degenerate neutrophils in a blood smear

These *degenerate* neutrophils contain paler, swollen nuclei, with fewer distinct segments (*karyolysis*) (Fig 4.6). In contrast, neutrophils displaying shrunken, rounded, very dense

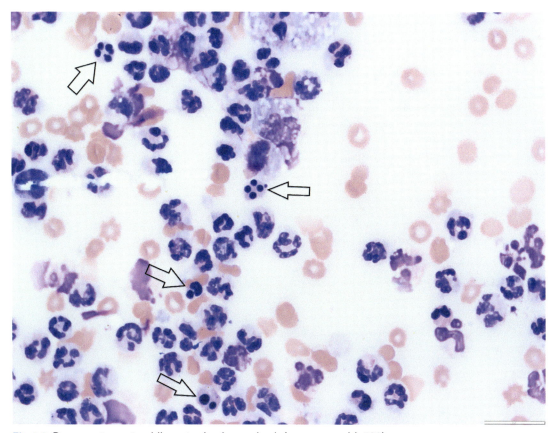

Fig 4.6 Degenerate neutrophils; note also *karyorrhexis* (open arrows) (×500)

nuclei (*pyknosis*) or nuclei fragmented into multiple small dense dots (*karyorrhexis*) with intact membranes are more likely to be ageing in situ rather than degenerating due to toxins. However, pyknotic neutrophils and those displaying *karyorrhexis* are often seen in low numbers amongst degenerate neutrophils.

When neutrophils are poorly preserved, especially when this is due to delayed processing of fluid samples, they can closely resemble degenerate neutrophils – for this reason, care should be taken in interpreting degenerate neutrophils in poorly-preserved samples.

Although bacteria should be considered in all predominantly neutrophilic inflammatory lesions, the presence of degenerate neutrophils should raise the cytologist's suspicions and prompt a search for bacterial organisms (see below) although note that some septic diseases (especially septic arthritis – see page 267) elicit almost no degenerate change.

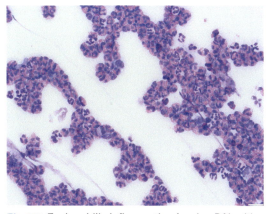

Fig 4.7 Eosinophilic inflammation (canine BAL with *Angiostrongylus* infection (not shown) (×500)

There are many other causes of neutrophilic inflammation, including necrosis, foreign body reactions (although this is more commonly associated with a mixed inflammatory pattern, including numerous macrophages), immune-mediated diseases, neoplasia (such as squamous cell carcinomas), trauma and ischaemia.

See Chapter 5 for more information on bacterial infections.

> **Key points**
>
> **Neutrophilic inflammation**
>
> - Neutrophilic inflammation is defined when >75% of leukocytes are neutrophils
> - Neutrophils usually indicate acute inflammation
> - Degenerate neutrophils raise suspicion for the presence of bacterial toxins

Eosinophilic inflammation

Eosinophils are a less common, albeit more flamboyant, leukocyte, and so their presence in smaller proportions is considered significant – when more than 10% of inflammatory cells are eosinophils, inflammation is described as eosinophilic (Fig 4.7). Recruitment of eosinophils is one of the chief functions of mast cells, and so they are commonly found together.

Eosinophils have large red cytoplasmic granules containing (among other things) major basic protein. This strongly basic protein has affinity for the eosin dye (which is acidic) and therefore they typically stain deeply red (although there are some exceptions – see Chapter 11 for more information). The granules are morphologically distinct between species – dogs have round granules, whereas cats have smaller linear granules (Fig 4.8).

If neutrophils are the foot soldiers of the immune system, eosinophils are the specialist troops. They are often seen in more unusual conditions, occasionally collectively called 'worms, wheezes and weird diseases' (Raskin, 2016). Eosinophils respond to parasitic infestations and are one of the key cells involved in type 1 hypersensitivity ('immediate hypersensitivity', including allergies). They can be found in eosinophilic plaques and are also one of the more common leukocytes found in neoplasia-related inflammation (*paraneoplastic inflammation*), usually associated with mast cell tumours (Fig 4.9), although several other neoplasms, notably some lymphomas, also attract eosinophils).

More rarely, eosinophils can be found in foreign body reactions and fungal infections.

> **Key points**
>
> - Eosinophilic inflammation is defined when >10 leukocytes are eosinophils
> - Often associated with hypersensitivity, parasites, and some tumours (mast cell tumour, lymphoma)

Macrophagic inflammation

Macrophages are the big guns of the inflammatory world. They have great versatility, able to phagocytose infectious organisms and debris, or secrete cytokines to aid in fighting infection or healing. Inflammation containing more than 50% macrophages are described is described as macrophagic or 'granulomatous', whereas mixtures of neutrophils (60–70%) and macrophages (20–30%) are described as neutrophilic/macrophagic or 'pyogranulomatous' (the author prefers the terms 'macrophagic' and 'neutrophilic/macrophagic' as 'granulomatous' and 'pyogranulomatous' conjure up images of granulomas – granulomas are a diagnosis which can only be definitively made histologically) (Fig 4.10).

The versatility of macrophages can make them harder to identify, as it gives them a varied appearance – they can occasionally be mistaken for neoplastic cells (see page 323 regarding the confusion macrophages can cause cytologically).

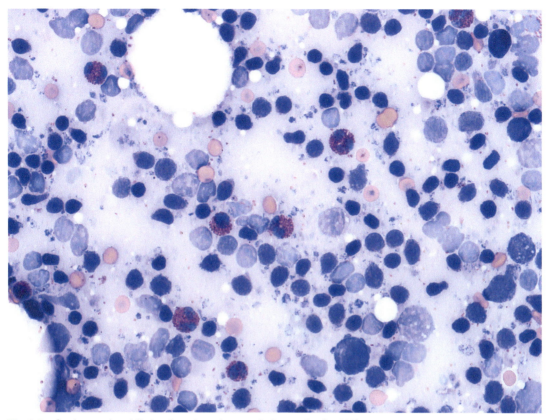

Fig 4.8a Canine eosinophils in a lymph node; rounded granules (×1000)

Most macrophages have pale grey cytoplasm, with variably-sized nuclei.

Inactivated macrophages

'Inactivated' macrophages and dendritic cells (antigen presenting cells, closely related to macrophages and cytologically identical to them) are often collectively described as '**histiocytes**' (Fig 4.11). They are smaller than macrophages and have small amounts of bland pale basophilic (blue) cytoplasm and are observed less commonly because most cases of clinical interest are more likely to active inflammation (although they are seen in high numbers in histiocytomas – see page 85).

Activated macrophages

'Activated' macrophages have more abundant cytoplasm, frequently containing vacuolation, and are found in chronic inflammatory lesions (Fig 4.12). Given their major role in phagocytosis, it can be rewarding to check the cytoplasm of activated macrophages to see if they contain leukocytes or infectious organisms.

The presence of phagocytosed leukocytes (leukophagia) confirms that inflammation is present, and this can be useful in heavily blood-contaminated preparations where it is not clear if the leukocytes present are from the tissue sampled or the blood (Fig 4.13).

In more intense or long-standing inflammatory lesions, macrophage cytoplasm sometimes darkens to a deep blue (Fig 4.14), and 'epithelioid' macrophages, which cluster together in a manner similar to epithelial cells (Fig 4.15), can be present. They can sometimes be very challenging to distinguish from epithelial cells – care should be taken in diagnosing epithelial

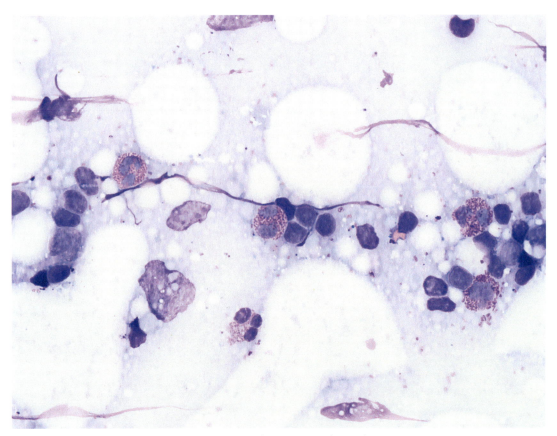

Fig 4.8b Feline eosinophils in a lymph node; linear/oval granules (×1000)

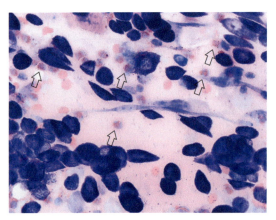

Fig 4.9 Eosinophils in a mast cell tumour (open arrows and other examples) (×500)

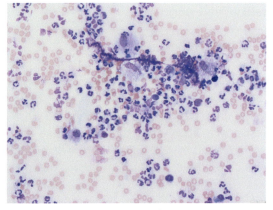

Fig 4.10 Pyogranulomatous inflammation; note frequent degenerate neutrophils and leukophagia (×500)

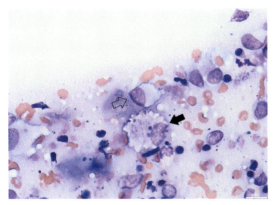

Fig 4.11 Histocyte (open arrow) next to a macrophage (closed arrow); note the histiocyte has smooth and relatively unvacuolated cytoplasm; the other similar cells nearby are probably also histiocytes, although they may also be mesenchymal cells given their slightly oval shape (×1000)

proliferation where significant macrophagic inflammation and multinucleate macrophages are also present.

Epithelioid macrophages are more associated with cytokine secretion than phagocytosis and can be easily confused with epithelial cells. Multinucleated 'giant' macrophages occur for similar reasons and are seen most commonly associated with foreign body reactions (such as stick injuries, ruptured keratin-containing lesions or suture reactions). These bizarre looking cells can be confused with atypical or neoplastic cells, although they usually have relatively uniform nuclei of roughly equal size (i.e. they exhibit minimal *anisokaryosis*) (Fig 4.16).

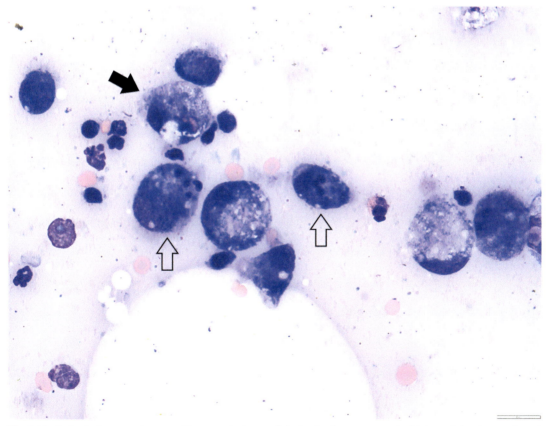

Fig 4.12 Activated macrophages with expanded vacuolated cytoplasm, some of which contain phagocytosed neutrophils (open arrows) and one of which contains a phagocytosed erythrocyte and other debris (black arrow) ×1000

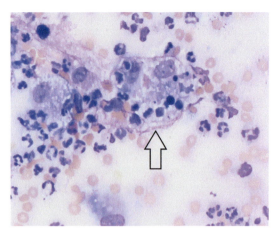

Fig 4.13 Marked leukophagia (open arrow) – this large multinucleate macrophage contains many phagocytosed neutrophils, ranging from larger cells still recognisable as neutrophils to small condensed unrecognisable cells

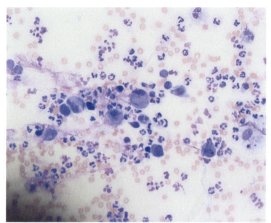

Fig 4.14 Activated macrophages displaying increased basophilia (bluer cytoplasm); they are mixed with neutrophilic inflammation (×500)

> **Key points**
>
> - Macrophagic inflammation defined when >50% of cells are macrophages
> - Indicators of more chronic inflammation
> - Epithelioid and multinucleate macrophages in intense inflammation can be mistaken for neoplastic cells – the context is important

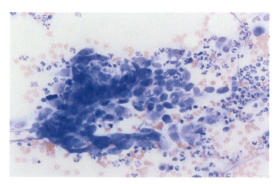

Fig 4.15 Epithelioid macrophages; note their abundant vacuolated cytoplasm and occasional phagocytosis of neutrophils – these features are not exclusive to activated macrophages but when found together with together with other macrophages they can help distinguish between macrophages and epithelium

Lymphocytic and lymphoplasmacytic inflammation

Lymphocytes perform a wide variety of key immune functions, mostly related to the acquired immune response. They're planners, regulators, manufacturers of ammunition (antibodies), as well as occasionally getting their pseudopods dirty on the front line. Primarily lymphocytic inflammation is relatively uncommon in dogs and cats – lymphocytes are found much more commonly in mixed inflammatory responses. Purely lymphocytic inflammation should be interpreted with caution, as lymphoma is also a consideration for the presence of high numbers of lymphocytes.

Lymphocytes are classified according to the size of their nucleus – small lymphocytes have nuclei smaller than a neutrophil (and roughly 1–1.5 erythrocytes in diameter) with dark, dense chromatin and no nucleoli, intermediate lymphocytes have nuclei about the same size as a neutrophil (about 1.5–2 erythrocytes) with more

General principles of cytology | Chapter 4   67

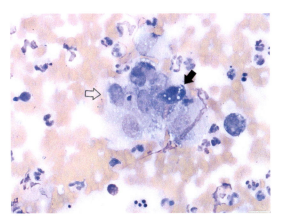

Fig 4.16 Multinucleate giant cell in a foreign body reaction (open arrow); it contains phagocytosed material resembling a neutrophil and an erythrocyte; a plasma cell is also embedded next to this cell (black arrow) (×1000)

'open' (paler) nuclear chromatin, and large lymphocytes have nuclei that are larger than a neutrophil (and usually 2.5–3.5 erythrocytes) with even more open chromatin and frequently containing nucleoli (Fig 4.17).

A genuinely reactive population of lymphocytes should contain predominantly small cells (>60% of observed cells), with progressively fewer intermediate and large lymphocytes (Fig 4.18). In contrast, a monomorphic population of similarly-sized cells (especially intermediate to large cells) raises concern for a clonal, and often neoplastic, population – lymphoma (see page 86 for more details).

Reactive populations often contain scattered plasma cells – these are mature B-lymphocytes which produce antibodies and are one of the

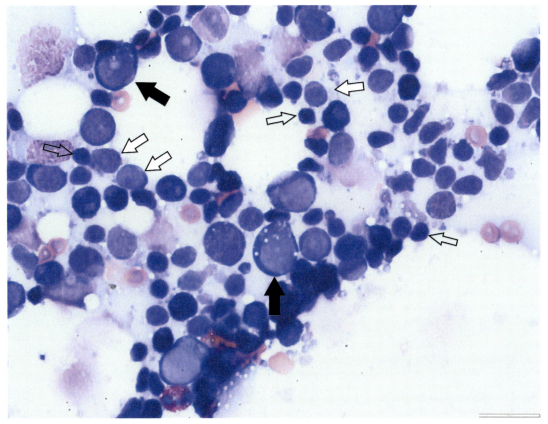

Fig 4.17 Examples of small (open arrows), intermediate (white arrows) and large (black arrows) lymphocytes – note that the nuclear chromatin becomes progressively paler as the cells mature and become more active (×1000)

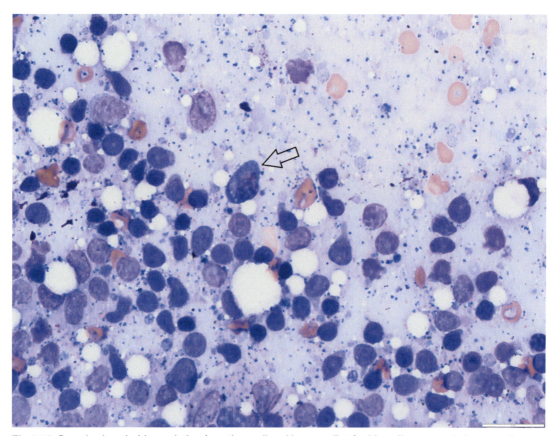

Fig 4.18 Reactive lymphoid population (mostly small and intermediate) with well-preserved plasma cell (open arrow). Note also melanin pigment granules in the background (melanin incontinence; common in nodes draining skin disease) (×500)

natural end points of a normally functioning lymphoid follicle (see below for more information). The complete absence of plasma cells amidst high numbers of lymphocytes again raises concern for lymphoma.

Common causes for true lymphocytic inflammation include antigenic stimulation – such antigens could originate from vaccines, foreign bodies, insect bites and viral infections, amongst many other sources. Lymphocytes are often also found in regressing histiocytomas (Fig 4.19) and type IV sensitivity reactions (delayed-type hypersensitivity).

> **Key points**
>
> **Pure lymphocytic inflammation is unusual in dogs and cats**
> - Lymphocyes in inflammation should be mixed and mostly (>60%) small cells
> - Monomorphic lymphocytes raise concern for lymphoma

Plasma cells (FIG 4.20)

Plasma cells are mature and fully differentiated B-lymphocytes specialised in the formation of antibodies specific to a single antigen. They are easily recognisable (and, in the author's opinion, extremely beautiful). They have densely

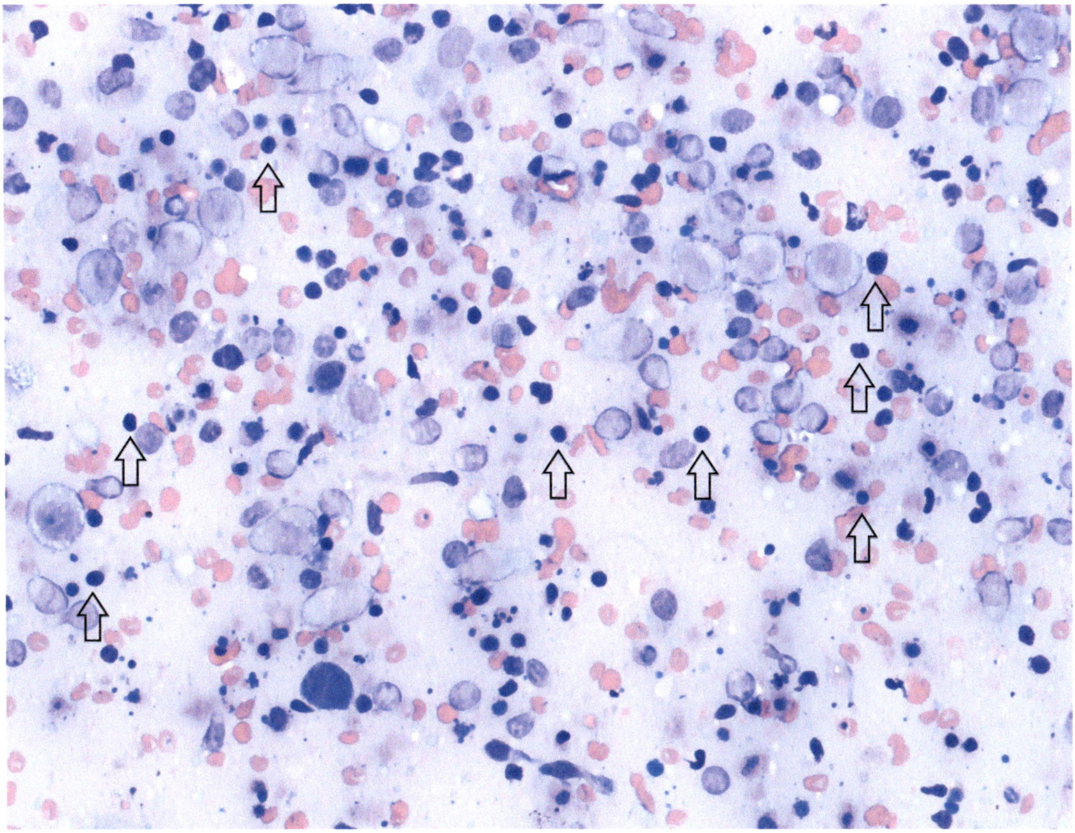

Fig 4.19 Histiocytoma (large blue cells are histiocytes) with lymphocytic inflammation (mostly small lymphocytes – open arrows and many other examples) (×500)

'clumped' chromatin (often described as appearing like a dried out river bed) with expanded deeply basophilic cytoplasm, often containing a clearer area adjacent to the nucleus. This paranuclear clear zone represents the well-developed Golgi apparatus that plasma cells possess in order to produce antibodies.

Mott cells are variants of plasma cells packed with pale basophilic or eosinophilic structures (Russell bodies), usually circular (although many different shapes can be observed) representing packets of immunoglobulins (Fig 4.21).

Mixed Inflammation

Mixed inflammatory patterns are amongst the most commonly encountered on cytology – many different leukocytes are present with no clear predominance (Fig 4.22). In these cases, differentials include all of the possibilities for different leukocytes present. Consideration of the history, location and the proportion of different inflammatory cells present will help to narrow the differential list in these cases.

Other cells present in inflammation

Aside from plasma cells, Mott cells and flame cells, fibroblasts are commonly seen, particularly in marked or long-standing inflammatory lesions. These cells are fusiform (spindle-shaped) mesenchymal cells and can be numerous (depending upon the degree of fibroplasia present) (Fig 4.23).

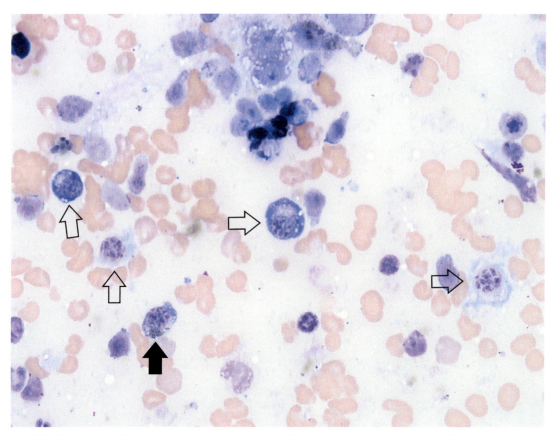

Fig 4.20 Plasma cells (open arrows); note one plasma cell contains low numbers of Russell bodies and is actually a Mott cell (black arrow; see below) (×1000)

As fibroblasts are highly active cells, they can display several criteria of malignancy (particularly pleomorphism and variable nuclear features) which can lead to a misdiagnosis of a neoplastic population (e.g. sarcoma). Mesenchymal cells are also found with angiogenesis, also common in inflammatory lesions.

Additionally, in the presence of significant inflammation, other cells (such as epithelial cells) can undergo dysplastic (reversible atypia) change, which can mimic malignancy (see page 177 for more information on cytological pitfalls such as these).

Cytology of neoplasia

When a lesion comprises predominantly tissue cells, neoplasia becomes a concern. To help establish this, a number of questions need to be answered.

- Are the tissue cells present appropriate for the tissue sampled? (e.g. hepatocytes present on liver aspirates).
- Is the number of cells appropriate for the tissue sampled? (e.g. aspirates from normal lung tissue are often very poorly cellular).
- Is the morphology of the cells normal for the tissue sampled?

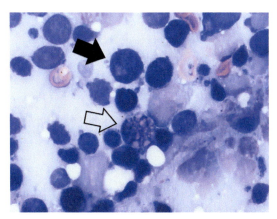

Fig 4.21 Mott cell (open arrow) with eosinophilic immunoglobulin packets. Note also plasma cell (black arrow) (×1000)

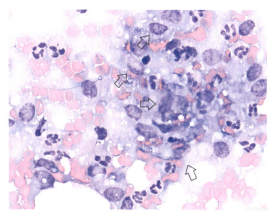

Fig 4.23 Poorly preserved mesenchymal cells (open arrows and other examples), interspersed with neutrophils, in reactive fibroplasia (×1000)

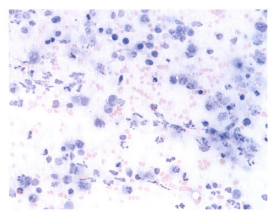

Fig 4.22 Very mixed (neutrophilic/macrophagic/eosinophilic/lymphocytic) inflammation in a vaccine reaction (poor preservation) (×500)

If the answer to any or all of these questions is 'no', then neoplasia is likely. At this stage, there are two more important questions to attempt to answer: 'What is the origin of the cells present? and 'Is this lesion likely to behave in a benign or malignant fashion?'

Cell origin – tissue types

Cytologically, neoplasms are grouped into four main groups according to their microscopic appearance (exceptions, of course, do occur). These groups are broad and varied (especially 'round cell' tumours) but are useful to help predict the clinical behaviour of the lesion. Table 4.2 summarises the cytological characteristics of the main groups and is followed by brief discussions of each group.

Epithelial neoplasms

Epithelial tumours arise from the cells lining organs, glands, and most other tissues. These cells are involved in protection, secretion and absorption, and generally have very tight cell-cell junctions – junctions that are often preserved during aspiration. For this reason, the cells are often found adherent to each other in dense clusters and flattened sheets in cytological specimens. Epithelial clusters usually have rounded, well-defined edges, containing tightly packed cells (Figs 4.24, 4.25). When found in fluids, they have a tendency to curl up into 'balls' of cells.

Epithelial tumours are described as '*adenomas*' when benign, or '*carcinomas*' when malignant; '*adenocarcinoma*' refers to a malignant neoplasm of glandular origin. Due to the preservation of cell junctions, architectural patterns reflecting the origin of the cells are most readily recognised in epithelial tumours.

Table 4.2 Characteristics of the tumour groups

	Epithelial	Mesenchymal	Neuroendocrine	'round' cell
Low power appearance (patterns)	Tightly cohesive 'clusters' and sheets of cells	Loosely cohesive 'aggregates'	Cohesive clusters with poorly defined borders and many bare nuclei	Individual cells with little cohesion, occasional groups
High power appearance (cell morphology)	Cuboidal, columnar, and squamous cells with distinct borders	Spindle, caudate or stellate cells with 'wispy' indistinct borders	Round but indistinct borders; often appear as bare nuclei within a sea of cytoplasm	Round or polygonal cells with distinct borders
Nuclear shape	Round nuclei	Slender to plump oval nuclei	Round nuclei, often bare nuclei	Round to polygonal nuclei
Tumour types	Adenoma, carcinoma	Sarcoma	Neuroendocrine adenoma, carcinoma	Variety (see below)

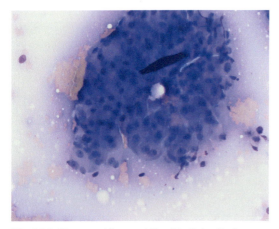

Fig 4.24 Cluster of 'hepatoid' epithelial cells from a perianal adenoma; the term 'hepatoid' refers to the finely granular eosinophilic cytoplasm, reminiscent of hepatic epithelium. Note the close cohesion of the cells and the smooth, rounded cluster edges (×500)

Low power appearance – patterns

Common patterns for epithelial neoplasms include:

Palisading – cells arranged in regular rows (like a picket fence); usually seen in basilar cell tumours (basal cell tumours) such as trichoblastomas or apocrine ductular adenomas (Fig 4.26)

Honeycomb – polygonal cells in a regular tessellating pattern (like a mosaic); seen most commonly in aspirates from the prostate or intestinal tract (particularly the stomach wall) (Fig 4.27)

Papillary – cells arranged in rows around a central vascular or stromal core (this core is not always apparent cytologically), usually with finger-like rounded projections; often seen in pulmonary and mammary epithelium (Fig 4.28)

Pavement – thin layers of polygonal and often angular cells; usually seen with squamous epithelium lining mucosae and skin (Fig 4.29)

Trabecular – branching and often wide cohesive clusters of cells; reminiscent of trabecular bone, and often seen in liver and perianal aspirates (Fig 4.30)

Glandular tumours (*adenocarcinomas*) often contain acinar structures – rings of cells around a central area, which may contain secretory product (Fig 4.31). Secretory products are variable but are often small patches or lakes of pale eosinophilic (occasionally basophilic) amorphous rounded material.

High power appearance – cell morphology

Epithelial cells usually have a round central nucleus with abundant cytoplasm (although see 'Features of malignancy', below). Where

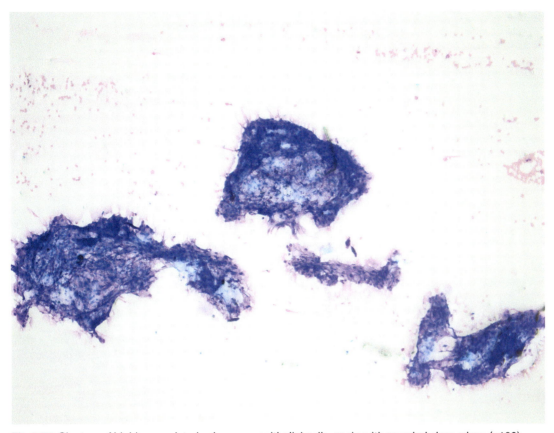

Fig 4.25 Clusters of highly vacuolated sebaceous epithelial cells, again with rounded clear edges (×100)

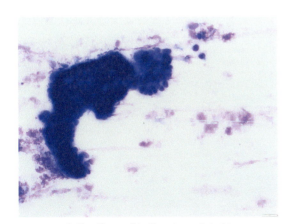

Fig 4.26 Palisading epithelium in a trichoblastoma (benign tumour of basal epithelium); cells are tightly packed and arranged with nuclei closely adjacent and often in rows, sometimes reminiscent of a picket fence (×500)

observable, the cell shape can also provide a clue to the origin of the cells:

- Cuboidal – small squarish, rounded or polygonal cells (Fig 4.32); found most often in renal aspirates, basilar epithelium or intact neuroendocrine neoplasms (see below)
- Squamous – larger irregular polygonal cells, angular when keratinised; seen usually in cutaneous or mucosal aspirates (Fig 4.33)
- Columnar – rounded rectangular cells with a 'basal' or paracentric nucleus (at one end of the cell); seen in respiratory epithelium (with cilia), intestine, prostate (cuboidal to columnar) and secondary to self-trauma in cutaneous lesions (a dysplastic change) (Fig 4.34)
- Transitional – cell shape varies between cuboidal (usually at the centre of clusters) to

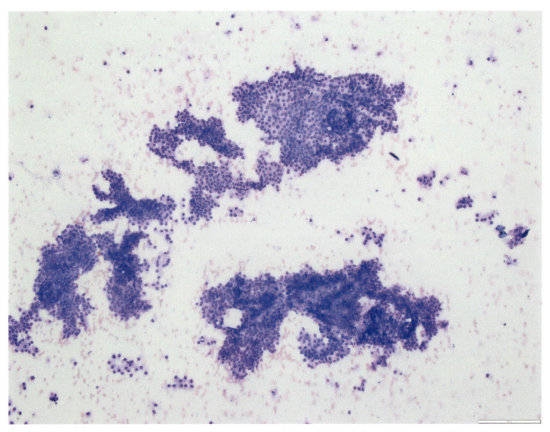

Fig 4.27 Distinctive honeycomb pattern of prostatic epithelium (cubiodal to columnar cells) (×100)

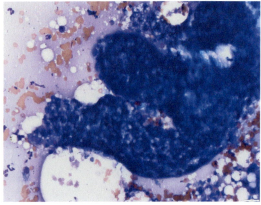

Fig 4.28 Papillary epithelial cluster in a pulmonary adenocarcinoma (×500)

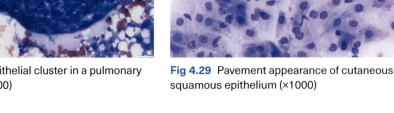

Fig 4.29 Pavement appearance of cutaneous squamous epithelium (×1000)

columnar or squamous (at the periphery); found lining the urethra, bladder and ureters. Individual cells from glandular neoplasms often contain vacuoles within the cytoplasm, usually clear; these can vary from multiple small 'punctate' vacuoles with clear borders to a large single vacuole, displacing the nucleus to the periphery of the cell ('sig-

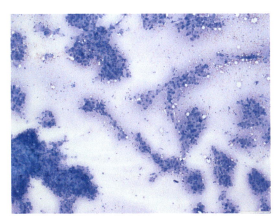
Fig 4.30 Trabecular pattern of hepatic epithelium (×100)

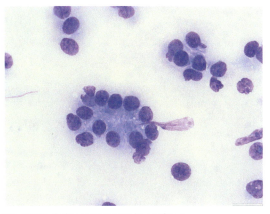
Fig 4.31 Acinar structure in anal sac adenocarcinoma (a neuroendocrine neoplasm, but epithelial acini appear similar; no central secretory product visible in this example) (×1000)

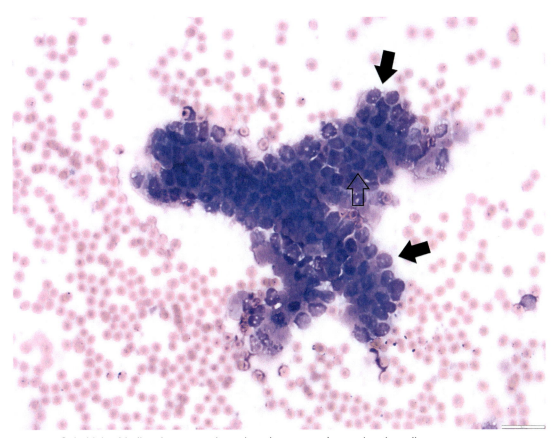
Fig 4.32 Cuboidal epithelium in a prostatic aspirate (open arrow); note that the cells assume a more columnar shape at the periphery of the cluster (black arrows) (this is characteristic of prostatic epithelium, usually described as 'cuboidal to columnar') (×500)

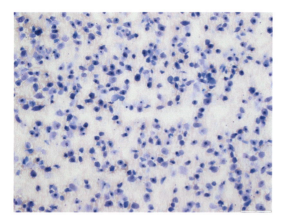

Fig 4.33 Individual keratinised squamous epithelial cells in a papilloma (×100)

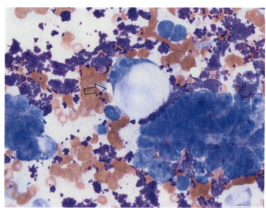

Fig 4.35 Large binucleate signet ring cell (centre of picture) in a pulmonary adenocarcinoma (×100)

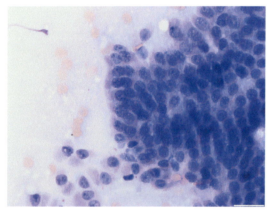

Fig 4.34 Columnar epithelial cells from small intestine; note the basal nuclei, most obvious at the edge of the cluster (×1000)

net ring' cells (Fig 4.35), a feature of malignancy (see below)).

The most commonly aspirated cutaneous epithelial neoplasms include basilar epithelial neoplasms (previously called 'basal cell tumours'), perianal ('hepatoid') neoplasms (see above for examples) and squamous cell carcinomas (Fig 4.36). More specific details about the most common neoplasms are found in Chapter 6.

Malignant epithelial neoplasms (carcinomas) often have high potential to metastasise – initially to local lymph nodes, and from there through the lymphatics to many other body tissues.

> **Key points**
>
> **Epithelial neoplasms**
> - Arise from lining and glandular tissue
> - Tightly cohesive – often exfoliate as 'clusters' or sheets with rounded/flattened edges and containing tightly packed cells, often forming distinctive patterns
> - Rounded nuclei with distinct cellular borders
> - When malignant, often metastasise via lymph nodes

Neuroendocrine neoplasms

These neoplasms derive from neuroendocrine tissue (such as the thyroid gland, the endocrine pancreatic cells, and chemotactic cells), and cytologically appear somewhat similar to epithelial tumours, in that they are often cohesive and contain round, dense nuclei. Unlike many epithelial tumours, they are extremely fragile and frequently rupture during aspiration, so that they often contain high numbers of bare nuclei. Again, unlike carcinomas, the cytoplasmic borders of these cells are indistinct. When

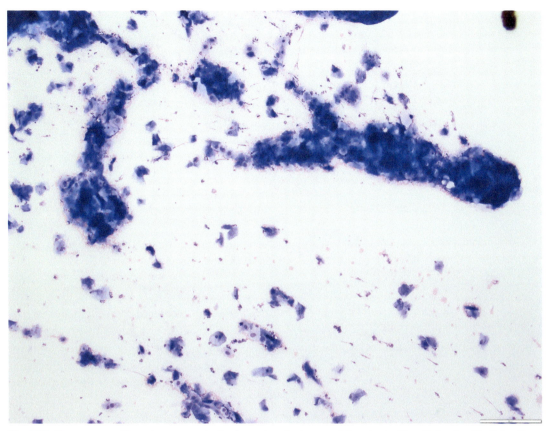

Fig 4.36 Squamous cell carcinoma – note the irregular clusters, and the atypical keratinised epithelial cells (with large prominent nuclei when they should instead be regressing) (×100)

intact, the clusters of cells look like free nuclei within a pool of pale cytoplasm (Fig 4.37).

Despite their often innocuous cytological appearance, neuroendocrine tumours often follow an aggressive clinical course and frequently metastasise. The most commonly encountered neuroendocrine-appearing tumours in dogs are anal sac apocrine gland adenocarcinomas* (see above) and thyroid tumours (Fig 4.38).

*These are not technically neuroendocrine cells (as the glands from which they are derived are apocrine, not endocrine), but appear cytologically identical to them and so are described as having a 'neuroendocrine-like appearance'

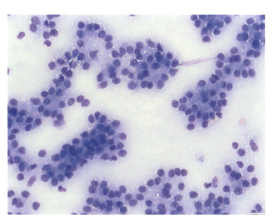

Fig 4.37 Neuroendocrine-appearing tumour (anal sac apocrine gland adenocarcinoma; epithelial-like clusters contain cells with indistinct borders and minimal malignant features (×500)

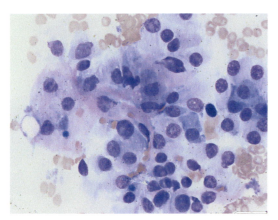

Fig 4.38 Thyroid carcinoma containing colloid (pale pink material interspersed with cells); again, malignant features are largely absent (×500)

> **Key points**
>
> **Neuroendocrine tumours**
> - Arise most commonly from thyroid gland and anal sac apocrine glands (especially dogs)
> - Appear similar to epithelial cells but with poorly-defined cell borders and often with high numbers of bare nuclei
> - Often behave aggressively despite relatively bland cytological appearance

Mesenchymal neoplasms

Mesenchymal cells form the connective tissues of the body – bone, cartilage, fibrous tissue, muscles, fat and vascular tissue. Although they are somewhat cohesive, the cell to cell junctions are not as strong as epithelial cells. Consequently, although their architecture is occasionally preserved on cytological samples, these looser *aggregates* form less distinctive patterns than those seen in epithelial tumours, and many individual cells are often concurrently present (Figs 4.39, 4.40).

Benign mesenchymal neoplasms carry the suffix '*-oma*', similar to some other benign tumours (and, confusingly, some more aggressive tumours such as lymphoma). Examples include lipoma (Fig 4.41), fibroma, myxoma, chondroma and haemangioma. Malignant versions are described as *sarcoma* (for more information on specific mesenchymal neoplasms, see Chapter 6, amongst others).

Cytology of mesenchymal neoplasms is complicated by the fact that fibroblasts and other mesenchymal cells proliferate as a response to inflammation or injury, and it can be challenging to distinguish between a reactive and neoplastic population of cells. In general, high numbers of mesenchymal cells with no evidence of inflammation and no previous history of trauma should raise the cytologist's suspicions for neoplasia.

Low power appearance – patterns

Cytologically, although mesenchymal aggregates can be dense and packed with cells, they have a rougher, more irregular outline, and give the imaginative pathologist the impression that they are attempting to 'spread out' on the slide.

A few recognised patterns include:

Storiform – cells arranged in loose bundles, with whorls and somewhat resembling a straw mat; most commonly noted in soft tissue sarcomas, but not a very specific pattern (Fig 4.42)

Perivascular – cells arranged irregularly around one or more small capillaries; seen in perivascular wall tumours and Leydig cell tumours (Fig 4.43)

Despite the looser cell-cell junctions, mesenchymal cells are usually well-embedded within their surrounding matrix, which can be abundant. Due to this, mesenchymal tumours are often grossly firmer than epithelial tumours, and generally do not exfoliate as well. Individual cells are elongated, with oval nuclei, and the cytoplasmic borders are indistinct (often described as 'wispy') and blend into the background (Fig 4.44).

General principles of cytology | Chapter 4 79

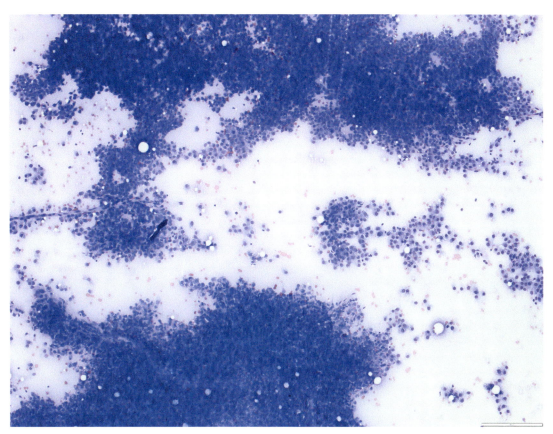

Fig 4.39 Mesenchymal aggregates in a soft tissue sarcoma; note the looser 'frayed' appearance and scattered individual cells (×100)

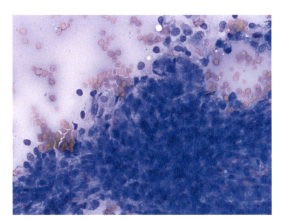

Fig 4.40 Higher power mesenchymal aggregate (×500)

High-power appearance – cell morphology

As with the low-power architecture, the individual cell shape is less specific in mesenchymal neoplasia, but some information can still be gained from a close inspection:

Fusiform – 'spindle' shaped cells, tapering at both ends with central nuclei (Fig 4.45); these are the most commonly observed mesenchymal cell, found in many sarcomas, but most often seen in soft tissue sarcomas

Stellate – like a star, with three or more tapering projections with central nuclei (Fig 4.46); again, not specific but often seen in soft tissue sarcomas

Caudate – eccentric nuclei, similar to columnar epithelial cells, although tapering to a

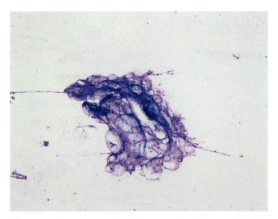

Fig 4.41 Aggregate of adipocytes in a lipoma (×500)

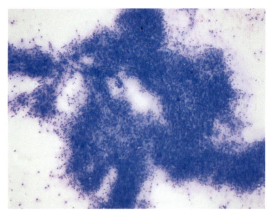

Fig 4.42 Storiform pattern of mesenchymal cells in a soft tissue sarcoma (×100)

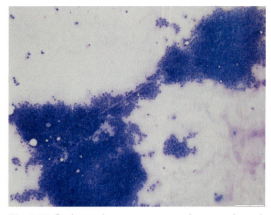

Fig 4.43 Perivascular arrangement of mesenchymal cells in a soft tissue sarcoma (×100)

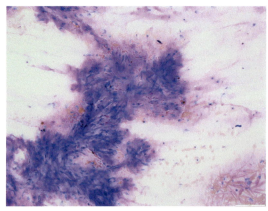

Fig 4.44 Marked matrix production in a mesenchymal neoplasm, probable chondrosarcoma; the blue mesenchymal cells are embedded in large amounts of bright pink matrix (×100)

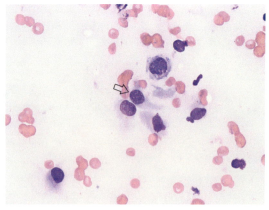

Fig 4.45 Fusiform mesenchymal cell (open arrow) (×1000)

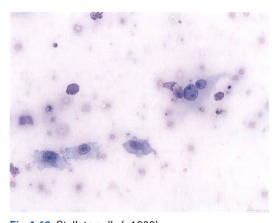

Fig 4.46 Stellate cells (×1000)

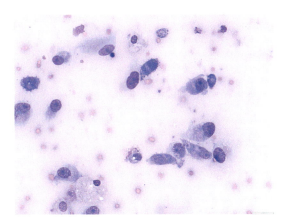

Fig 4.47 Caudate cells (×1000)

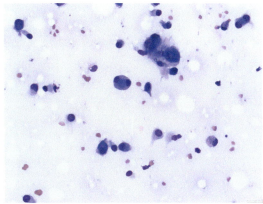

Fig 4.48 Individual mesenchymal cells (fusiform and caudate) with indistinct borders from a soft tissue sarcoma (STS); note the indistinct borders and the binucleate 'alien head' cell (centre of picture), commonly seem in STS (×500)

rounded end or point opposite the nucleus (Fig 4.47); seen most commonly in osteoblasts and chondroblasts (the neoplastic cells in osteosarcomas and chondrosarcomas respectively)

Soft tissue sarcomas (Fig 4.48) often behave in a similar clinical fashion – they are locally invasive but slow to metastasise. Other sarcomas vary in their metastatic potential. When metastasis occurs, it is usually via invasion of blood vessels, in contrast to the lymphatic spread most commonly seen in carcinomas and round cell tumours. Metastasis to lymph nodes is very rare for sarcomas.

It is often difficult to distinguish between different types of sarcomas cytologically, but their morphology (which can indicate if the cells are higher grade) can be a useful predictor for their clinical behaviour (see features of malignancy, below).

The most commonly encountered mesenchymal neoplasms presenting as skin and subcutaneous masses are lipomas and soft tissue sarcomas (including haemangiopericytomas and peripheral nerve sheath tumours; distinguishing between them has no prognostic value).

Extracellular matrix

Aspirates from mesenchymal cells often include the extracellular matrix they produce. This is composed of lakes and clumps of granular or fibrillar (containing thin strands of fibrils) material, and the mesenchymal cells are often closely associated or embedded within it (Figs 4.49, 4.50).

The colour and appearance of the matrix varies with its nature; it is most commonly pink to eosinophilic, although can vary from a reddish appearance (in fibromas/fibrosarcomas), pink fluidly material resembling joint fluid (in myxomas/myxosarcomas), intense pinkish-purple (chondroid from chondromas/

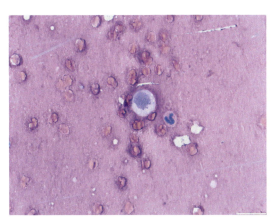

Fig 4.49 Granular pink matrix with embedded mesenchymal cell ("lacuna") from a chondrosarcoma (×1000)

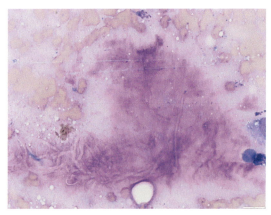

Fig 4.50a Osteoid in an osteosarcoma (no cells visible) (×1000)

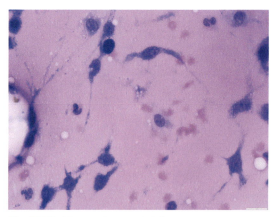

Fig 4.50b Myxomatous matrix in a myxosarcoma (×1000)

chondrosarcomas), or intense pink (osteoid from osteomas/osteosarcomas), although sarcomas can produce matrix atypical for their original cell line.

The presence of material resembling matrix lends support for mesenchymal neoplasia but is not absolutely specific – secretory material from glandular epithelial tumours, basement membrane associated with basilar epithelial cells and amyloid from plasma cell tumours can all closely resemble matrix on Romanowsky stains.

> **Key points**
>
> **Mesenchymal neoplasms**
>
> - Arise from connective tissue
> - Present in loose 'aggregates' with 'frayed' or 'ragged' borders, or individual cells
> - Individual cells are elongated with oval nuclei and indistinct borders
> - Can be very challenging to distinguish from reactive fibroplasias (so take care when diagnosing neoplasia when inflammation or a known history of trauma is present)
> - Metastasis usually occurs via blood vessels – metastasis to lymph nodes is rare

Round cell neoplasms

Tumours in this broad and slightly unsatisfying category vary greatly in clinical behaviour and prognosis. Rather than being defined by their origin, they are linked by their cytological appearance. Round cell tumours are a collection of tumours containing, unsurprisingly, round cells, with round nuclei. The cells are found individually and are not usually cohesive (although they may appear in groups due to high numbers). They mostly exfoliate well – specimens often contain high numbers of discrete cells with distinct cell borders.

Due to the varied appearance and behaviour of the neoplasms in this section, it is easier to discuss them separately, rather than as a whole group.

Mast cell tumour

Mast cells are readily recognisable on cytological specimens, as they usually appear as rounded cells packed with distinctive purple granules (Fig 4.51) (although note that cytoplasmic granules, including mast cell granules, stain unreliably using aqueous Romanowsky stains (such as Diff-Quik)).

Mast cells appear in low numbers as part of normal inflammatory processes and trafficking

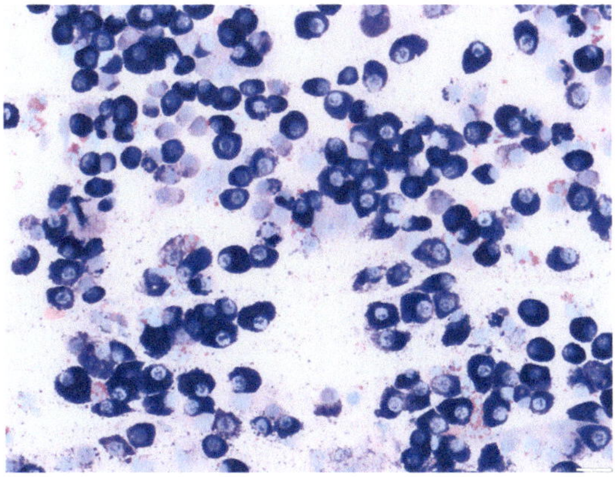

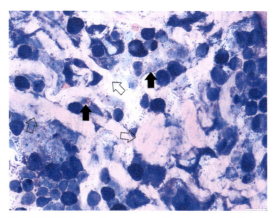

Fig 4.51 Mast cell tumour, canine, probable low-grade (×500)

Fig 4.52 Collagen (open arrows) and eosinophils (black arrows) in a mast cell tumour (×500)

(passage through other organs such as lymph nodes, liver or spleen, without causing inflammation), but their presence in high numbers is strongly suggestive of aspiration of a mast cell tumour (MCT); these tumours are a common cytological diagnosis in aspirates from skin and subcutaneous tissues (more commonly in dogs), but are also encountered in the viscera (especially the spleen, liver and GI tract; the spleen is a relatively common site of primary mast cell tumours in cats, whereas visceral mast cell tumours in dogs are usually secondary). Boxers, Staffordshire bull terriers, golden retrievers and Labradors are reported to have an increased incidence of MCTs. Siamese cats are reported to have increased occurrences of cutaneous MCTs, whereas other cat breeds more commonly suffer from visceral disease.

Due to the cytokines which mast cells produce, MCT aspirates also frequently contain significant numbers of eosinophils. Many MCTs also contain mesenchymal cells, representing the supporting stroma of the tumour – these mesenchymal cells can be markedly pleomorphic (variably-shaped) and atypical-appearing, due to their high activity. Aspirates from MCTs can also contain ribbons of collagen due to the collagenolytic activity of mast cells (Fig 4.52) (this is slightly suggestive of lower-grade neoplasia – see below).

The grade of mast cell tumours is of great clinical importance in mast cell tumours; unfortunately, grading has historically been unreliable based on cytological appearance alone. Recent work, however, has identified several key features which correlate well with high grade **canine** neoplasms on histopathology (Fig 4.53). These features are:

- granulation
- mitotic index
- binucleation/multinucleation
- anisokaryosis (>50% i.e. some cells with nuclei 50% larger than others)
- nuclear pleomorphism (variably-shaped nuclei).

Of these features, poor granulation is the most likely to be correlated with higher-grade tumours, although this can occasionally be challenging to assess with poorly preserved cells and in mast cells that have degranulated during sampling (such cells often contain clear cytoplasmic vacuoles).

For well-granulated tumours, if two of the other four features above are present, then a higher-grade tumour should also be suspected. The presence of collagen appears to be slightly more associated with lower-grade tumours. Note: these features are not consistent or

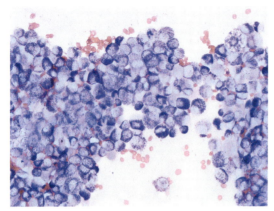

Fig 4.53a Reduced granulation, mast cell tumour (×500)

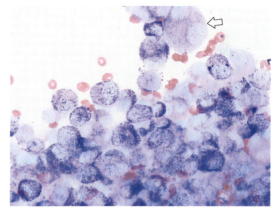

Fig 4.53c Anisokaryosis and binucleation (open arrow), mast cell tumour (×1000)

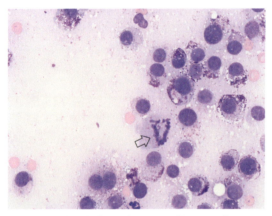

Fig 4.53b Mitotic figure in mast cell tumour (open arrow) (×1000)

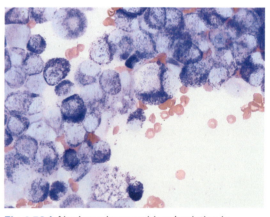

Fig 4.53d Nuclear pleomorphism (variation in nuclear shape), mast cell tumour (×1000)

confirmed in feline mast cell neoplasia, although higher numbers of mitotic figures appears to be related to higher-grade tumours in cats.

Where higher-grade mast cell tumours are suspected (Fig 4.54), further staging is recommended – aspiration of local lymph nodes, and, if possible, the spleen and liver, are commonly carried out to further investigate metastasis. Examination of a peripheral blood film (or, potentially, a buffy-coat preparation) to assess for the presence of mast cells (*mastocythaemia*) is also recommended. Circulating mast cells can occasionally be found in dogs (usually when there is marked systemic inflammation), but the presence of circulating mast cells in cats is almost always associated with neoplasia.

Key points

Mast cell tumour

- Distinctive appearance but granules do not stain well with aqueous Romanowsky stains (such as Diff-Quik)
- Granulation, binucleation, pleomorphism and mitotic figures are a guide to the grade, but histopathology is needed for definitive grading

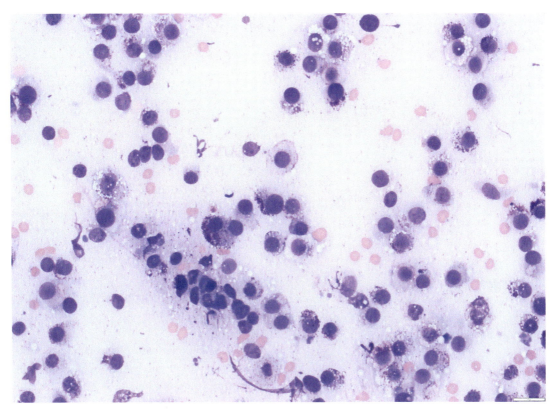

Fig 4.54 High-grade canine mast cell tumour; note poor granulation, frequent binucleation and anisokaryosis (×500)

Histiocytoma

These are common benign lesions of dogs, frequently occurring in young patients, arising from dendritic cells in the epidermis (large mononuclear cells related to macrophages but more involved with antigen recognition and presentation than phagocytosis). They are usually solitary raised, rounded and frequently reddened lesions (sometimes called 'button tumours'), often found around the head and pinnae. They generally spontaneously regress within three months.

Aspirates are often highly cellular, and frequently have a deeply basophilic background. Individual cells usually have large (1.5–3 erythrocyte diameters) central nuclei with round, indented or kidney-shaped nuclei, occasional nucleoli and abundant pale cytoplasm – often they have a characteristic 'fried egg' appearance (Fig 4.55).

Although most cells are individual, the cells can occasionally be found in groups which appear quite cohesive (presumably via mechanisms similar to those involved in the formation of epithelioid macrophages). There is often some mitotic activity present. When well-preserved with their classical appearance, they are a relatively simple cytological diagnosis but, in some cases, they can appear surprisingly similar to plasmacytomas. Additionally, epitheliotropic lymphoma (see page 145) can on first examination appear very similar, although the differences are apparent on close inspection (lymphoma usually has a higher nuclear to cytoplasmic ratio, with denser chromatin).

Histiocytomas are often inflamed, which can complicate the cytological pattern – frequently, they contain lymphocytes (probably cytotoxic

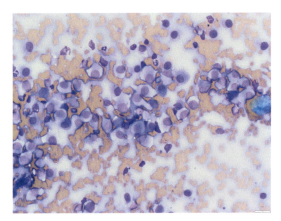

Fig 4.55 Canine histiocytoma with frequent "fried eggs"; note the basophilic background and occasional small lymphocytes present (×500)

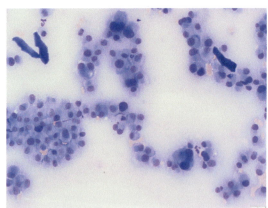

Fig 4.56 Canine plasmacytoma; differences from histiocytoma include eccentric nuclei, clumped chromatin and occasional binucleation (×500)

lymphocytes involved in regression of the lesion), which can occasionally outnumber the histiocytes.

> **Key points**
>
> **Histiocytoma**
>
> - Often have a basophilic (blue) background, cells have a 'fried egg' appearance
> - Cells are often mixed with small lymphocytes

Plasma cell tumour (plasmacytoma)

These neoplasms are more common in older dogs, and generally appear as single raised cutaneous lesions, frequently on pinnae or the lips. Single cutaneous plasmacytomas are usually benign, although local recurrence has been reported following surgical excision.

Cytologically, they usually contain high numbers of plasma cells, although they often contain high numbers of binucleate cells, and can display quite marked variation in cell size (anisocytosis). Nuclei are usually eccentric, and the presence of eccentric nuclei and moderate numbers of binucleate cells can help to distinguish them from histiocytomas in less clear-cut cases (Fig 4.56) (also, plasmacytomas more commonly have eosinophilic or clear backgrounds, rather than basophilic, which is more common in histiocytomas).

Some plasmacytomas (approximately 10%) also contain small patches of amyloid protein, due to immunoglobulin production. This usually appears as a small smooth purple wispy clump of material (Fig 4.57).

> **Key points**
>
> **Plasma cell tumour**
>
> - Cells have eccentric nuclei, are often binucleate and can display marked variation in cell size and shape

Lymphoma

Lymphoma is covered in more detail in later chapters, but when present as a cutaneous mass, lymphoma can have a very variable appearance. Cutaneous lymphoma is not automatically epitheliotropic lymphoma – this is a specific subtype of lymphoma (also called *mycosis fungoides*) with a characteristic appearance somewhat similar to histiocytomas (see histiocytoma section for a summary of the differences, and page 145 for further discussion).

Melanocytic tumours (melanocytoma/melanoma)

Although melanocytes are technically mesenchymal cells, they are often included in the round cell category due to their cytological appearance. Melanocytes are the great imitators of cytology. When the lesions are benign (melanocytomas) the diagnosis is more straightforward, as the cells appear as heavily pigmented individual cells within which cytological details cannot be observed. These 'black holes' are quite easy to identify although it can be challenging to distinguish them from melanophages – macrophages packed with melanin granules, which are often also present (Fig 4.60).

However, malignant melanocytic tumours ('melanomas', confusingly – they are often called 'malignant melanomas' for clarity) are sometimes very challenging to identify. Their appearance can vary greatly from individual round cells to aggregates of cells and even occasionally cohesive clusters. When melanin is observed within the cytoplasm, the diagnosis can be made more confidently, but in poorly-pigmented tumours the melanin is often present only as a light dusting in a few cells – and is sometimes not present at all. They often have a quite open ('stippled') chromatin pattern (see page 38), and many cells have a single large nucleolus, often larger than an erythrocyte (*macronucleoli* – a feature which is strongly correlated with malignancy (see page 31, Fig 3.5c below)).

Given that malignant melanomas are one of the most aggressive neoplasms encountered in veterinary medicine, with frequent metastasis to lymph nodes and distant sites, it is frustrating that they can be difficult to identify. Poorly-pigmented melanoma should be on the differential list for any cutaneous or mucocutaneous lesion which is otherwise challenging to classify cytologically (Fig 4.61).

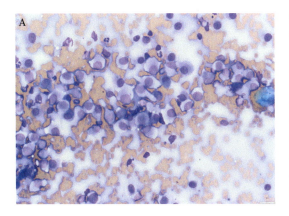

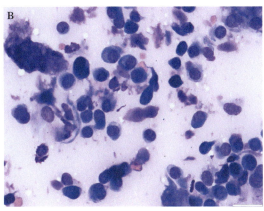

Fig 4.57 Plasmacytoma including amyloid (purple amorphous and slightly wispy material) (×1000)

When large cell lymphoma is present, the diagnosis is relatively simple – the appearance is similar to the disease observed within lymph nodes (Fig 4.58) (see chapter 10 page 236). When small cells predominate the diagnosis is challenging and hard to distinguish from lymphocytic inflammation (Fig 4.59). Further investigation (such as histopathology or PARR analysis) is often required in these cases.

> **Key point**
>
> **Lymphoma**
> - Key finding is a MONOMORPHIC population of cells – a variety of sizes and shapes of lymphocytes is more suggestive of reactivity

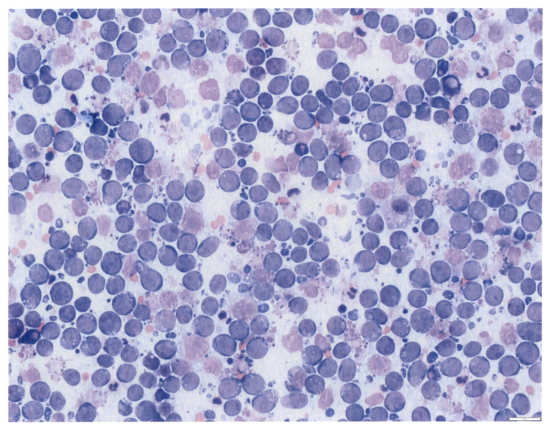

Fig 4.58 Large cell lymphoma in canine lymph node (×500)

> **Key points**
>
> **Melanocytic tumour**
> - Distinctive 'black holes' when benign, very varied appearance when malignant
> - Most reliable features in malignant tumours – 'open' or 'stippled chromatin', single large nucleolus (larger than an erythrocyte)
> - Melanoma should be a consideration for any round cell tumour otherwise difficult to classify cytologically

Histiocytic sarcoma

These aggressive histiocytic neoplasms can present as localised or generalised disease – local lesions appear as firm cutaneous or subcutaneous masses, frequently on the limbs. Despite the name 'sarcoma', they are round cell tumours, although occasional aggregates of cells can be found. Cytologically, the cells often display extreme pleomorphism, and often contain very large multinucleate cells. Chromatin is open and frequently 'ropy' (see below), and mitotic figures are frequent (Figs 4.62, 4.63)).

It can sometimes be challenging to distinguish between histiocytic sarcomas and intense granulomatous inflammation, although in histiocytic sarcomas there are usually occasional cells displaying features too atypical for even markedly reactive macrophages. Malignant features are common (see below and images in 'features of malignancy' section). These neoplasms frequently metastasise to local nodes. Localised disease is more common in dogs,

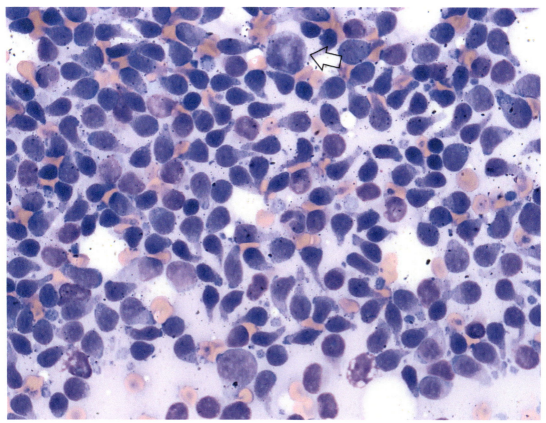

Fig 4.59 Small cell lymphoma, canine; a monomorphic population of small to intermediate (smaller than a neutrophil to roughly neutrophil size) lymphocytes. Many of the cells have prominent uropods (triangular cytoplasmic projections, also called 'hand mirror' forms); a mitotic figure (open arrow) is also present (×500)

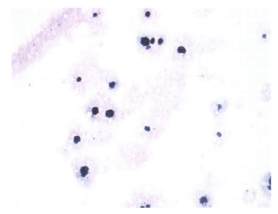

Fig 4.60a Melanocytoma at low power – the 'black holes' are cells packed with melanin (×100)

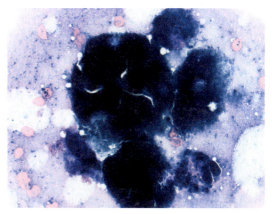

Fig 4.60b Melanocytoma at high power – it is not possible to assess the cytological details of the cells; note also the many small melanin pigment granules in the background (×1000)

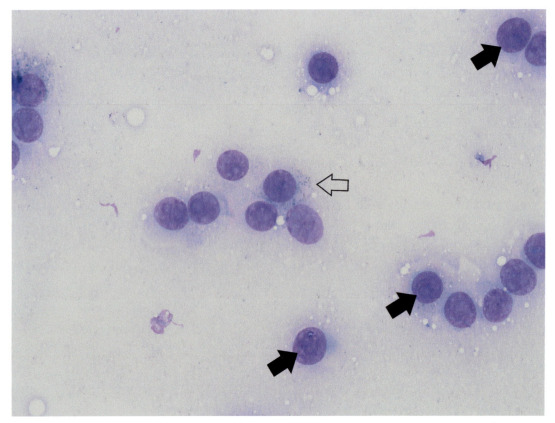

Fig 4.61 'Classic' malignant melanoma; note the open chromatin and large, usually single nucleoli (black arrows), and the scattered melanin pigment in the central cell (open arrow) (×1000)

generalised in cats. Bernese mountain dogs and flat coat retrievers are strongly predisposed to these lesions, and histiocytic sarcoma should be considered as a differential in any granulomatous-appearing lesion from these patients.

> **Key points**
>
> **Histiocytic sarcoma**
>
> - Flat coat retrievers and Bernese mountain dogs strongly predisposed
> - Highly pleomorphic appearance
> - Can be difficult to distinguish better-differentiated tumours from macrophagic inflammation

Transmissible venereal tumour

This is a rarely diagnosed canine tumour in northern Europe, the UK and the USA, usually found in imported patients. These tumours are a rare fascinating example of infectious neoplasia, in which the tumour cells are transplanted into a new host via direct contact with the previous patient. Due to the nature of these tumours, they are usually found in the genital region, but they are occasionally found on the nose or other areas of skin.

They generally exfoliate well on both aspirates and impression smears and have a characteristic cytological pattern. They contain high numbers of round cells with a central nucleus and abundant pale cytoplasm, somewhat similar to histiocytomas, but the cells contain high numbers of round, clear and distinct vacuoles (Fig 4.64).

General principles of cytology | Chapter 4 | 91

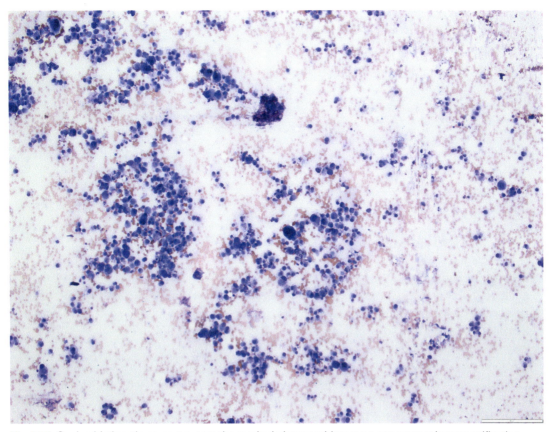

Fig 4.62 Canine histiocytic sarcoma; note the marked pleomorphism even apparent at low magnification (×100)

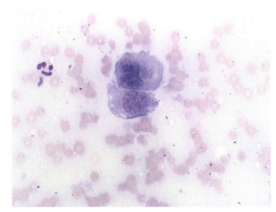

Fig 4.63 Higher power histiocytic sarcoma – cells with multiple nucleoli and variation in nuclear size/shape (×1000)

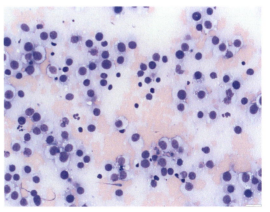

Fig 4.64 Transmissible venereal tumour; the cytoplasmic vacuolation is characteristic of this neoplasm (×500)

> **Key points**
>
> **Transmissible venereal tumour**
> - Rare in the northern Europe, the UK and the USA but seen in imported animals
> - Characteristic appearance: round cells with round central nuclei, pale cytoplasm and small clear vacuoles

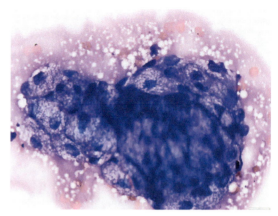

Fig 4.65 Well-differentiated sebaceous epithelium in a sebaceous adenoma (×500)

Features of benign and malignant tumours

Once a lesion has been identified as neoplastic, the most important question to answer is whether the tumour is likely following a benign or malignant clinical course. The following section describes the typical features of benign and malignant neoplasms, although there are many exceptions to these general rules – most notably, neuroendocrine tumours (such as thyroid carcinomas and anal sac adenocarcinomas) can have relatively benign appearance but are often extremely aggressive biologically. Similarly, lymphoma *usually* appears as a uniform collection of cells, rather than the markedly pleomorphic population that characterises many other malignant neoplasms.

General features of benign tumours

Benign tumours display only limited changes from their tissue of origin, and typically closely resemble the original tissue. The cells present are usually homogenous, and a similar size to normal cells from the original tissue.

Benign cells often have a low nuclear to cytoplasmic ratio (N:C ratio); that is, they usually have small nuclei with moderate to abundant amounts of cytoplasm, although there are exceptions in tumours derived from cells with a naturally high N:C ratio (such as basal epithelium). Their nuclei are usually small and uniform with dense chromatin. If nucleoli are present, they also tend to be small, uniform, well defined, with similar numbers and shapes in each nucleus (Fig 4.65). Binucleate and multinucleate cells are usually uncommon (exception: plasmacytomas and benign tumours of liver tissue – normal hepatocytes commonly display binucleation).

> **Key points**
>
> **Benign tumours**
> - Cells usually uniform appearance, minimal anisocytosis/anisokaryosis/pleomorphism
> - Usually resemble tissue of origin

General features of malignant tumours

As cells accrue mutations which move them genetically, behaviourally and (crucially, from a cytological perspective) morphologically further away from their original tissue, they tend to behave more aggressively. Cells become more individualised and less uniform; variations in shape (*pleomorphism*) and the size of both cells (*anisocytosis*) and their nuclei (*anisokaryosis*) become more common.

Malignant features can be broadly divided into changes noted within three categories: cellular, nuclear and cytoplasmic.

Cellular criteria for malignancy

Abnormal location: cells found in a location distant to their original tissue, such as cutaneous

lymphoma (high numbers of dermal lymphocytes) or epithelial/neuroendocrine cells found within a lymph node)
- **Variations in cell size and shape**: *anisocytosis* (varied cell size) and *pleomorphism* (varied cell shape). Benign lesions often display mild anisocytosis, but twofold or larger variations are more suggestive of malignancy (Figs 4.66, 4.67)
- **Loss of cohesion**: one feature of more aggressive neoplastic behaviour is decreased cell-cell adhesion, which increases the chance of metastasis; this leads to increased sample cellularity, and epithelial and mesenchymal tumours often exfoliate in smaller clusters or aggregates, with more individual cells
- **Disorderly arrangement**: as cells change size, shape and lose cohesiveness, the overall appearance of the groups becomes more disordered. Epithelial clusters become crowded and disorganised, with nuclear moulding occasionally visible (nuclei become 'moulded' around the shape of larger adjacent nuclei; this can occur between adjacent cells or within multinucleate cells); the presence of nuclear moulding is a feature of malignancy (Fig 4.68)

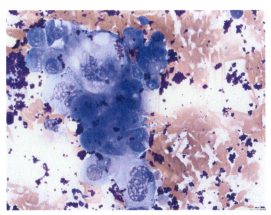

Fig 4.66 Marked cytomegaly (increase in cell size) in an anaplastic cutaneous canine neoplasm (×500)

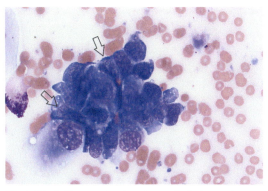

Fig 4.68 A disorganised and crowded cluster from a pulmonary adenocarcinoma; many nuclei appear "squeezed" by adjacent cells (nuclear moulding – open arrows and other examples) (×1000)

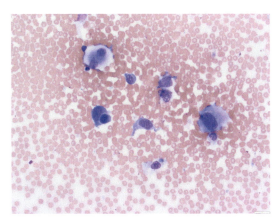

Fig 4.67 Pleomorphic cells from a canine transitional cell carcinoma; note also the poor cohesion of these cells (×500)

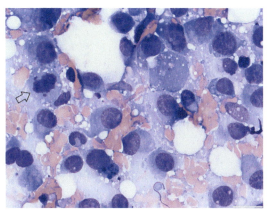

Fig 4.69 multiple variably-sized nucleoli in cells from a histiocytic sarcoma; note also the irregular 'ropy' chromatin; an atypical mitotic figure (open arrow) is present (×1000)

Nuclear Criteria for Malignancy

Variations in nuclear size and shape: *anisokaryosis* (varied nuclear size), nuclear pleomorphism (varied nuclear size) and *macronucleosis* (large nuclei) are all features of malignancy, and lead to variations (usually increases) in the N:C ratio (Fig 4.69)

Nucleolar changes: nucleoli are the site of ribosome construction within the nucleus and are therefore more prominent and more numerous in active cells; as neoplastic cells are usually highly active, they frequently display increased numbers of them. Variations in the size, shape and number of nucleoli are also criteria for malignancy (Fig 4.69). The presence of *macronucleoli* (nucleoli larger than a red blood cell) is a feature strongly associated with malignancy

Mitotic figures: mitotic figures are visible as cells replicate DNA ready for division – a population of cells containing mitotic figures indicates actively replicating tissue; small numbers may be seen in reactive or hyperplastic tissues such as lymph nodes or mesothelial cells, but high numbers are more commonly associated with malignancy (Fig 4.70). In addition, the presence of atypical mitotic figures (tripolar or multipolar division, 'scattered' chromatin due to fragments lagging behind the axis of division, asymmetry – see appendix G) raises significant concern for a malignant tumour

Chromatin changes: dense chromatin with no discernible pattern (commonly seen in small lymphocytes or basal epithelium) indicates

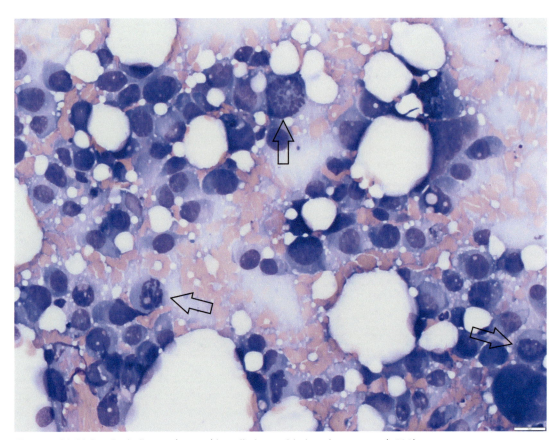

Fig 4.70 Multiple mitotic figures (arrows) in cells from a histiocytic sarcoma (×500)

tightly packed chromosomes and, usually, inactivity; the more 'open' the chromatin (i.e. paler with discernible patterns), the more active the cell; malignancy is associated with 'coarse' or 'ropy' chromatin, with irregular patches and clumps visible within the nuclei (Fig 4.69)

Cytoplasmic criteria for malignancy

Of the three criteria, these changes are the least specific – the changes below indicate increased cellular activity, including hyperplasia, reactivity, and benign neoplasia, not necessarily malignancy.

- **Cytoplasmic basophilia**: as cells accrue organelles, synthesise protein and secretory products, their cytoplasm becomes more basophilic (blue); in contrast, cells with shrunken eosinophilic cytoplasm are likely to be inactive, or potentially apoptotic or necrotic
- **Cytoplasmic vacuolation**: proteins and other products can accumulate in vacuoles within the cytoplasm, especially when production is excessive or aberrant (Fig 4.71); vacuoles are most commonly found in the perinuclear area (as this is the location of the Golgi apparatus); 'signet ring' cells are found within adenocarcinomas and are cells with a large single vacuole containing secretory product, displacing the nuclei to the side of the cell (Fig 4.72).

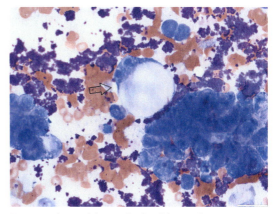

Fig 4.72 Large 'signet ring' cell in a pulmonary adenocarcinoma (×1000)

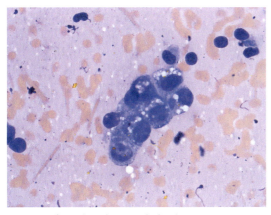

Fig 4.71 Cytoplasmic vacuolation in a cutaneous carcinoma (×1000)

> **Key points**
>
> **malignant tumours**
> - Cells generally become more individualised, and overall lesions appear disorganised with variations in cell size and shape
> - Changes in three areas – cellular, nuclear and cytoplasmic
> - Cellular changes: cells present in abnormal locations, variations in cell size and shape, disordered appearance and loss of cohesion
> - Nuclear changes: nucleus often increases in size, increased N:C ratio, variation in size and chromatin pattern, increased mitosis
> - Cytoplasmic changes (least specific): increased vacuolation, changes in colour (often increased basophilia/deeper blue colour)

Cytology of non-inflammatory and non-neoplastic lesions

Not every pathological process is inflammatory or neoplastic – there are a variety of other causes for fluid-filled or solid masses, many of which can still be recognised or at least suspected on cytological examination. Here are some of the most commonly encountered lesions, as well as other cellular and acellular material that may be present.

Cellular lesions and material

Hyperplasia

Hyperplasia is a reversible non-neoplastic proliferation of tissue, usually epithelial tissue, in response to stimuli. The cells have normal morphology, and hyperplasia cannot be definitively confirmed cytologically, but the presence of high numbers of morphologically unremarkable cells in an enlarged organ or tissue is strongly suggestive. Hyperplasia of the prostate gland (Fig 4.73) and lymph nodes are the most commonly seen hyperplastic tissues. In cutaneous lesions, sebaceous epithelial hyperplasia and mammary hyperplasia can be challenging to distinguish from well-differentiated neoplastic lesions, such as sebaceous and mammary adenomas.

Necrosis (and degeneration)

Necrosis is more 'formerly cellular' than cellular, comprising the remains of degenerate non-viable cells. Necrosis appears as greyish-blue amorphous material, found in wide swathes, often containing indistinct and blurred necrotic cell ghosts, or degenerating clusters or aggregates of cells. Neutrophils and macrophages are often embedded, as necrosis stimulates an inflammatory response (Fig 4.74).

Apoptotic cells (cells undergoing controlled cell death) or early necrotic cells are more challenging to assess – they still retain their cellular structure but are condensed, with small dense nuclei and small amounts of pale cytoplasm, slightly resembling epithelium. Apoptotic cells

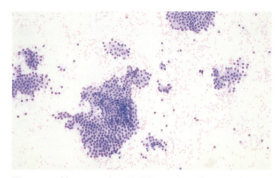

Fig 4.73 Clusters of well-differentiated prostatic epithelial cells in prostatic hyperplasia (×1000)

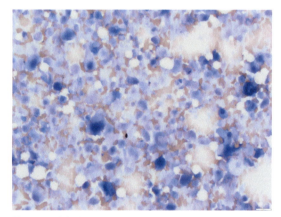

Fig 4.74 Marked necrosis within a prostatic carcinoma; note the blurred/smudged indistinct shapes which were once living cells (×500)

are frustrating to find cytologically, as the preparations initially appear to be cellular enough for successful diagnosis, but closer inspection reveals that the cells have lost most of their unique structure and appearance, and they generally cannot be identified.

Necrosis is not a specific finding, as it can be caused by intense inflammation or infarction, but the otherwise unexplained presence of necrosis in a lesion often raises concern for underlying neoplasia.

Occasionally, highly degenerate material, as opposed to necrosis, is observed – for instance, in degenerate benign epithelial neoplasms in cats, or markedly degenerate keratin (Fig 4.75). It can be very challenging to distinguish between this degenerate material and necrosis, which is frustrating as necrosis is associated with more severe diseases (malignant neoplasia, severe chronic inflammation) than degenerate material. Sometimes it is impossible to decide between the possibilities, but necrosis generally triggers neutrophilic/macrophagic inflammation, whereas degenerate material typically doesn't. As will be repeated through the course of this book, the context is important and must be considered.

Squames

'Squames' are large anucleate keratinised squamous epithelial cells. They are the surface layer of skin, constantly shed from the body, and are a common finding in aspirates from the skin but are also found on many other specimens due to contamination (from dust or fingerprints). They are also the main finding in aspirates from the prostate when it has undergone squamous metaplasia (usually secondary to hormone production from Sertoli cell tumours).

Cytologically, they are large angular pale blue cells, missing a nucleus (Fig 4.76).

Acellular lesions and material

Keratin-filled lesions

Although there are significant histological differences between the many adnexal lesions which contain keratin, they are cytologically identical, and have a good prognosis – excision is expected

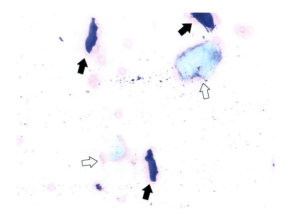

Fig 4.76 Anucleate squames (open arrows) (alongside rolled 'bars' of keratin – black arrows) (×1000)

to be curative, when required. Aspiration of these lesions usually produces variable amounts of thick off-white material which, when examined cytologically, is a mixture of keratin, keratin bars and scrolls, and cholesterol crystals.

Keratin is angular, anucleate and palely to deeply basophilic, or (less commonly) slightly purple (Fig 4.77). Keratin bars and scrolls are small linear angular structures with pale (scrolls) or deep (bars) basophilic staining. Cholesterol crystals are formed from the breakdown of cell membranes and are clear, square or rectangular. 'Ghost cells' are also commonly encountered – these are anucleate cellular shape-structures

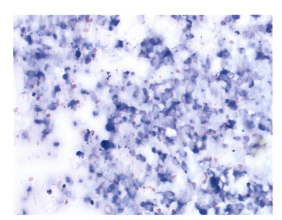

Fig 4.75 Degenerate non-necrotic material from a keratinising cyst (×500)

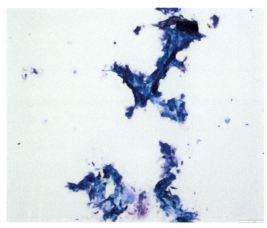

Fig 4.77 Clumps of keratin (×100)

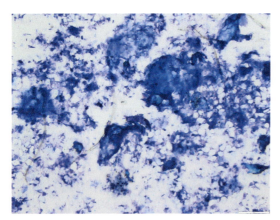

Fig 4.78 Keratin and embedded "ghost cells", associated with pilomatricomas (×100)

with pale central areas and have been associated with pilomatricomas (benign hair follicle tumours) (Fig 4.78).

Keratin is also a common contaminant of cytological specimens – see page 48 for a discussion of this and suggestions of how to distinguish between contamination and truly keratinised specimens.

Keratin is irritant to surrounding tissue – when these lesions rupture, they commonly produce a marked neutrophilic, macrophagic or mixed inflammatory pattern, often with multinucleate macrophages (consistent with a foreign body reaction – see above). Ruptured keratin-containing lesions can be challenging to resolve medically, and surgical excision often proves the fastest route to resolution in these cases. However, care should be taken when interpreting inflamed lesions containing keratin, as the cytological appearance of squamous cell carcinomas can be similar to ruptured keratinising cysts, particularly where high numbers of neutrophils are present (Fig 4.79).

Apocrine cysts

These common lesions form due to occlusion of apocrine (sweat) glands. They are firm dermal masses filled with pale yellow to brown fluid. Cytologically, this fluid is usually acellular with a clear to slightly pink background (Fig 4.80).

Seromas/haematomas and protein clefts

The cytological appearance of these lesions is somewhat similar – both contain low to moderate numbers of macrophages, usually activated, within a fluid background. Seromas contain proteinaceous fluid, which appears cytologically as a markedly stippled pale-to-mid eosinophilic or amphophilic background, often with protein clefts – crescent-shaped folds within the fluid (Fig 4.81). Haematomas usually have a far less stippled, often eosinophilic, background and contain moderate to high numbers of erythrocytes with evidence of previous haemorrhage (see below).

Blood contamination versus previous haemorrhage

When cytological samples yield large amounts of blood, it is valuable to distinguish between fresh blood contamination during sampling and bleeding prior to sampling. Platelets are only present for a very short time (always less than an hour and typically less than a few minutes) following haemorrhage, and their presence on cytology almost always indicates accidental contamination.

In lesions with pre-existing haemorrhage, macrophages are often seen containing phagocytosed red blood cells or (after several days) red cell breakdown products – haemosiderin (dark granular pigment) (Fig 4.82) or haematoidin (golden-brown rhomboid crystals) (Fig 4.83). Note that red cell phagocytosis (erythrophagia) can occur while fluids are in sample tubes, which is why it is important to make fresh fluid preparations as soon as possible after sampling.

Calcinosis

Dystrophic mineralisation is often readily recognisable grossly on cytological specimens. *Calcinosis circumscripta* is seen in pressure points and areas of repeated trauma, seen uncommonly in dogs and rarely in cats. *Calcinosis cutis* is more usually seen in dorsal regions, especially over the neck,

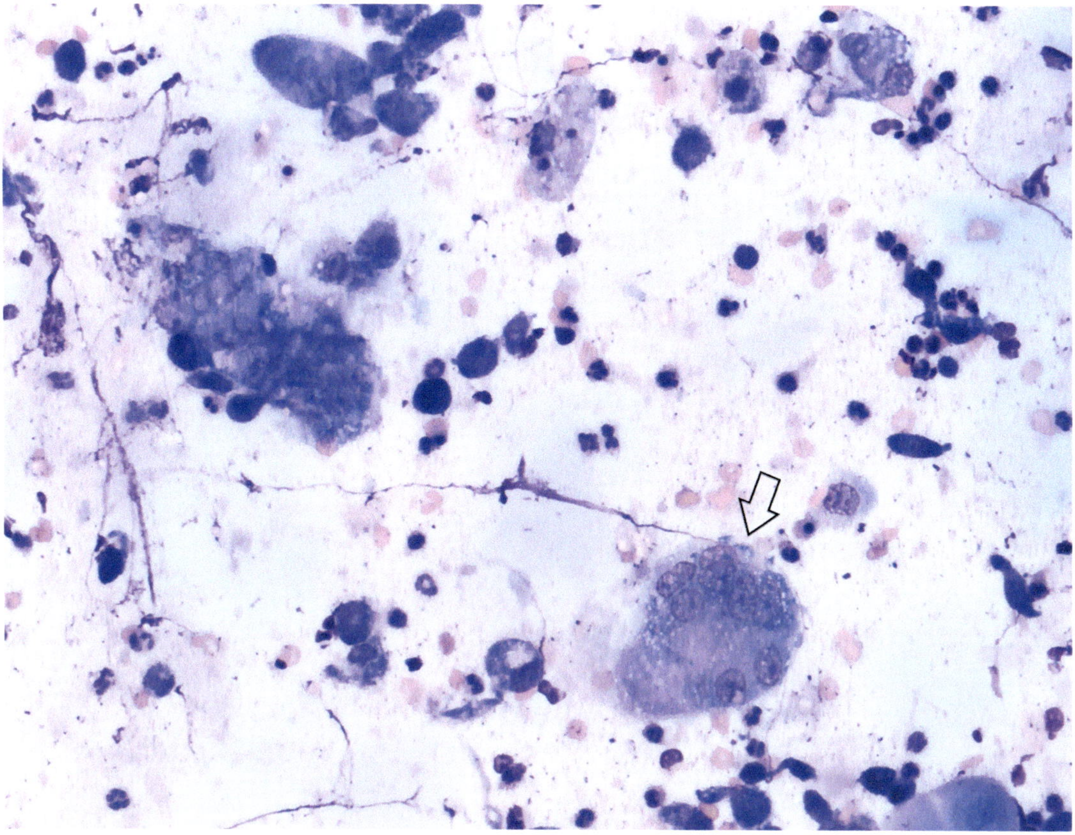

Fig 4.79 Ruptured keratin cyst with neutrophilic/macrophagic inflammation; note the large multinucleate macrophage (open arrow), a common feature in foreign body reactions

Fig 4.80 Acellular fluid aspirated from an apocrine cyst (×500)

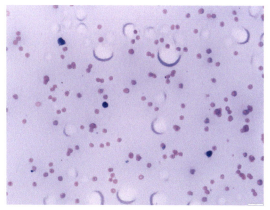

Fig 4.81 Stippled purple fluid with protein clefts (the crescent-shaped objects), indicative of high-protein fluid (×500)

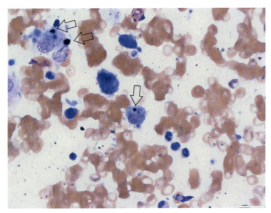

Fig 4.82 Macrophages containing haemosiderin (arrows), indicating haemorrhage prior to sampling (×1000)

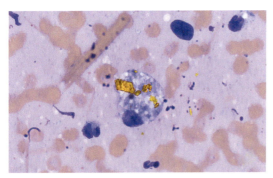

Fig 4.83 Macrophages containing haematoidin crystals (golden-yellow crystals, also free in background) (×1000)

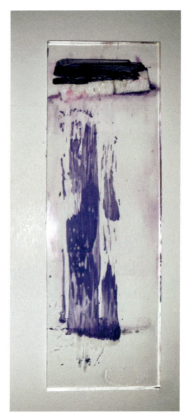

Fig 4.84 Gross 'chalky' appearance of mineralised specimens

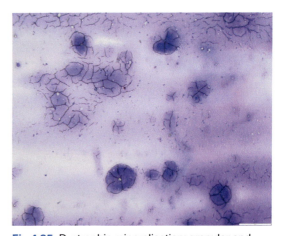

Fig 4.85 Dystrophic mineralisation; granular and brownish-purple background (×100)

and is associated with glucocorticoids (and therefore is occasionally seen in Cushing's disease).

The conditions appear cytologically identical – on the slides, the stained material often has a chalky pale blue to lilac appearance (Fig 4.84). Under the microscope, the material has a darker and often brownish appearance, with a granular irregular background, sometimes containing rounded calcium carbonate crystals (Fig 4.85). This background (and the crystals) dissolves when immersion oil is applied to the slide. Due to of the irritation associated with mineralisation, macrophages, sometimes multinucleate, are often seen, as well as other leukocytes and fibroblasts.

When unexpected mineralisation is found in a cytological preparation, evaluation of the patient's serum calcium may be prudent.

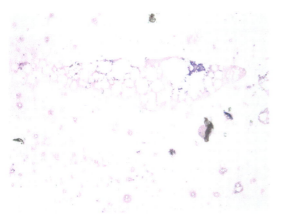

Fig 4.86 Low power appearance of fat droplets (×100)

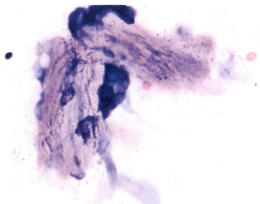

Fig 4.87 Collagen ribbons in a mast cell tumour (×500)

Fat

In Romanowsky-stained specimens (i.e. most in-house and lab-stained samples), extracellular fat is dissolved by the methanol fixative, and therefore is not visible. Instead, fatty specimens will have many non-staining clear circular spaces (Fig 4.86) – checking whether a slide appears greasy or not prior to staining (and possibly noting this on the slide in some way, such as a 'G' inscribed on the corner) is helpful.

Collagen

Collagen is sometimes found scattered in cutaneous samples, and also features prominently in several lesions: mast cell tumours (due to the collagenolytic activity), fibroadenaxal hamartomas and keloidal fibroma/sarcoma (Fig 4.88).

Cytologically, collagen appears as small smooth ('hyaline') ribbons of pale pinkish material, found in characteristic whorls and convoluted shapes in keloidal fibrosarcomas (Fig 4.87).

Melanin

Melanin is a common finding in cutaneous aspirates, often embedded within surface squames, or free in the background. It is also present within cells in pigmented epithelial tumours and melanocytic tumours (melanocytomas and melanomas), sometimes phagocytosed within macrophages (melanophages), and can be found in the background of lymph nodes reacting to areas of skin inflammation (melanin incontinence).

Melanin is usually found in brownish-black lozenge shaped granules (Fig 4.89). When phagocytosed within macrophages or present within melanocytes, it is usually darker and found in more variably-sized globules. Poorly-pigmented melanomas may only contain a fine sandy scattering within their cytoplasm.

Amyloid

Amyloid is a collection of misfolded protein which accumulates within tissues and is often highly relevant when observed. Amyloid deposits can be found within the spleen, liver and kidney in animals with *amyloidosis* (particularly in Shar Peis, and Abyssinian, Rex, and Siamese cats). It can also be found in small amounts in some plasmacytomas (where it represents immunoglobulins).

Cytologically, it appears as small clumps of fluffy material, resembling clouds or candy floss, but usually deeply purple in colour. It slightly resembles extracellular matrix but is not fibrillar (Fig 4.90). Special cytological stains (most commonly *Congo red*) confirm its presence.

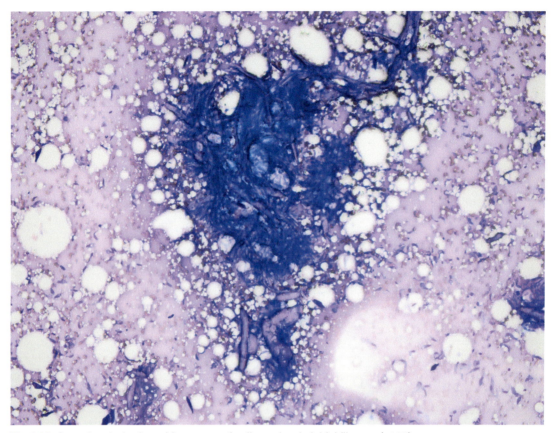

Fig 4.88 Convoluted whorls and fragments of collagen in a keloidal fibroma (×100)

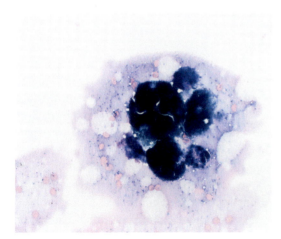

Fig 4.89 Melanin embedded in the background of a melanocytoma (×500)

Matrix

Extracellular matrix is usually produced by mesenchymal cells, often in response to inflammation (part of fibroplasia) but some mesenchymal tumours also produce matrix, and in some lesions (such as myxosarcoma or chondrosarcoma), the matrix is the predominant finding.

Matrix appears cytologically as an amorphous patch of red, pink or purple material, often (but not always) in association with mesenchymal cells. It is often *fibrillar* – that is, it has the appearance of having small fine fibres within it, rather than appearing completely featureless (Fig 4.91). The colour and amount of extracellular matrix should be noted. It is discussed more on page 81 (above) in the context of mesenchymal neoplasia.

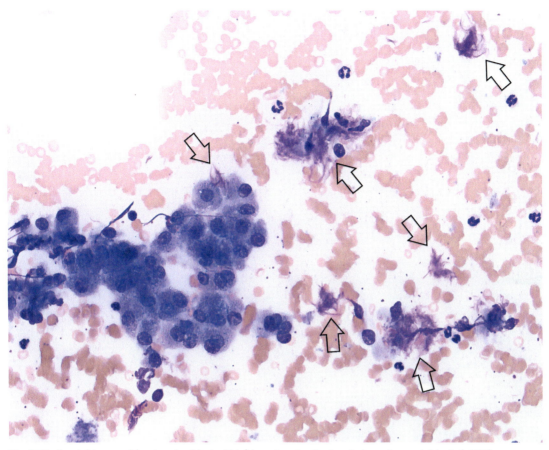

Fig 4.90 Amyloid around (and embedded within) hepatocyte clusters in hepatic amyloidosis (×500)

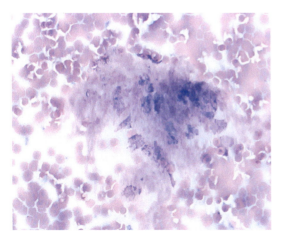

Fig 4.91 Fibrillar purple extracellular matrix from a gastrointestinal stromal tumour (GIST) (×100)

Crystals and crystal fragments

Small fragments of crystalline material can be found in debris, but larger intact crystals (usually larger than an erythrocyte) should be examined as they may be relevant; the colour and shape of crystals helps to identify them, and some of them help to identify the lesion. See appendix D for more detail.

> **Key points**
>
> **Non-neoplastic lesions**
> - Necrosis typically induces neutrophilic/macrophagic inflammation, as opposed to degenerate or apoptotic material
> - Keratin is highly irritant to surrounding tissue when exposed to it (in ruptured cysts) and can trigger a strong neutrophilic /macrophagic inflammatory response. The macrophages can be large, multinucleate or clustered like epithelial cells, which can be mistaken for malignancy
> - Further care should be taken when interpreting inflamed lesions containing keratin, as the cytological appearance of squamous cell carcinomas can be similar to ruptured keratinising cysts
> - Platelets are only present for a short time following haemorrhage, and their presence on cytology almost always indicates accidental contamination
> - Collagen can feature prominently in several lesions: mast cell tumours, fibroadenaxal hamartomas and keloidal fibrosarcomas

Some final points on general cytology

A note on signalment and context

It is useful to remember whilst examining specimens that cytology is a highly contextual discipline. Our samples comprise low numbers of cells, unexpectedly removed from their surroundings and presented to us divorced from their environment. This missing context can only be usefully found with knowledge of the exact location of the area sampled, the history of the lesion ('Did it arrive recently?' 'Has it grown rapidly?' 'Have similar lesions been sampled before?'), and the signalment.

As an example, consider a slide containing aggregates of fat cells. The slide alone can only indicate to the cytologist that fat has been sampled. If the sample was taken from a smooth, subcutaneous mass in a middle-aged dog, then it is likely that a lipoma has been aspirated. If it was taken from a red cutaneous mass which has only been present for a week in a young cat, then it is highly likely that the sample represents inadvertent aspiration of subcutaneous fat, rather than the lesion itself. If the aspirate was from a nodule in the spleen, then a myelolipoma starts to become a consideration.

This becomes especially important when examining specimens for colleagues, or when submitting specimens for external laboratories. Shorn of context, the interpretation of cytological specimens becomes much more limited.

Exceptions to general principles: Common pitfalls and useful points to remember

Cytological specimens are full of traps for the unwary cytologist. This chapter has outlined many general points and principles of cytology, but there are many exceptions to these rules. Here are some of the most common.

- Inflammation causes hyperplasia and dysplasia in tissues, which can mimic neoplasia – be cautious when diagnosing tumours in the presence of inflammation.
- Degeneration of cells within fluid (particularly urine) can also mimic malignant features, as cells swell variably and so appear chaotic and disorganised – be cautious when diagnosing neoplasia based on poorly preserved cells within fluid.
- The prognosis of many tumours depends upon their grade; because grading of tumours often involves examining their invasiveness to adjacent tissues, cytological schemes for grading have not been established; histopa-

thology is required for the grading of many neoplasms.
- Despite the general guidelines for the appearance of malignant tumours, several tumours (particularly neuroendocrine tumours such as thyroid carcinomas and anal sac apocrine gland adenocarcinomas) behave much more aggressively than their cytological appearance suggests.
- Similarly, the behaviour of complex tumours – particularly mammary tumours – is often poorly correlated with their appearance on cytology preparations, and mammary neoplasia may be better examined histopathologically than cytologically.
- Fibroblasts present due to reactivity can display many features consistent with malignancy and are often extremely challenging to distinguish from poorly-cellular aspirates from sarcomas, particularly when inflammation is also present.
- Similarly, due to their highly plastic nature, macrophages can appear very variable in cytological specimens, displaying anisocytosis, anisokaryosis, multinucleation and pleomorphism; examining the N:C ratio can be helpful in these cases as the larger active cells will usually also have expanded cytoplasm, keeping the N:C ratio low, but macrophages provide a constant challenge even for experienced cytologists.
- Reactive mesothelial cells, which can be found in areas lined with mesothelium (i.e. the pleural, pericardial and peritoneal cavities) can also take on multiple features of malignancy, particularly if an effusion is longstanding or markedly inflammatory. Mesothelial cells can be challenging to distinguish from exfoliating carcinomas in effusions; mesothelial cell harvests can be particularly high in pericardial effusions, or in pleural effusions from patients with histories of pericardial disease or pericardectomy (see later).

Chapter 4 – take home messages

- A systematic approach is the most useful way to assess cytological specimens.
- Specimens are broadly classified as inflammatory or neoplastic.
- Inflammation is then further categorised into type: neutrophilic, macrophagic, lymphocytic, eosinophilic, mixed, etc.
- Similarly, neoplasms are categorised as epithelial, mesenchymal, 'round cell', neuroendocrine.
- For inflammatory lesions, further assessment looks for infectious agents, foreign material or underlying neoplasia.
- For neoplasia, further assessment identifies whether the lesion is likely to benign or malignant.

Chapter 5

Infectious agents

The diagnosis of infection is one of the key strengths of cytology. Lesions which appear grossly similar (such as an abscess or necrotic tumour) can be quickly differentiated cytologically, and whilst further testing is sometimes required for confirmation, the presence of infectious agents leads to a rapid presumptive diagnosis.

Contamination of preparations with infectious agents and the presence of commensal organisms can lead to confusion, however. The most useful method to distinguish between contamination/commensals and genuine infection is the presence of inflammation (Fig 5.1). Contaminants or commensals do not elicit an inflammatory response, as they were not present before sampling.

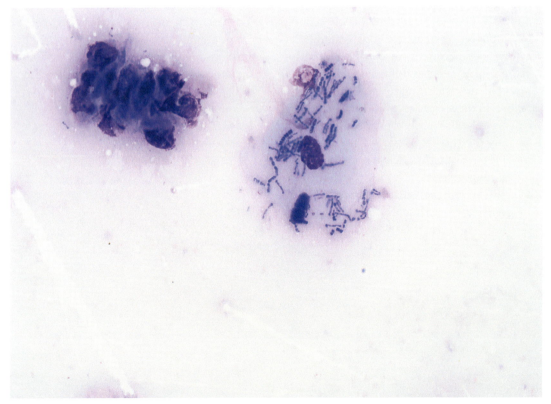

Fig 5.1a Mixed bacterial commensals embedded within an anucleate squame without inflammation present (×1000)

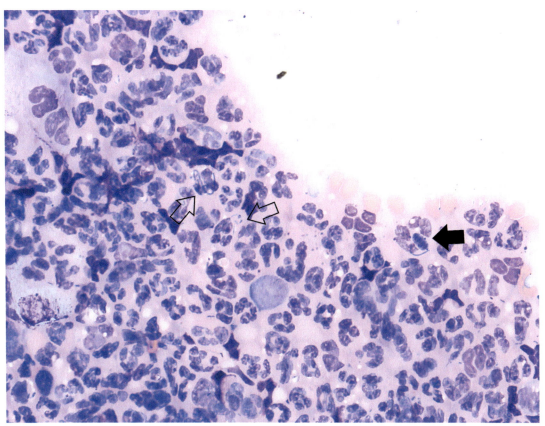

Fig 5.1b Mixed bacterial infection; there is marked inflammation and bacteria are phagocytosed within neutrophils (open arrows); note there is also a colony of *Conchiformibius* present – this is a commensal organism and unlikely to be involved in the infection (black arrow) (×1000)

Pathogens generally elicit strong inflammation, and the pattern of inflammation is often indicative of the type of organism (for instance, neutrophilic for bacteria, macrophagic for fungi, eosinophilic for parasites) although there is some overlap (for instance, chronic or secondary bacterial infections can also contain high numbers of macrophages), and hypersensitivity reactions to bacterial toxins (particularly *Staphylococcus*) can lead to an influx of eosinophils.

There are exceptions; sometimes pathogens elicit only weak inflammatory responses, or the patient's immune response may be weakened, and contaminants can also be found in already inflamed lesions. The presence of infectious organisms phagocytosed within leukocytes, however, is extremely strong cytological evidence for infection (Fig 5.2).

The rest of this chapter comprises a brief discussion of several infectious organisms. This discussion is not exhaustive – a complete list of infectious agents of the dog and cat is already the subject of several entire textbooks – but covers the organisms most commonly encountered cytologically, as well as the form that these organisms are most often observed in.

Bacteria

Bacteria are by far the most common organism found on cytological specimens, both as

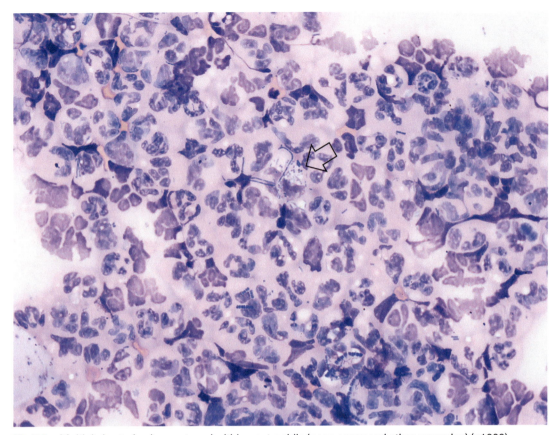

Fig 5.2a Multiple bacteria phagocytosed within neutrophils (open arrow and other examples) (×1000)

contaminants and as pathogens. Whilst culture is required for definitive identification of bacteria, the morphology and variety of bacteria can give important clues as to the type and even the origin of infection.

It is important to try to get samples prior to starting antibiotics – the chance of finding bacteria rapidly reduces after commencing antimicrobial therapy. Failing to find bacteria on cytology does not exclude bacterial infection, and culture should be carried out on all suspect samples.

Given their size, searching for most bacteria is only realistically possible on higher magnifications (using at least ×50 and usually ×100 objectives).

A note on stain precipitate

Stain precipitate is made up of small dense blobs of dye, formed within the dyeing solution. It can be confusing because on occasions it can strongly resemble bacterial cocci (Fig 5.3), although there are several differences which help distinguish between the two.

- Stain precipitate is often refractile (it will change in colour and intensity as the focus is slightly altered) – true bacterial organisms usually aren't.
- Stain precipitate is often slightly variable in size – true bacteria (of the same species) are usually nearly identical size, staining intensity and shape.

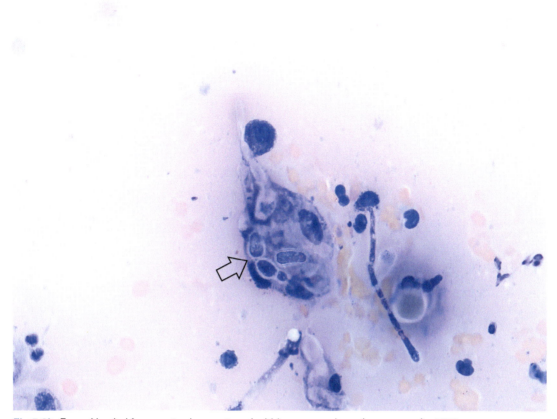

Fig 5.2b Fungal hyphal fragments phagocytosed within a macrophage (open arrow) ×1000

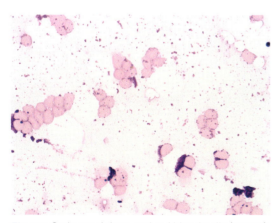

Fig 5.3 Stain precipitate and red blood cells (×1000)

- Bacteria are often found in chains, pairs or small colonies, whereas stain precipitate is usually distributed randomly across the slide.

In genuine infection, bacteria are often found in the areas of the preparation where the neutrophils appear most degenerate. Again, the presence of bacteria phagocytosed within neutrophils (Fig 5.4) (or occasionally eosinophils or macrophages) is diagnostic of bacterial infection, although care must be taken not to confuse karyorrhexis (an ageing change of neutrophils) with bacterial organisms (see page 107, Fig 5.1b). It is also worth noting that in cases where all bacteria are observed within neutrophils with no free organisms present, culture can often be negative despite the cytological appearance. Finally, remember that in fluid samples, limited bacterial phagocytosis can occur within the sample if there is a delay in processing.

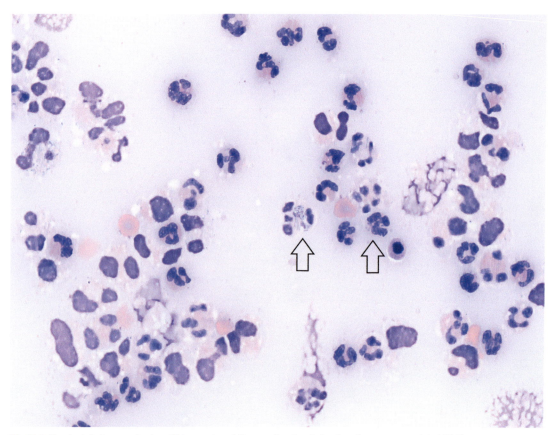

Fig 5.4 Bacterial phagocytosis within neutrophils, confirming infection (open arrows) (×1000)

Cocci

Cytologically, these appear as small dense dots, of the same size (Fig 5.5), and these are the most common commensal organisms on the skin. *Staphylococcus*, the most commonly encountered, is generally slightly larger and often found in pairs (diplococci) or small groups, whereas *Streptococcus* (slightly less common) is usually smaller and found in chains, although the species cannot be reliably determined cytologically.

Bacilli

Bacilli vary widely in size and shape, from short thick rods to longer, slender rods forming chains (Fig 5.6). Bacilli form the majority of bacteria found within the gastrointestinal tract, where a large variety of bacteria are found (very

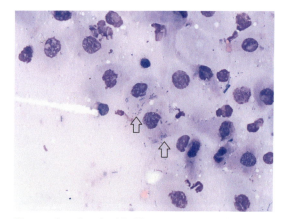

Fig 5.5 Cocci embedded in a squamous epithelial cell (open arrows) (×1000)

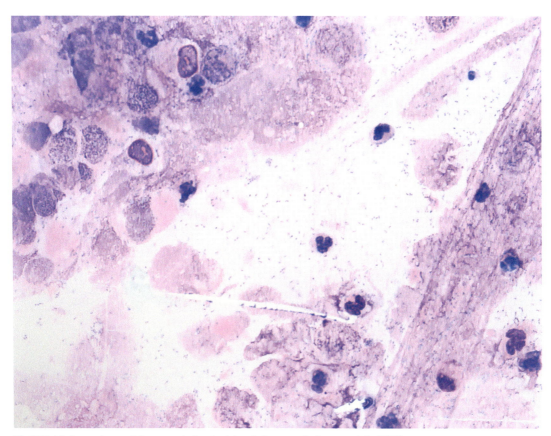

Fig 5.6 High numbers of degenerate bacterial rods in a respiratory wash (×1000)

few cocci are found within the intestinal lumen in a normal situation). Bacterial rods observed on cytological specimens from the external ear raise suspicion of (but are not specific for) *Pseudomonas* infection.

Conchiformibius (previously Simonsiella)

These highly distinctive bacteria are a useful finding cytologically. At first glance they appear to be large tablet-like organisms, but in fact are colonies of bacterial rods arranged parallel to each other (Fig 5.7). Their utility is that they are oral commensal organisms, almost never pathogenic, and their presence on a specimen (i.e. on a skin lesion, or a respiratory wash) indicates the presence of some oropharnygeal contamination.

Spirochaetes (FIG 5.7A)

Slightly harder to spot, but no less distinctive than *Conchiformibius*, spirochaetes are spiral-shaped organisms, usually found within the gastrointestinal system. Their presence on cytology preparations can indicate oral contamination, as above. They are also prevalent on stomach aspirates (their presence does not necessarily indicate *Helicobacter* infection, although it is a clue to the presence of the organism; as with many bacteria, the significance of finding them also depends on whether inflammation is also present). *Leptospira* is a spirochaetal organism but is rarely identified on cytological specimens. Similarly, *Borellia sp.* (which include *B. burgdoferi*, the causative agent of Lyme disease, and *B. turocatae*, causing tick-borne relapsing fever) are rarely

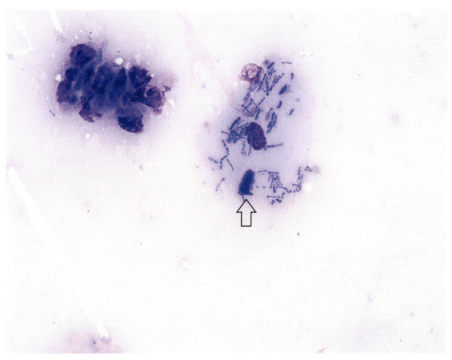

Fig 5.7 A colony of *Conchiformibius* embedded in a squamous epithelial cell (open arrow) along with other mixed bacteria (×1000)

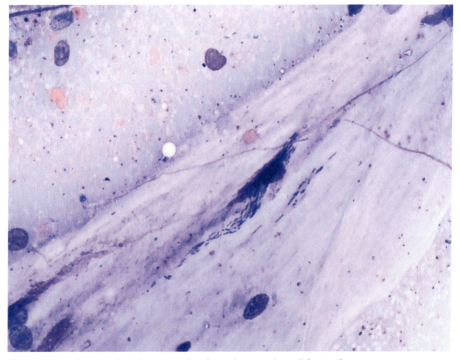

Fig 5.7a Spirochaetes in a cytobrush preparation from the gastric wall (×1000)

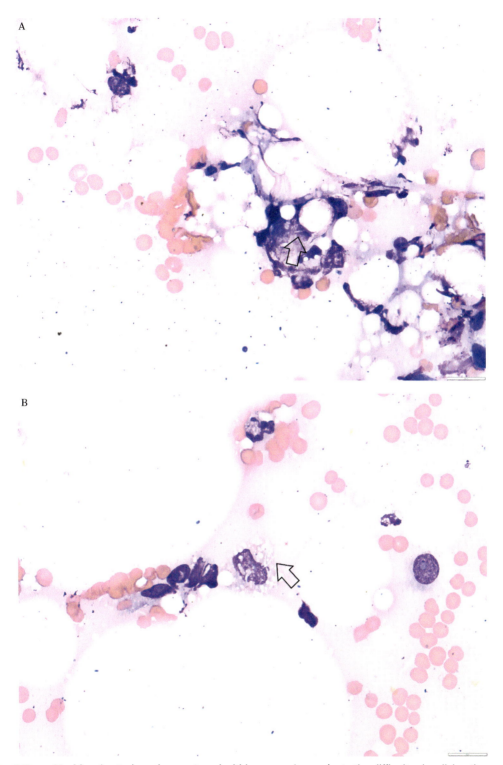

Figs 5.8a and b *Mycobacterium* phagocytosed within macrophages (note the difficulty visualising these negative staining organisms) (×1000)

encountered cytologically, although it is worth noting that spirochaetes observed on peripheral blood smears are far more likely to be *B. turicatae* than *B. burgdoferi*. *B. turicatae* has a much more limited distribution than *B. burgdoferi*, however, and is mostly found only in the western United States, Florida and Mexico.

'Negative staining' organisms

These are organisms that stain poorly with Romanowsky stains; if they appear at all, it is as a faint outline within the background. All of these organisms are clinically important, most notably *Mycobacterium*, which stain poorly due to their thick lipid walls. They appear as short slender rods or, more accurately, as clear spaces in the shape of short slender rods and are often present in high numbers phagocytosed within macrophages (within which they survive and multiply) (Fig 5.8). Acid-fast stains (such as Ziehl-Neelsen (ZN) stain) highlight them (Fig 5.9). Great care should be taken with patients and samples where *Mycobacterium* is suspected due to the zoonotic potential of the organism. Any samples submitted to external labs should be clearly labelled as suspected of *Mycobacterium*.

Mycobacterial infections often (but not always) elicit macrophagic inflammation, unlike many other bacteria.

Actinomyces and *Nocardia* species are also often negative-staining, but the organisms are long and branching (resembling fungal hyphae) and are often found in thick dense mats. They are usually introduced via foreign bodies. *Nocardia* can sometimes stain positively with acid-fast stains, but *Actinomyces* usually doesn't.

Mycoplasma

Mycoplasmas are a group of obligate intracellular bacteria, much smaller than most bacterial organisms, and consequently much harder to identify, but which occasionally cause respira-

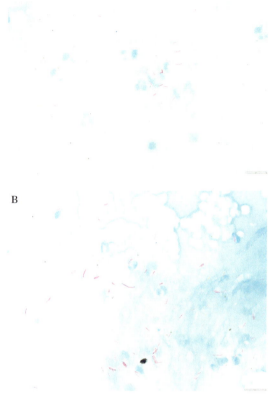

Figs 5.9a and b *Mycobacterium* highlighted with Ziehl-Neelsen stain (pink rods) (×500)

tory disease in cats. They do not grow on standard culture and are most easily identified by molecular testing (PCR).

Similarly, haemomycoplasmas – most notably *Mycoplasma haemofelis* – are bacteria which reproduce on the surface membrane of red blood cells, triggering lysis of the cells (feline infectious anaemia). Cytologically the organisms can be found adhered to the surface red blood cells, but their small size and similarity in appearance to stain precipitate makes them challenging to find. *Mycoplasma haemofelis*, the most pathogenic of the haemomycoplasmas, can appear as rings or chains of tiny cocci across the surface of erythrocytes (Fig 5.10). Fresh blood smears represent the best chance of finding them – they often detach in stored or anticoagulated blood, making them almost impossible to find. Again, molecular testing is more sensitive for these organisms than visual examination.

Other bacteria

There are a variety of other less common bacteria with varying size and shape, often encountered in samples from the gastrointestinal tract, or with faecal or oral contamination. As with the above organisms, their significance usually depends on whether there is concurrent inflammation. Other organisms such as the obligate intracellular parasites of blood cells (the rickettsial organisms, *Ehrlichia* and *Anaplasma*, both spread via tick bites), which can be found as groups of organisms in small pale blurry circles called *morulae*, can be difficult to spot cytologically (Fig 5.11).

Ehrlichia Canis (mostly found in monocytes) has a worldwide distribution except Australia, although it is rarely seen in the UK. *Ehrlichia ewingii* (mostly neutrophils) is confined to parts of the United States, mostly Missouri, Oklahoma and Arkansas. *Anaplasma phagocytophilium* (mostly neutrophils) is found throughout the northern hemisphere (again, rarely in the UK), and *Anaplasma platys* (platelets) has been reported in the United States, southern Europe, Asia, South America, the Middle East, Australia, the Caribbean and Africa.

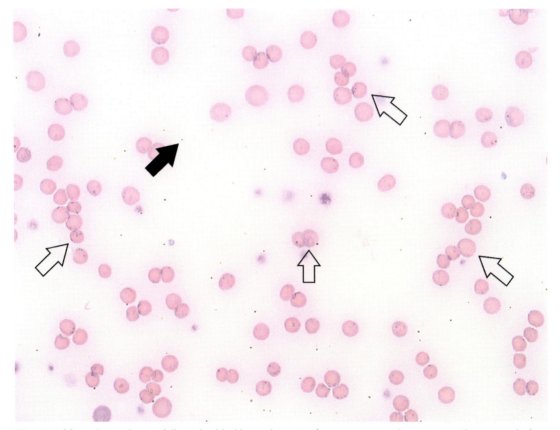

Fig 5.10 *Mycoplasma haemofelis* embedded in erythrocytes (open arrows and numerous other examples); note difficulty distinguishing from stain precipitate (black arrows) which appear darker and in a slightly different plane (slightly out of focus) (×1000)

> **Key points**
>
> **Bacteria**
>
> - The most useful method to distinguish between contamination and genuine infection is the presence of inflammation
> - The presence of infectious organisms phagocytosed within leukocytes, is extremely strong cytological evidence for infection
> - The presence of *Conchiformibius* (formerly *Simonsiella*) on a specimen (i.e. on a skin lesion, or a respiratory wash) indicates the presence of at least some oropharnygeal contamination
> - Mycobacterial infections often (but not always) elicit macrophagic inflammation, unlike many other bacteria

Fungi

Fungal organisms are encountered less commonly than bacteria (particularly in cooler or dryer climates) but they have the potential to cause very severe disease. With the severe infections, dogs are more prone to systemic disease, whereas cats more commonly have single and often cutaneous lesions, although there are, again, exceptions to this general rule. Fungal organisms usually elicit macrophagic inflammation – in chronic cases (common in fungal infections as they are often challenging infections for the immune system to combat), macrophages are often large and stuffed with high numbers of organisms. The macrophages may be the predominant cell present or may be mixed with neutrophils or occasionally lymphocytes (and plasma cells). Other patterns of inflammation (such as primarily neutrophilic or eosinophilic) are much rarer in fungal infections.

Although many fungi are visible using Romanowsky stains, stain update is unpredictable. Special stains such as Periodic acid-Schiff (PAS) (Fig 5.12) and Grocott's Methenamine Silver (GMS) are used in laboratories to highlight fungi, where suspected.

Fungi exist in a wide variety of forms, from long branchlike multicellular hyphae to small individual yeasts – whether they form yeasts or hyphae depends on a variety of factors, most notably temperature. The majority of fungi encountered on cytology specimens exist in one form or the other and are listed here in their most commonly encountered form, but cytologists should be aware that exceptions do occur (for instance, *Aspergillus* can sometimes be encountered predominantly as a yeast, and *Candida* can be found as yeast, hyphae and pseudohyphae simultaneously).

Hyphae

The fungal hyphae of many different species share a lot of morphological characteristics and coupled with the relatively uncommon nature of mycotic disease (making them less familiar to many cytologists), this makes the species of hyphal organisms challenging to identify (Fig 5.13). When examining hyphae, the cytologist should note the width of the organism (see page 34 for information on identifying the size of cytological objects in comparison to neutrophils and

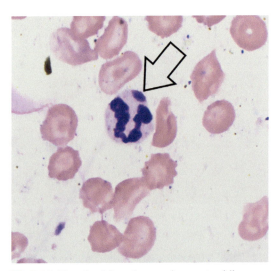

Fig 5.11 Morule of *Anaplasma phagocytophilum* within a neutrophil (open arrow) ×1000

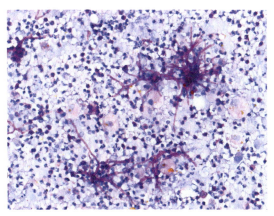

Fig 5.12 Fungal hyphae highlighted with PAS stain (×500)

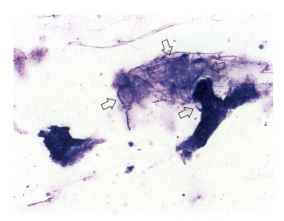

Fig 5.13 Poorly-preserved fungal hyphal fragments in nasal wash (open arrows) (×500)

erythroctyes), whether it branches and at what angle (i.e. right angled, acute, obtuse, irregular), whether their walls are parallel or non-parallel, and whether they are septate (i.e. they have hyphae divided into sections by small thin walls (*septa*) or non-septate. These features can help identify organisms – *Aspergillus*, the most commonly encountered of the pathogenic hyphal fungi, is usually septate, with parallel walls and right-angled branches (Fig 5.14) – but for most cytologists, the morphological findings alone are not specific enough for identification and culture or PCR examination is generally required.

As mentioned above, *Aspergillus* is the most commonly encountered pathogenic hyphal organism. Many other organisms are opportunistic saprophytic organisms (such as *Alternaria*) and cause fungal mycetomas (a chronic slow-growing inflammatory lesion, usually found in cats, present as cutaneous or subcutaneous lesions) due to their accidental introduction into a wound. Such cases are often both surgically and medically challenging to treat.

Yeasts

Yeasts are the unicellular form of fungal organisms, and they vary widely in size and shape. The organisms discussed here are predominantly found as yeasts, but as with the hyphae, exceptions do occur and some organisms are present as hyphae or pseudohyphae (sometimes concurrently with yeasts, as with *Candida*).

When examining yeasts, the important features to note are the size and shape of the organisms, whether they are surrounded by a capsule and how large the capsule is). Careful examination for the type of budding the organism exhibits is also useful; budding is the process of yeast reproduction where a new yeast 'buds' off another. In 'narrow-based' budding, there is an obvious narrowing (resembling a waist) between the organisms, whereas with 'broad-based' budding, the new yeast emerges from the old without an obvious narrowing/waist.

In general practice, the yeast most commonly encountered cytologically is *Malassezia*, usually found on preparations from cases of otitis externa or skin fold dermatitis. Although *Malassezia* can be found in a variety of forms, the most common is one resembling a footprint or a peanut – a small basophilic (deep blue) organism comprising two adjacent circular ends joined by a slightly narrow waist.

Although ringworm (usually *Trichophyton* or *Microsporidium species*) is a common infection in dogs and cats, it is a relatively uncommon finding on cytological specimens, probably because the organism is mostly adhered to

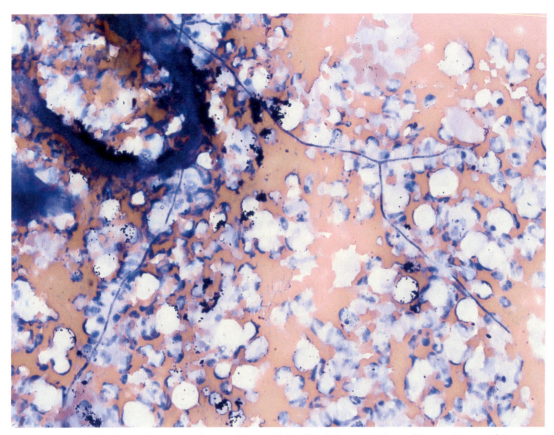

Fig 5.14 *Aspergillus* in respiratory wash: note the parallel walls, right-angled branching and septae (clear divisions between hyphal segments) (×500)

hair follicles, although occasionally the infection has extensive dermal involvement, and in some cases a raised dermal lesion known as a **kerion** can be present. The yeasts are small round to slightly oval structures, 2–3μm wide, with a thin clear capsule, often found in dense aggregates (Fig 5.15). Large clumps of them may be seen attached to hair shafts. Hyphae are rare and often negatively staining.

Persian cats are predisposed to *dermatophytic pseudomycetoma* – ringworm which penetrates deep into the subcutaneous layer. These lesions usually require wide surgical excision, as with true mycetomas (see page 179, Fig 6.77).

Other yeasts are relatively uncommon, depending on the geographic location – in general, warmer and wetter climates are more supportive of fungal infections. Of those most commonly encountered, *Blastomyces* is the main organism to exhibit broad-based budding. The yeasts are medium in size (10–20μm) with thick double walls.

Narrow-based budding yeasts include the small (1–4μm) yeasts *Sporothrix* and *Histoplasma*, which are distinguishable because *Histoplasma* yeasts are uniformly round to slightly oval (Fig 5.16), whereas *Sporothrix* also contain fusiform (spindle-shaped) yeasts; the medium yeast *Cryptococcus* (often distinctive due to the thick capsule surrounding them, which can comprise the majority of the width of the organism (5–15μm not including the capsule, 20–40μm including it) (Fig 5.17), and organisms

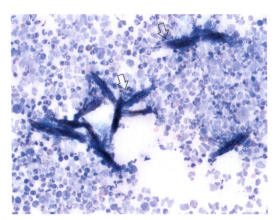

Fig 5.15a Ringworm (open arrows and numerous other examples) adhered to hair shafts (×500)

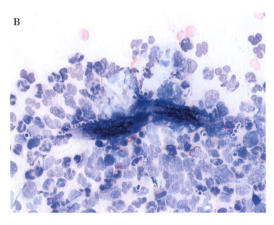

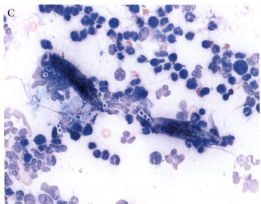

Figs 5.15b and c Ringworm at higher power (×1000)

which form very large (100–200μm) spherules, packed with much smaller endospores, such as *Coccidioides* and *Rhinosporidium* (although this is technically classified somewhere between a fungus and an animal).

Many of the above organisms can cause extremely severe systemic disease and some of them (such as *Coccidioides* and *Sporothrix*) are zoonotic.

Finally in this category is *Pneumocystis* – this is classified as fungi but displays some characteristics of a protozoan. It is rarely seen except in immunocompromised animals; in particular, Cavalier King Charles spaniels and miniature dachshunds are genetically predisposed to immune disorders leaving them vulnerable to *Pneumocystis*. The organism forms small (5–10μm diameter) cysts containing up to eight small dots (intracytoplasmic bodies), slightly resembling a tiny clock or wheel, as well as very small (1–2μm) trophozoites, which can easily be mistaken for platelets.

> **Key points**
>
> **Fungi**
> - Fungal organisms usually elicit macrophagic inflammation
> - They exist in a wide variety of forms, from long branchlike multicellular hyphae to small individual yeasts
> - Fungi are *usually* only found in one form (yeasts or hyphae) within lesions, but there are exceptions
> - *Aspergillus* is the most commonly encountered of the pathogenic hyphal fungi; it is usually septate, with parallel walls and right-angled branches
> - *Malassezia* is the most commonly encountered pathogenic yeast; its most common form resembles a footprint

Protozoa

Protozoa are single-celled eukaryotes (as opposed to bacterial prokaryotes, which lack nuclei and many organelles) and a number

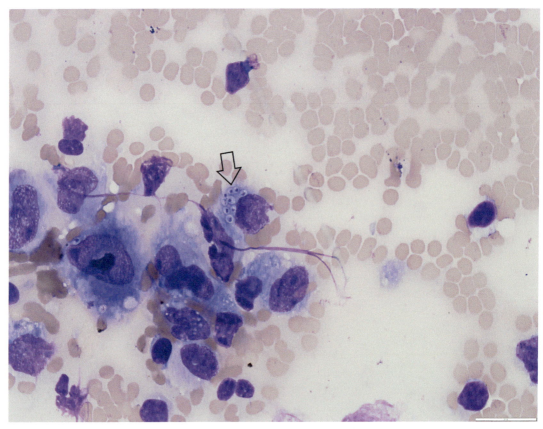

Fig 5.16 *Histoplasma* yeasts within a macrophage (open arrow) (×1000)

of organisms cause disease in the domestic species commonly (or, at least, relatively commonly, which is to say much less commonly than bacteria). The life cycle of protozoans varies from species to species; this book focuses on the stage of organisms most commonly encountered in clinical infection.

Toxoplasma/neospora

These are coccidian organisms usually encountered in their definitive hosts (cats for *Toxoplasma*, dogs for *Neospora*). They have a somewhat complex life cycle but are usually encountered as tachyzoites cytologically. The tachyzoites are morphologically similar in both organisms (as are the tachyzoites of a handful of other coccidians such as *Hammondia* – further testing such as PCR is required to distinguish between them) and appear as crescent or banana-shaped structures, 4–8μm long, with a single central nucleolus (Fig 5.18).

Leishmania

Leishmania infantum is endemic in southern European countries and large parts of South America. It is spread from sandflies to dogs (rarely cats) and causes disease which can be controlled with medication but usually not eliminated; the organism stimulates the immune system to produce antibody complexes which cause chronic systemic disease, especially causing hyperglobulinaemia and renal disease. It is a potential zoonosis.

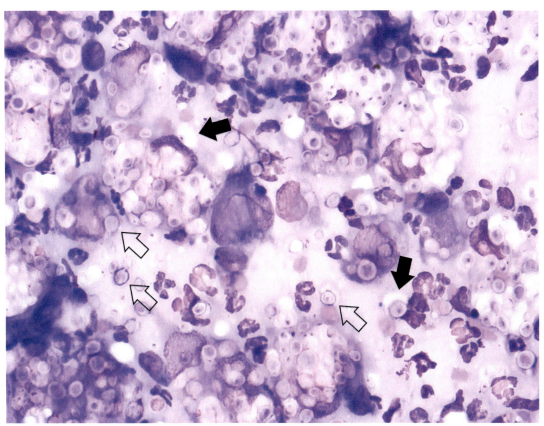

Fig 5.17 *Cryptococcus* yeasts from a feline nasal flush (open arrows and many other examples); note the presence of a pale thick capsule around some organisms (black arrows and many other examples) (×1000)

Many patients have cutaneous lesions and/or lymph node enlargement, and aspirates from these areas are most likely to contain the organisms. *Leishmania* elicits predominantly macrophagic/lymphocytic/plasmacytic inflammation – the presence of significant numbers of plasma cells in a cutaneous lesion from a dog with a history of travel to endemic areas should elicit a search for the organism. *Leishmania* organisms are usually encountered as amastigotes – small (2–5μm) oval structures, with a small but distinctive kinetoplast (short and rod-shaped, protruding at right angles approximately halfway along the organism) (Fig 5.19). They usually stain dark purple (occasionally dark blue) with Romanowsky stains and can be found free in the background or densely packed within macrophages, within cutaneous lesions, lymph nodes and, occasionally, the spleen, of infected patients.

Other protozoan organisms (FIG 5.20)

There are many other protozoan diseases, notably *Babesia Canis*, which causes haemolytic anaemia, and *Cytauxzoon Felis*, a commonly and rapidly fatal disease of cats, again via haemolysis. Intestinal parasites such as *Giardia* and *Tritrichomonas* are most commonly found on faecal examination but are occasionally found on aspirates from the gastrointestinal tract, or (rarely) pancreas or bile.

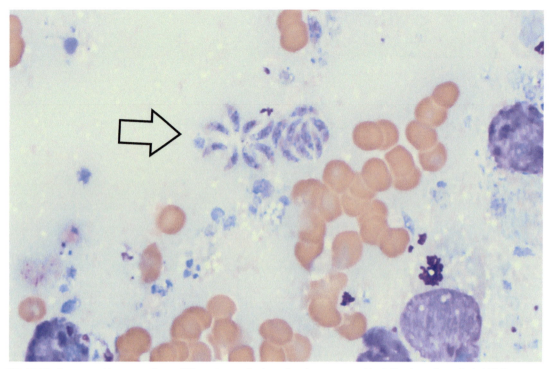

Fig 5.18 A group of banana-shaped *Toxoplasma* tachyzoites (open arrow) in feline lymph node (×1000)

> **Key points**
>
> **Protozoans**
> - They usually elicit macrophagic inflammation
> - Toxoplasma/neospora tachyzoites (the most commonly encountered life stage) are crescent or banana-shaped structures, 4–8μm long, with a single central nucleolus
> - Leishmania amastigotes are small (2–5μm) oval structures, with a small but distinctive kinetoplast (short and rod-shaped), protruding at right angles approximately halfway along the organism

Multicellular parasites

Nematodes

The larval stage of the lungworms *Angiostrongylus vasorum* and *Crenosoma vulpis* (in dogs) and *Aelurostrongylus abstrusus* (in cats) are the most commonly encountered nematodes on cytological specimens (Fig 5.21). They are usually found within respiratory wash samples, although they can occasionally be found on direct lung aspirates. The larval stages are large pale blue worm-like structures, often tightly coiled, most easily found on low power (4× or 10×) magnification. They are morphologically similar; in theory, close examination of the end of the tail can help to identify the organisms: *Aelurostrongylus* has a characteristic 'kink' at the tip of the tail, *Angiostrongylus* has indentations on either side whereas *Crenosoma* has a pointed tail with no indentations. However, in the author's experience, the organisms are frustratingly coy creatures and are usually curled in such a way as to obscure their salient anatomical features. PCR testing is more reliable to identify the organisms.

Lungworm larvae are usually accompanied by significant eosinophilic inflammation, and

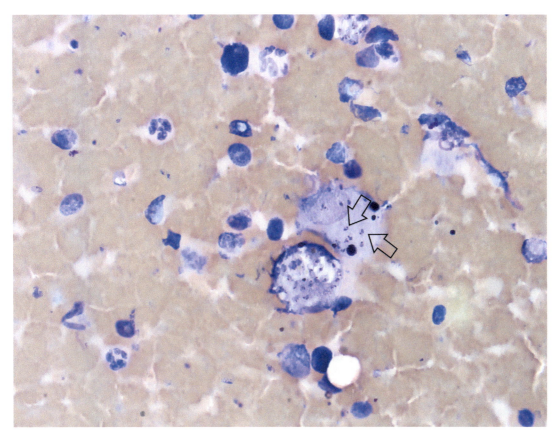

Fig 5.19 *Leishmania* amastigotes phagocytosed within macrophages (open arrows and many other examples)

indeed this finding should precipitate a search for the organisms.

Other less commonly encountered nematodes in the respiratory tract include *Filaroides* (previously *Oslerus) Osleri* and *Eucoleous* species (previously *Capillaria*). *Filaroides* are usually found as larvae and appears similar to the other lungworms, whereas *Eucoleus* is most commonly encountered as large (80x50μm) oval egg.

Microfilariae are early larval stages of large nematodes, the most clinically significant of which is *Dirofilaria immitus* – the canine heartworm, transmitted (as microfilariae) by mosquitos. The microfilariae are observed cytologically on peripheral blood smears and, occasionally, in aspirates from bloody organs such as the liver and spleen and haemorrhagic effusions. They are, again, long slender worm-like structures, not usually found coiled, more slender and darker in colour than lungworm (Fig 5.22).

Microfilaria of the parasite *Dirofilaria repens* are occasionally found on aspirates from skin and subcutaneous lesions (again, usually in dogs) – they are morphologically very similar to *D. Immitis* – PCR testing is most useful to differentiate between them. The clinical disease caused by *D. Repens* is less severe, but it has a much greater zoonotic potential than *D. Immitis*.

Although other nematodes, particularly gastrointestinal, are common in dogs and cats, they are very uncommonly encountered cytologically.

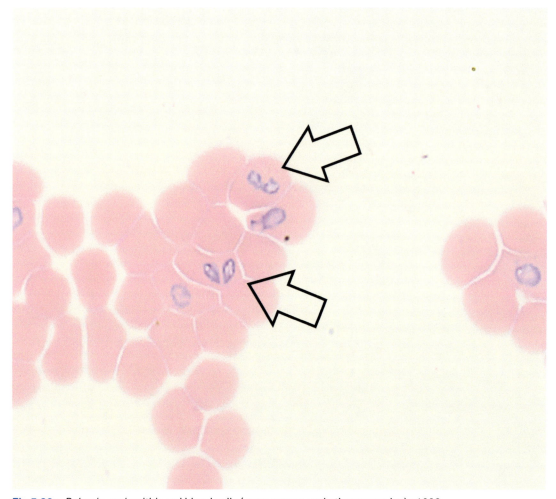

Fig 5.20a *Babesia canis* within red blood cells (open arrows and other examples) ×1000

Cestodes and trematodes

These organisms are very rarely found on cytology specimens. The most clinically significant cestodes (albeit extremely rarely diagnosed ones) are the *Echinococcus* and *Taenia* species, most notably *E. Multilocularis*. Unlike the more common and largely clinically insignificant tapeworms, *Echinococcus* form large cystic structures within the abdomen, aspiration of which can yield high numbers of large tapeworm scolices – the bulbous and hooked head of the parasites. Larval fragments can also contain calcareous corpuscles – small refractile crystalline concentrations of calcium which are thought to be a production of the organism's metabolism.

Perhaps the most significant trematode is *Nanophyetus salmincola*, which transmits *Neorickesttsia heminthoeca*, the cause of salmon poisoning. This and other flukes are most likely to be encountered as large egg structures within the liver, bile or pancreas of infected animals. Such cytological findings are rare, however, and confined to the north western United States, mostly northern California and Washington State.

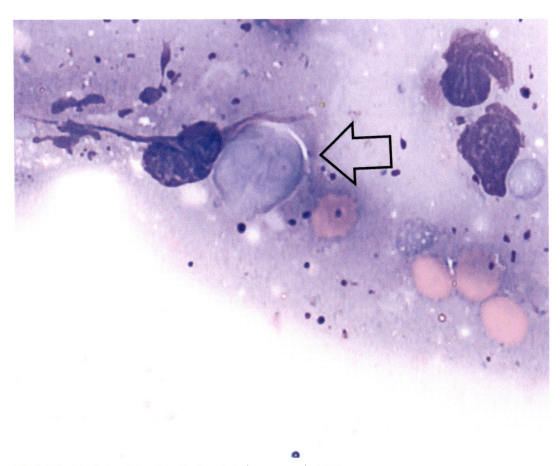

Fig 5.20b *Giardia* in a feline intestinal aspirate (open arrow) ×1000

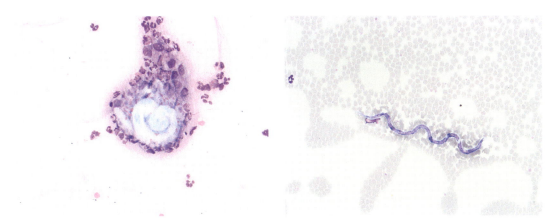

Fig 5.21 *Angiostrongylus* larva surrounded by eosinophils in canine BAL; as is typical, the larva is curled making definitive identification challenging (species was confirmed by PCR in this case) (×500)

Fig 5.22 Microfilaria of *Dirofilaria immitus* in a canine blood film (×100)

> **Key points**
>
> **Multicellular parasites**
>
> - Often elicit eosinophilic inflammation
> - Lungworms are the most commonly encountered, usually on BAL or tracheal wash, rarely on direct lung aspirates
> - Their larval stages are large pale blue worm-like structures, often tightly coiled, most easily found on low power (4x or 10x) magnification
> - Microfilariae are early larval stages of large nematodes such as *Dirofilaria Immitis* (heartworm); they are long slender worm-like structures, not usually found coiled, more slender and darker in colour than lungworm, usually found in blood smears

Viruses

Viruses are too small to be identified cytologically, but occasional intracellular inclusion bodies can be observed. The most clinically relevant inclusion bodies are those of distemper, found within blood cells. They are most commonly seen in polychromatophils (larger and bluer early red blood cells) and are most easily identified with aqueous Romanowsky stains (such as Diff-Quik), with which they stain red, and appear as small irregular reddish blobs within the affected cells.

Other inclusion bodies have been reported with papilloma virus, canine adenovirus, and others, but are relatively rare cytological findings.

Other organisms

As recent history has taught humanity, evolution has created a vast array of organisms capable of ruining the day of other organisms, and a complete list is beyond the scope of this book. Other organisms which have been identified cytologically include the algae *Prototheca zopfii* and *wickerhamii*, which appear cytologically as small jelly-bean like structures.

> **Key points**
>
> **Viruses**
>
> - Too small to be seen cytologically, but occasional inclusion bodies are found
> - *Distemper* is the most clinically relevant, found most often within polychromatophils
> - Unusually, *Distemper* inclusions stain more prominently with aqueous Romanowsky stains (such as Diff-Quik)

> **Chapter 5 – take home messages**
>
> - Organisms found cytologically can reflect pathogens or contaminants; the most useful method for distinguishing is the presence or absence of inflammation.
> - The presence of infectious organisms phagocytosed within leukocytes is extremely strong cytological evidence for infection.
> - Searching for bacteria is usually only possible on higher magnifications (using at least ×50 objectives).
> - Common (but not exclusive) inflammatory patterns for organisms: neutrophilic for bacteria, macrophagic for fungi, eosinophilic for parasites.
> - *Mycobacterium* does not stain well with Romanowsky stains, and the organisms appear as 'negatively staining' rods, or clear spaces within the specimen.

Part two
Cytology of specific locations

Chapter 6

Skin and subcutaneous lesions

The skin and associated underlying tissues comprise the largest organ of the body and have a correspondingly wide variety of cytological appearances. Skin lesions and subcutaneous masses in pets are often quickly noticed by owners, and are relatively easily and safely sampled, meaning that the skin and subcutis are the most commonly aspirated areas of our domestic companions.

A note: cutaneous/dermal versus subcutaneous/subdermal

This is an important distinction cytologically, and the knowledge of whether a lesion is cutaneous (that is, confined to the dermis) or subcutaneous (that is, present in the underlying tissue and not present within the dermis) has implications for interpretation (Fig 6.1). For example, the presence of fat cells on a preparation is likely to be interpreted as a lipoma if a lesion is subcutaneous, whereas if a lesion is cutaneous the cytologist is likely to conclude that the sample represents inadvertent sampling of subcutaneous fat (as cutaneous lipomas are very rare).

Similarly, a cutaneous mass containing clusters of unusual vacuolated epithelial cells in the submandibular region could represent a sebaceous proliferative lesion if cutaneous, or a salivary neoplasm if subcutaneous.

Unfortunately, it can be challenging to distinguish if a lesion is cutaneous or subcutaneous by visual examination and palpation. For cytological purposes, if a mass is visible on the surface of the skin, or (even if not visible on the surface) palpable within the dermal layer, it should be described as cutaneous. If the skin cannot be lifted without lifting the lesion, then it is, at least partially, cutaneous. If the skin can be lifted off it, it should be described as subcutaneous. If the skin can be mostly lifted off with some attachment, it should be described as subcutaneous with some potential cutaneous involvement. Lesions with significant attachment or clearly present in both layers should be described as such.

'Normal' cytological appearance

As with other locations, 'normal' skin is rarely sampled, for obvious reasons. As a general rule, the skin and subcutaneous tissues do not exfoliate well when aspirated, and samples from 'normal' tissue often have very low cellularity. Some amount of blood is usually present, as well as platelet clumps and scattered leukocytes associated with the blood (usually neutrophils). With cutaneous aspirates, there may be occasional ribbons of collagen, small amounts of anucleate squames (although clumps of keratin are usually not present).

Epithelial cells other than squames are not usually harvested from normal skin, but occasionally small scraps of basal epithelium or sebaceous epithelium are found (see page 132 below for a description of these).

Aspirates from subcutaneous tissue usually harvest low numbers of adipocytes (see page 133 below for a description of these).

130 Part two | Cytology of specific locations

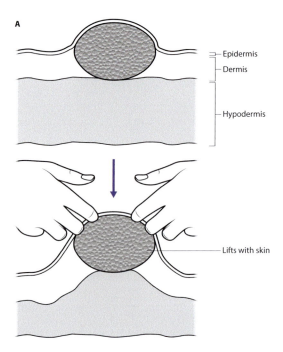

Fig 6.1a Cutaneous mass – the lesion is lifted as the skin is lifted

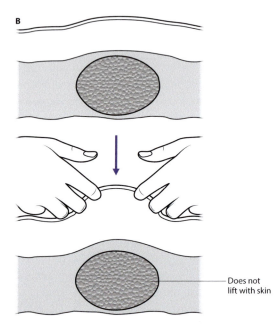

Fig 6.1b Subcutaneous mass – the lesion remains underneath the skin as it is lifted

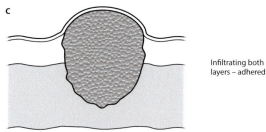

Fig 6.1c Infiltrating both layers – the lesion adheres the skin to the underlying subcutaneous layer

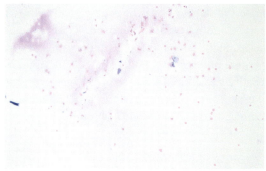

Fig 6.2 'normal' skin – blood with a few scattered anucleate squames (×100)

In summary, aspirates from 'normal' skin are likely to contain mostly blood, with occasional scattered adnexal elements and fat cells (Fig 6.2).

Impression smears (FIG 6.3)

Although ulcerated and inflamed lesions are amenable to sampling via impression smear, in the author's experience the results are often disappointing. The majority of impression smears from such lesions contain high numbers of anucleate squames, keratin bars, and often high numbers of neutrophils. Surface commensal bacteria are often present, often confusing the cytological picture, but infection can be confirmed if bacteria are seen phagocytosed within leukocytes.

In some lesions the pattern of inflammation is instructive (for instance, plasma cells with

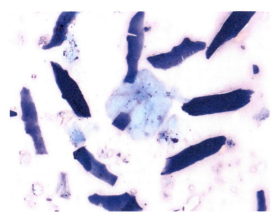

Fig 6.3 Anucleate squame surrounded by thick blue keratin 'bars' (rolled squames), typical of impression smear

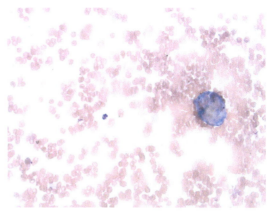

Fig 6.4 Erythrocytes and a keratinised squames from a cutaneous aspirate

Leishmania, or lymphocytes with cutaneous lymphoma and histiocytoma) and occasionally high numbers of acantholytic cells are present which raises strong suspicion for immune-mediated disease. Some significant infectious agents can occasionally be sampled and very rarely, neoplastic cells can be harvested this way. Most of the time, however, impression smears harvest only very superficial inflammation and infection. Direct aspirates from lesions are usually more diagnostically rewarding.

Common cytological findings on skin aspirates

There follows a list and brief description of the most commonly encountered cells and structures from skin lesions. Descriptions of specific entities are discussed later in the chapter; the purpose of the list is to help cytologists rapidly identify material common material (and therefore hopefully to also highlight any less common material concurrently present).

Blood (FIG 6.4)

Red blood cells, platelet clumps, fibrinocellular aggregates (blood clots), associated leukocytes (mostly neutrophils) – see page 59. Mixtures of fresh blood (indicated by the presence of platelets) and old haemorrhage (indicated by macrophages containing red-cell breakdown products such as haematoidin) are sometimes a feature of vascular lesions like vascular hamartomas or haemangiomas (see page 144).

Collagen (FIG 6.5)

Ribbons of pink (on Romanowsky stains) protein – see page 27. Collagen can be present on any samples from the dermis, although it is a particular feature of mast cell tumours (page 135), fibroadnexal hamartomas (page 137) and keloidal fibromas.

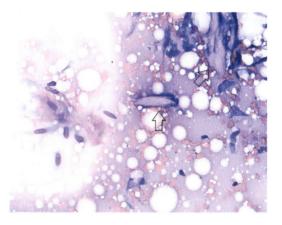

Fig 6.5 Collagen ribbon fragments (open arrow) in a keloidal fibroma (×1000)

Keratin (FIG 6.6)

Anucleate squames, as well as flakes and bars of keratin, can be found on almost any aspirate. Large clumps of keratin, however, are not typical, and are a feature of epidermal inclusion cysts (see page 179).

Basal Epithelium

Basal epithelial cells are dense, tightly cohesive cells which form the base of the surface squamous epithelium. They are found in deeply basophilic (dark blue) cohesive clusters, with uniform small round nuclei, usually 1.5 erythrocytes in diameter, no visible nucleoli and a small amount of pale- to mid-basophilic cytoplasm (Fig 6.7). The clusters are very rounded and sometimes have small amounts of pink extracellular material attached at the periphery, somewhat resembling extracellular matrix (more usually produced by mesenchymal cells). This is believed by some to represent the basement membrane of the epithelium.

Basal epithelium is sometimes found in small amounts from aspirates of normal skin, fibroadnexal hamartomas (see page 137), or from the lining of epidermal inclusion cysts (see page 179). Found in greater amounts, it is more commonly associated with cutaneous basilar epithelial neoplasms (basal cell tumours (see page 138) or, occasionally, sebaceous epitheliomas (usually mixed with other epithelial cells (see page 137).

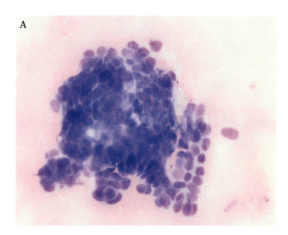
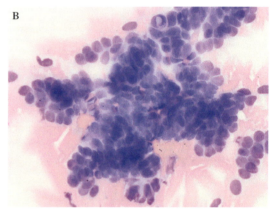

Fig 6.7a and b Basal epithelium at ×1000 and ×1000 magnification

Sebaceous epithelium (FIG 6.8)

These are secretory epithelial cells, and their nature is clearly marked in their morphology – they have similar small dense nuclei to basal epithelial cells, but these nuclei are surrounded by large amounts of clear cytoplasm filled with high numbers of uniform vacuoles; they are distinguishable from adipocytes, which usually have abundant smooth pink cytoplasm rather than multiple vacuoles. They can be sometimes challenging to distinguish from highly activated macrophages (which also have large amounts of vacuolated cytoplasm) or (rarely) highly vacuolated mesenchymal cells (such as those aspirated from a liposarcoma).

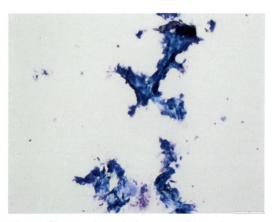

Fig 6.6 Clumps of keratin from an epidermal inclusion cyst (×100)

Skin and subcutaneous lesions | Chapter 6   133

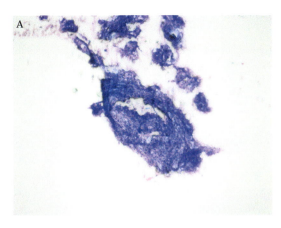

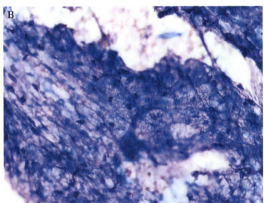

Fig 6.8a and b Sebaceous epithelium at ×100 and ×500 magnification; note the high numbers of regularly-sized vacuoles within the cytoplasm

Sebaceous epithelium is often accompanied by its sebaceous secretion, which appears cytologically as keratin often mixed with a waxy substance which does not stain well. It can be found in proliferative sebaceous lesions, such as sebaceous hyperplasia (often adjacent to a separate neoplastic or inflammatory lesion), or sebaceous neoplastic lesions (such as sebaceous adenomas, epitheliomas or fibroadnexal hamartomas, see page 137).

Adipocytes

Fat cells are an extremely common denizen of cytological specimens from many different locations. They are mesenchymal cells, but distorted by large fat droplets which fill most of their cytoplasm. They appear cytologically as large pink balloon-like cells with a small unremarkable nucleus and are found both individually and in large aggregates (Fig 6.9).

When fat is inflamed the cells can appear quite different; they collapse and become much more basophilic (bluer); collapsed aggregates of adipocytes can confused inexperienced cytologists, as they can somewhat resemble necrosis or degenerate keratin.

Adipocytes can be found in any locations which contain fat; adipocytes from lipomas (see page 150) are cytologically identical to those from normal fat, and therefore some interpretation of the location and gross appearance of

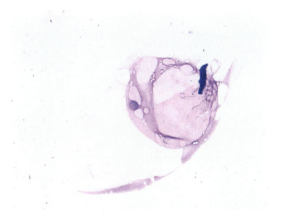

Fig 6.9a Individual adipocyte (×500); a keratin bar is overlying

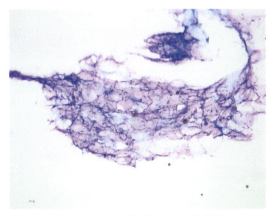

Fig 6.9b An aggregate of adipocytes (×100)

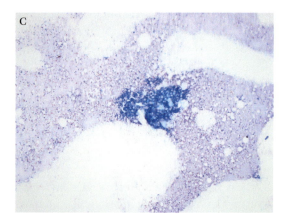

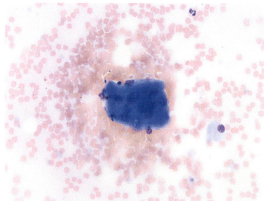

Fig 6.10 Aggregate of skeletal muscle; note the deeply basophilic (blue) cytoplasm and striations (×500)

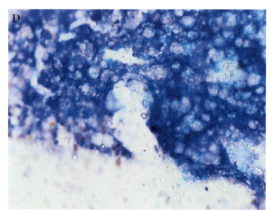

Fig 6.9c and d Collapsed adipocytes from inflamed fat; note the much more basophilic (bluer) cytoplasm (×100 (c) and x500 (d))

the sampled lesion is required for definitive diagnosis.

Skeletal Muscle

Skeletal muscle often exfoliates poorly, but small aggregates are not infrequently found in aspirates from deeper lesions. Aggregates of skeletal muscle are deeply basophilic (dark blue) with dense oval nuclei, hard to discern within the cytoplasm (Fig 6.10). At higher magnifications (×50 or ×100 objectives), the presence of skeletal muscle can be confirmed by the presence of very fine striations, visible (but very indistinct) as close faint parallel lines within the dark blue background. This can help distinguish skeletal muscle from the collapsed aggregates of adipocytes occasionally found on samples from inflamed fat. The presence of skeletal muscle and fat within a deep lesion could reflect sampling of an infiltrative lipoma, a benign but locally invasive variant of lipomas (see page 151).

> **Key points**
>
> **Skin and subcutis introduction**
> - It is important to clearly distinguish between cutaneous and subcutaneous lesions (where this is possible)
> - Cytology of 'normal' skin is generally poorly cellular but can include blood, collagen, keratin, sebaceous epithelium or basal epithelium
> - Cytology of 'normal' subcutaneous tissue usually comprises fat

Neoplasia of the skin and subcutis
Neoplastic lesions – cutaneous

The following section contains a list of commonly sampled cutaneous/dermal neoplastic lesions (that is, lesions which usually have an obvious cutaneous/dermal component) in rough order of commonality (so the lower down this list you travel, the less common the lesion and the less likely the diagnosis). The sections include a brief description of the most relevant non-cytological signalment factors which may aid diagnosis (such as common locations, age and breed) and the typical cytological features present on sampling. The focus of this book is on diagnosis; for up-to-date information on treatment, other sources should be consulted.

Mast cell tumour (FIGS 6.11, 6.12)
Neoplasm type: round cell
Age: risk increases with age, but can occur in very young patients (have been described in puppies as young as two weeks old)
Location: can occur anywhere; usually cutaneous but can be subcutaneous; slight predilection for hindlimbs; possible slight trend for higher-grade tumours on the scrotum and inguinal areas
Gross appearance: usually solitary masses but occasionally multiple simultaneous skin masses (not necessarily associated with higher-grade tumours); appearance can vary greatly – they most commonly present as small raised hairless masses, sometimes reddened, but nodular rashes, ulcerated lesions and diffuse swellings are all reported
Species/breed predispositions: usually dogs (most commonly sampled cutaneous neoplasm in dogs), less common in cats; dog breeds most commonly affected include boxers, pugs (on average, slightly lower grade neoplasms), Shar Peis (on average higher grade), Staffordshire

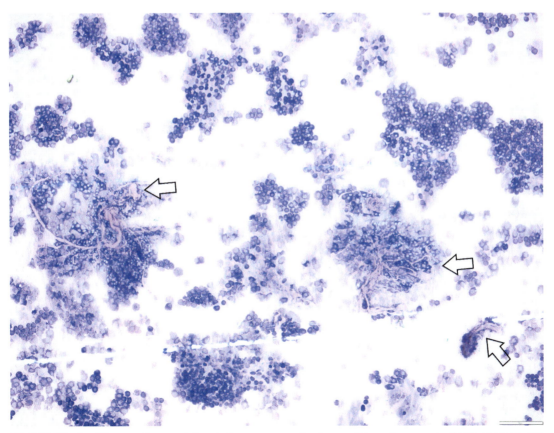

Fig 6.11 Mast cell tumour (low grade); note the presence of collagen ribbons (open arrows) interspersed with the mast cells (×100)

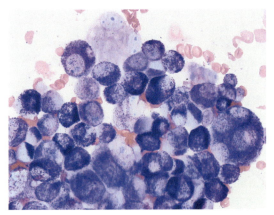

Fig 6.12 Mast cell tumour (high grade); granulation is reduced and the cells display multinucleation and multiple nucleoli

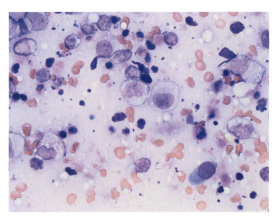

Fig 6.13 Histiocytoma (×1000); note the slightly indented nuclei of the central two cells

bull terriers, golden retrievers and Labradors, as well as Persian cats

Cytological appearance/further comments: similar to mast cell tumours elsewhere on the body (see page 82 for full description and information on grading); as well as mast cells, aspirates often contain eosinophils, pleomorphic mesenchymal cells (which can sometimes appear highly atypical) and/or ribbons of collagen.

Note that mast cell granules can stain quite poorly with aqueous Romanowsky stains (such as Diff-Quik).

Mast cell tumours generally exfoliate relatively well cytologically, and even when ruptured the presence of mast cells can often be guessed because of the distinctive purple granules scatted in the background, but it is worth remembering that mast cells can also form part of the 'normal' inflammatory response; the presence of relatively few mast cells interspersed with other inflammatory cells is more typical of mixed inflammation than a mast cell tumour.

Histiocytoma (FIG 6.13, 6.14)

Neoplasm type: round cell
Age: usually less than 4 years old (but any age can be affected)
Location: any cutaneous location but head and pinnae most commonly
Gross appearance: classic 'button tumour' – a small, smooth, pink, raised, hairless and often erythematous mass; they are occasionally ulcerated
Species/breed predispositions: dogs, breeds include boxers and flat coat retrievers
Cytological appearance/further comments: see page 85 for full description. The classic 'fried egg' histiocytes are commonly accompanied by a pale-blue background and low numbers of small lymphocytes, both features which can help differentiate from other round cell tumours (such as plasmacytomas) when the round cells are poorly preserved, or few in number.

There are a number of related histiocytic diseases, such as cutaneous and systemic histiocytosis in the dog, and progressive histiocytosis in the cat, which can be challenging to distinguish from histiocytomas cytologically (at least initially); however, they are much less common (and it is worth remembering that histiocytomas have not currently been reported in cats).

Histiocytic sarcoma is related but has many cytological differences from histiocytoma; distinguishing between the two is not usually a diagnostic challenge.

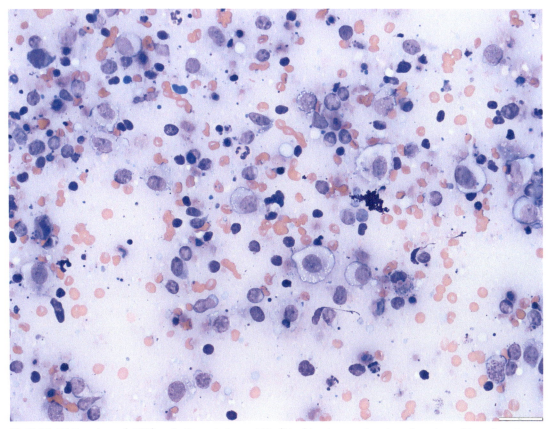

Fig 6.14 Histiocytoma (×500); note the pale basophilic (blue) background and scattered small lymphocytes

Sebaceous proliferation (adenoma, epithelioma, fibroadnexal hamartoma) (FIG 6.15)

Neoplasm type: epithelial
Age: middle age to older (peak broadly 7–13 years old for adenoma and hamartoma, slightly older for epithelioma)
Location: any cutaneous location but predilections for – head (dogs), back, tail, head (cats)
Gross appearance: elevated nodular skin masses, sometimes alopecic, pigmented or ulcerated
Species/breed predispositions: adenomas are common in dogs and uncommon in cats; epitheliomas and fibroadnexal hamartomas are usually only found in dogs
Cytological appearance/further comments: these lesions are not directly related but all share a similar cytological appearance, hence their grouping together here. Representative aspirates from all of these lesions contain well-differentiated sebaceous epithelial cells and associated secretions (see page 132 for full description of these). Finding keratin mixed

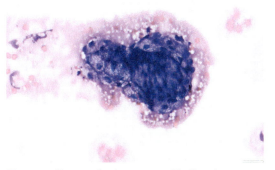

Fig 6.15 Cluster of sebaceous epithelium from a sebaceous adenoma (×500)

with a non-staining waxy substance significantly increases the suspicion of aspiration of a sebaceous proliferation, although this cannot be confirmed without finding the sebaceous epithelial clusters.

Sebaceous epitheliomas generally exfoliate well and usually contain a mixture of sebaceous epithelium and basal epithelium (see page 132). Sebaceous adenomas exfoliate moderately well and usually contain only sebaceous epithelium. Fibroadnexal hamartomas often exfoliate very poorly and often contain a mixture of skin adnexal elements, which can include keratin, collagen, basal and sebaceous epithelial cells, low numbers of mesenchymal cells and low numbers of mast cells.

Sebaceous adenomas and fibroadnexal hamartomas are essentially benign; sebaceous epitheliomas are usually very-low grade malignancies. All are expected to be cured by complete local excision, and histology should distinguish between them following excision. The presence of clusters of sebaceous epithelial cells on cytological examination usually indicates aspiration of one of these lesions; sebaceous hyperplasia is another consideration, although this usually appears grossly as diffuse thickening rather than a discrete lesion.

Basal cell tumour (cutaneous basilar epithelial neoplasm) (FIG 6.16)

Neoplasm type: epithelial
Age: any age (cats as young as 1 year old reported) but usually middle (4–10 years), common in dogs and cats
Location: slight predilection for head and neck
Gross appearance: well circumscribed dermal masses (often extending into the subcutaneous layer), sometimes haired but usually alopecic
Species/breed predispositions: common in both dogs and cats; long-haired cats more at risk, as are Kerry Blue Terriers, Bichon Frise and Bedlington Terriers; slight predilection for male dogs, no sex predilection in cats

Cytological appearance/further comments: 'basal cell tumour' is an outdated term, replaced by a number of more specific terms for lesions, all falling under the wordy umbrella of 'cutaneous basilar epithelial neoplasm'. They all share similar cytological features and all are usually benign or very low-grade malignancy; aspirates from these lesions are usually moderately cellular, but they sometimes exfoliate poorly. They comprise dense clusters of basal epithelial cells (see page 132 for a full description of these), sometimes associated with pink material resembling extra-cellular matrix (this may be the tightly adhered basement membrane of the cells).

The dark blue round clusters are generally easy to identify cytologically, but when the cells have separated from the clusters they often have a very spindloid appearance and can be surprisingly challenging to distinguish from mesenchymal cells (Fig 6.17) – when aspirates contain high numbers of individual cells and pink basement membrane they can sometimes be mistaken for sarcomas or fibrosis; this should be kept in mind when interpreting the presence of mesenchymal cells alongside clusters of basal epithelium.

Occasionally, aspirates from feline basilar epithelial neoplasms contain highly degenerate cells, similar to degenerate keratin or necrosis, although significant inflammation is not usually present (see page 327 for more details on degenerate lesions).

The most common of these lesions are trichoblastomas, found in both dogs and cats. Histopathology is required to distinguish between them but they are usually slow-growing and complete excision is expected to be curative for most of them.

Squamous cell carcinoma (FIG 6.18)

Neoplasm type: epithelial
Age: middle-aged to older
Location: cats – ear tips, eyelids, nasal planum most common; dogs – head, perineum, digits most common

Skin and subcutaneous lesions | Chapter 6 | **139**

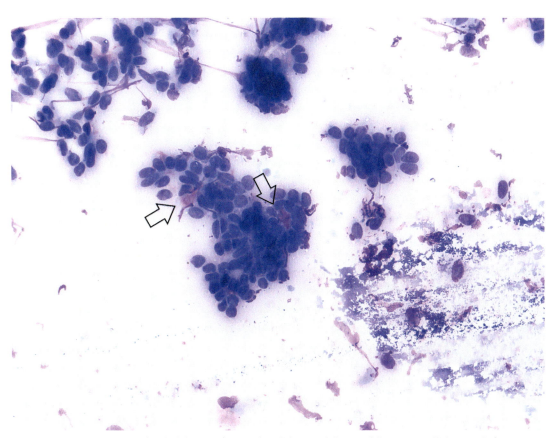

Fig 6.16 Basal cell tumour (trichoblastoma); note the pink material resembling extracellular matrix (open arrows) (×500)

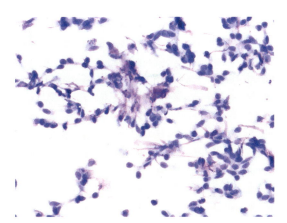

Fig 6.17 Cells ripped from clusters of basal epithelium, strongly resembling mesenchymal cells (×500)

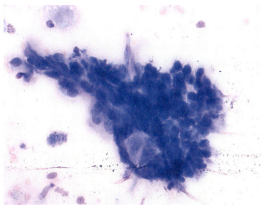

Fig 6.18a Atypical basal epithelium from a squamous cell carcinoma; cells are pleomorphic, display mild-moderate anisocytosis and anisokaryosis, and occasional binucleate cells are present

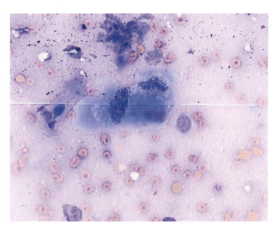

Fig 6.18b Atypical squamous cell from a squamous cell carcinoma; the nucleus is much bigger than expected for a mature keratinised cell, and has a bizarre shape; the vacuolation around the nucleus is characteristic of squamous epithelium

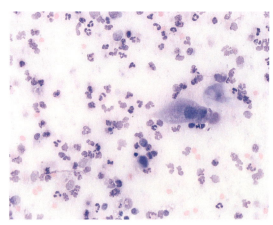

Fig 6.18c Atypical squamous cell from a squamous cell carcinoma; note also the marked neutrophilic inflammation (the neutrophils are poorly preserved here), typical in squamous cell carcinomas

Gross appearance: crusting lesions progressing to deep ulcerated erosive masses, often purulent exudate on the surface

Species/breed predispositions: the most common malignant cutaneous epithelial neoplasm in dogs and cats; more common in sites affected by UV radiation, and so more common in white-coated and short-coated animals

Cytological appearance/further comments: although relatively common, these can be challenging lesions to diagnose, not least because they are often markedly inflamed (typically neutrophilic) and secondary infection is not uncommon.

The atypical cells have a varied cytological appearance; most commonly there is a combination of atypical-appearing basal epithelium (atypical features often include pleomorphism, anisocytosis and anisokaryosis, multiple nucleoli and increased mitosis) and atypical keratinised squamous epithelial cells.

The keratinised cells generally display *nuclear: cytoplasmic asynchrony.* In a normal situation, as squamous cells mature, the keratin within the cytoplasm increases and the nucleus begins to degrade, ultimately producing an anucleate squame (see page 97). In squamous cell carcinoma, the nucleus often fails to degrade, leading to large angular keratinised cells with prominent nuclei. The nuclei often display atypical features (see page 92 for general details on malignancy), including binucleation. Large 'tadpole cells' are sometimes found. Keratinisation (cells displaying increasing size, angularity and basophilia (blueness) can sometimes be seen within the clusters of basal epithelium, often at the periphery; occasionally the clusters contain clumps of keratin).

The presence of both atypical basal epithelium and atypical keratinised squamous epithelial cells is strongly suggestive of squamous cell carcinoma. However, when only one or the other is present it can be challenging to distinguish between a carcinoma and dysplastic epithelium secondary to the marked inflammation that is often concurrently present (particularly ruptured keratinised cysts, which often contain large amounts of inflammation, keratin, and occasionally small amounts of basal epithelium and low numbers of nucleated squamous epithelial cells – see page 328 for more information on distinguishing between these possibilities).

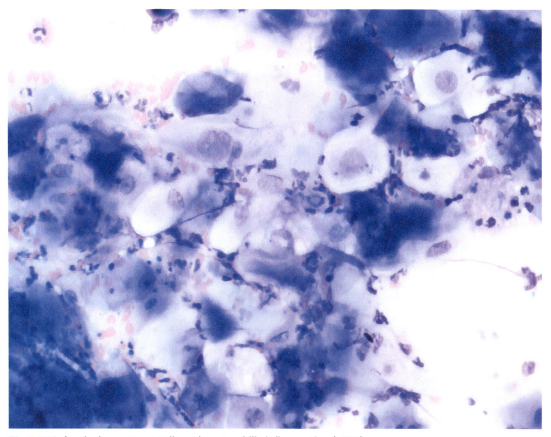

Fig 6.18d Atypical squamous cells and neutrophilic inflammation (×500)

As well as the inflammation, a further complication is that other epithelial neoplasms can occasionally undergo keratinisation, and therefore cytological resemble squamous cell carcinoma. Not for the last time in this textbook, the context will aid the cytologist here, taking into account the location and gross appearance of the lesion.

Melanocytic tumours: melanocytoma and malignant melanoma (FIGS 6.19, 6.20)

Neoplasm type: technically mesenchymal but appearance varies; most commonly appear as round cells

Age: melanocytoma dogs 7+ years (rarely reported in very young dogs); cats 4+
Melanoma: both usually older than six years
Location: melanocytoma: head, especially eyelids in dogs

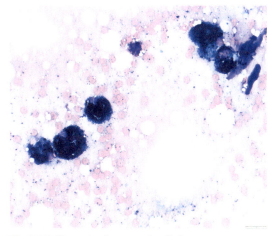

Fig 6.19 Densely pigmented cells in a melanocytoma; further cytological details are hard to see; melanin pigment is scattered in the background (×500)

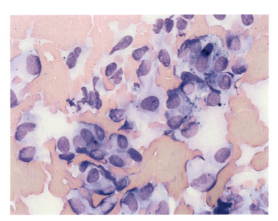

Fig 6.20 Poorly pigmented cells from a melanoma; some cells contain a fine dusting of melanin (×1000)

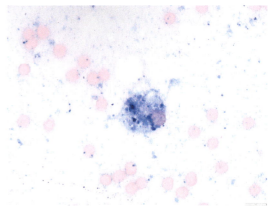

Fig 6.21 A melanophage containing phagocytosed melanin; note the rounded clumps of irregular pigment, as distinct from the fine pigment in Fig 6.20 (×1000)

Melanoma: dogs usually oral cavity or lips, occasionally dermal (dermal melanomas are often less malignant than oral); cats more commonly dermal (lips, nose and back)

Gross appearance: vary in pigmentation and size but usually small dark symmetrical dermal capsules; not possible to distinguish between melanocytoma and melanoma grossly

Species/breed predispositions: common in dogs, rare in cats. Breeds at risk include vislas, schnauzers, chow chow, Shar Pei and Irish setters.

Cytological appearance/further comments: see page 87 for a full description. The benign variant of this lesion, melanocytomas, contain normal and heavily pigmented melanocytes – round cells full of black pigment, obliterating further cytological details. Finding moderate numbers of these 'black holes' in aspirates from a pigmented lesion raises suspicion for sampling of a melanocytoma. Melanin pigment may also be present in the background (see page 101 for full description). It is also worth noting the heavily pigmented cells do not exclude the possibility of a malignant lesion, they only make it less likely.

As discussed in the full description, malignant melanomas are more difficult to diagnose, and are the 'great imitators' of cytology; at lower power they can appear mesenchymal, epithelial or as round cell tumours, and although they have a 'classic' appearance (round cells with stippled chromatin and single macronucleolus (larger than an erythrocyte), their appearance in the wild can deviate widely from this.

Melanophages (macrophages containing phagocytosed melanin pigment) may be present in both tumours (as well as in any aspirate from pigmented areas). It is sometimes possible to distinguish between the melanin present in melanophages (which tends to be found in irregular black rounded blobs, varying in size – very similar to haemosiderin) (Fig 6.21) and melanin present within less heavily-pigmented melanocytes, where it is found as a fine dusting or in small oval brownish-black granules. This is not a completely reliable indicator, however, and where melanocytes are densely packed with pigment, they are indistinguishable from well-fed melanophages.

Poorly pigmented melanomas are among the most biologically aggressive neoplasms encountered in veterinary medicine, and if their presence is suspected then further staging (aspiration of local lymph nodes, liver, spleen, imaging of the chest and abdomen) is recommended.

Plasmacytoma (FIGS 6.22 TO 6.24)
Neoplasm type: round cell
Age: 5+ in dogs; rare in cats

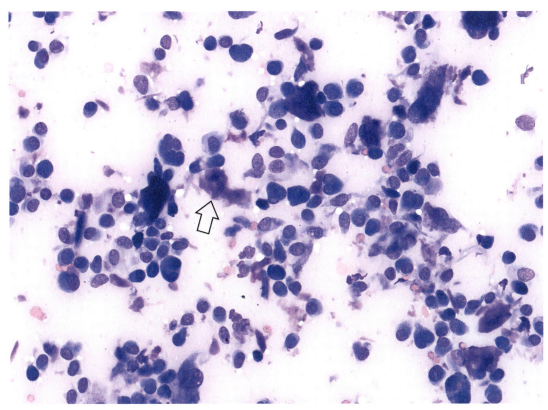

Fig 6.22 Plasmacytoma; note the eccentric nuclei and frequent multinucleation. Scraps of amyloid (purple irregular material, open arrow) are also present (×500)

Location: pinnae and digits most common, occasional oral cavity, rectum
Gross appearance: raised dermal mass, often alopecic and occasional ulcerated
Species/breed predispositions: terriers, cocker spaniels, standard poodle; rare in cats
Cytological appearance/further comments: see page 86 for full description.

Plasmacytomas are also (along with melanomas) lesions which can have a widely varying cytological appearance. Although they are tumours of plasma cells, the cells present are much more pleomorphic than typical plasma cells (in fact, the presence of high numbers of more normal-appearing plasma cells raises more concern for the malignant version of this lesion – multiple myeloma – than plasmacytoma, although plasmacytic inflammation is more likely in a cutaneous mass).

The lesions can sometimes be challenging to differentiate from other round cell tumours, particularly histiocytomas (see above), but they also share some cytological similarities to osteoblasts (both cells generally have eccentric nuclei and deep blue cytoplasm), further complicated by the fact that amyloid (sometimes present in plasma cell tumours as a result of immunoglobulin production) appears similar to osteoid, sometimes present in osteosarcomas (both appear as wispy purplish extra-cellular material).

To distinguish plasmacytomas from histiocytomas, the most reliable features in the author's experience are: multinucleation (plasma cell tumours often have a much higher number of binucleate cells as well as occasional multinucleate cells) and the presence of a pale or eosinophilic (reddish) background, as opposed to the basophilic (blue) background seen with histiocytomas. Eccentric nuclei are also more commonly seen in plasmacytomas, and the presence of amyloid can also help to identify them.

Features which help distinguish plasmacytomas from osteosarcomas include: cell and nuclear shape – cells in plasmacytomas tend to be rounder, with round nuclei and clearly-defined borders, whereas osteoblasts are more oval, also with oval nuclei and more indistinct borders. Granulation – osteoblasts sometimes contain fine red granules, assumed to be osteoid – this can occur in plasmacytomas but is less common. Nuclear features – although plasmacytomas can contain moderately pleomorphic cells, osteoblasts harvested from osteosarcomas tend to display more atypical features, with more marked pleomorphism, nuclear variation, and prominent multiple often variably-sized nucleoli, none of which are commonly a feature of plasmacytomas (Fig 6.23).

Unlike histiocytomas, plasmacytomas do not commonly regress spontaneously, but single cutaneous plasmacytomas usually follow a benign clinical course and complete excision is curative for most of them.

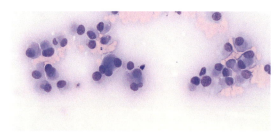

Fig 6.24 Plasmacytoma displaying frequent binucleation (×500)

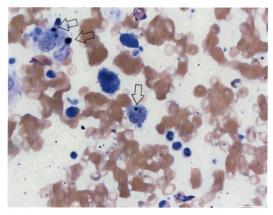

Fig 6.25 Macrophages containing haemosiderin alongside platelets (×1000)

Vascular hamartoma/haemangioma (FIG 6.25)

Neoplasm type: mesenchymal
Age: variable, vascular hamartomas more common in younger patients, haemangioma middle-aged to older
Location: any dermal or subcutaneous location (can occur internally, but rarely)
Gross appearance: raised well-demarcated masses varying from bright red to dark brown (darker ones can look very similar to melanocytic tumours)
Species/breed predispositions: common in dogs, rare in cats
Cytological appearance/further comments: both lesions are benign and usually slow growing neoplasms of vascular endothelium, and both have a very similar appearance cytologically. These lesions exfoliate poorly and the neoplastic endothelial cells are very rarely present. Instead, aspirates from these masses generally

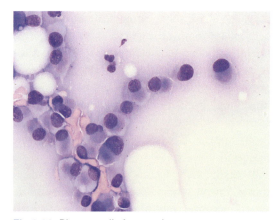

Fig 6.23 Plasma cells from a plasmacytoma resembling osteoblasts (note the lack of granulation (the small dots are stain precipitate) and relatively minimal atypical features, as distinct from osteosarcoma (×1000)

contain a mixture of fresh blood and evidence of old haemorrhage. The preparations mostly contain high numbers of red blood cells, and the presence of platelets or platelet clumps confirms fresh blood.

The presence of macrophages containing phagocytosed erythrocytes or, ideally, dark pigment resembling haemosiderin (see page 98 for more information on this) indicates bleeding prior to sampling. Therefore, finding large amounts of blood, platelet clumps and low numbers of macrophages containing red blood cells or dark pigment is suggestive of aspiration of a vascular hamartoma or haemangioma. This pattern is not specific, however – recent haematomas with iatrogenic blood contamination during sampling or poorly exfoliative haemangiosarcomas (or other underlying neoplasia) can appear similar cytologically. Histopathology is needed to assess these masses further and is generally recommended when this mixture is found on aspirates.

Cutaneous lymphoma (FIG 6.26, 6.27)

Neoplasm type: round cell
Age: usually middle-aged to older
Location: solitary lesions around mouth/lip or multiple lesions, more common on head/ventrum
Gross appearance: thickened areas, rarely discrete masses
Species/breed predispositions: uncommon in dogs and cats (see below)
Cytological appearance/further comments: not all cases of cutaneous lymphoma are epitheliotropic; they can be B-cell or T-cell, epitheliotropic or non-epitheliotropic, although the most common cutaneous lymphoma is T-cell epitheliotropic (also known as *mycosis fungoides*). Cytologically, cutaneous lymphoma appears similar to lymphoma found elsewhere, in that the aspirates contain a monomorphic population of lymphocytes (see page 86). In the skin, these lesions often also contain some degree of neutrophilic or pyogranulomatous (neutrophilic/macrophagic) inflammation, and

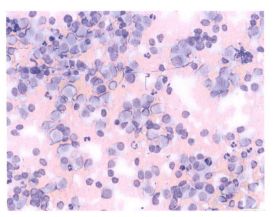

Fig 6.26 T-cell epitheliotropic lymphoma, slightly resembling histiocytoma but displaying more pleomorphism and with mostly eccentric nuclei (×500)

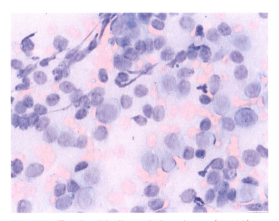

Fig 6.27 T-cell epitheliotropic lymphoma (×1000)

bacteria may be present (either commensals or as a secondary infection).

T-cell epitheliotropic lymphoma often has a distinct cytological appearance – the cells are large and often have abundant pale cytoplasm – at first glance this tumour can somewhat resemble a histiocytoma, although the cells have denser cytoplasm and a greater degree of anisokaryosis.

Sézary syndrome occurs when the neoplastic cells from T-cell epitheliotropic lymphoma are found on a blood smear, indicating stage V disease.

Papilloma (FIG 6.28, 6.29)
Neoplasm type: epithelial
Age: young (viral induced) to middle-aged
Location: usually head
Gross appearance: wart-like lesion, may be single or multicentric
Species/breed predispositions: more common in dogs
Cytological appearance/further comments: papillomas are often virally-induced (by papillomaviruses), hence their appearance in younger patients, although middle-aged to older patients can also be affected. They have a distinctive cytological appearance, mostly comprising large nucleated squamous epithelial cells – these cells can raise concern for squamous cell carcinoma. In contrast to squamous cell carcinoma, however, papilloma cells have patchy nuclei often with a crumbling or disintegrating appearance (this appearance may be due to viral inclusions within the nucleus).

The cytoplasm is usually purplish rather than pale blue, and many cells often contain laminar striations, like an onion, or irregular vacuoles – these squamous cells are sometimes called koilocytes. They are often inflamed due to trauma and sometimes contain bacteria. Lymphocytic inflammation is occasionally seen within them (possibly related to regression).

These are benign lesions and virally-induced papillomas will sometimes spontaneously regress, but there are also reports of transformation to squamous cell carcinoma.

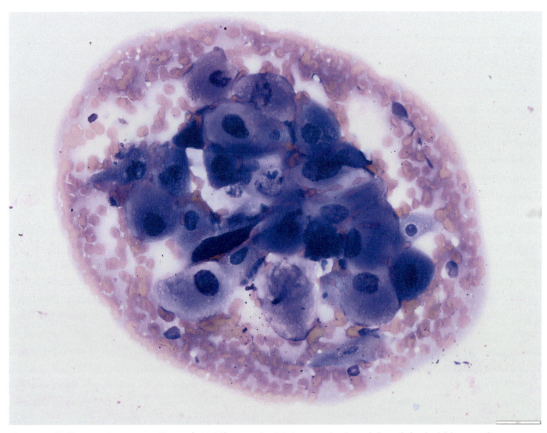

Fig 6.28 Koilocytes from a papilloma (×1000); note the 'disintegrating' nuclei, and the bubbly cytoplasm

Skin and subcutaneous lesions | Chapter 6

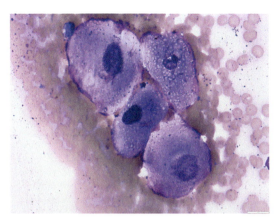

Fig 6.29 Koilocytes (×1000); note the purplish striated cytoplasm

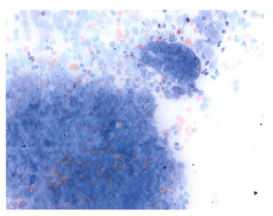

Fig 6.30 Malignant trichoblastoma (×500); cells are much more pleomorphic than normal basal epithelium, and the clusters are crowded and disorganised

Malignant epithelial neoplasms: sebaceous carcinomas, apocrine carcinomas and basal cell carcinomas (FIG 6.30)
Neoplasm type: epithelial
Age: usually middle-aged to older (10+ most common)
Location: any cutaneous region, head and neck more common in dogs, perineum in cats
Gross appearance: elevated nodular skin masses, sometimes ulcerated
Species/breed predispositions: cavalier King Charles (sebaceous carcinoma)
Cytological appearance/further comments: these are malignant variants of the more benign neoplasms already discussed above. They are rarer than their benign counterparts and are sometimes challenging to distinguish from them cytologically. Where the benign versions are uniform, however, the malignant versions usually display at least some features of malignancy (pleomorphism, anisokaryosis, multiple nucleoli etc… see page 92 for more examples of malignant features).

Sebaceous carcinomas, in particular, can be challenging to distinguish from both macrophages and liposarcomas – all three lesions contain loosely-connected cells with large amounts of vacuolated cytoplasm although macrophages at least generally do not display much nuclear variation.

Any cutaneous mass containing epithelial cells displaying atypical features should be considered for surgical biopsy and histopathological examination. If multiple atypical features are found, then further staging (with aspiration of any enlarged lymph nodes and imaging of the chest and abdomen) is probably sensible.

Haemangiosarcoma (FIG 6.31)
Neoplasm type: mesenchymal
Age: usually older
Location: most common limbs/trunk (especially ventral abdomen) (dogs), head, axilla, groin (cats)
Gross Appearance: hairless thickened mass, sometimes raised profile, dark red-black in colour, often ulcerated
Species/breed predispositions: short-haired and lightly pigmented breeds
Cytological appearance/further comments: cutaneous haemangiosarcomas are much less common than visceral lesions but appear cytologically similar. They often contain large amounts of blood, as well as haemosiderophages (macrophages containing phagocytosed red-cell breakdown products, indicating bleeding prior to sampling –

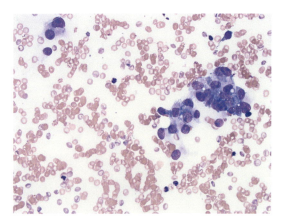

Fig 6.31 Large atypical mesenchymal cells from a cutaneous haemangiosarcoma

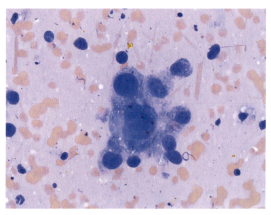

Fig 6.32 Cutaneous metastasis of carcinoma (suspected renal origin) (×1000)

see page 98). Actual neoplastic cells are often very few in number (although occasional neoplasms exfoliate high numbers of cells). The cells are usually fusiform (spindle-shaped), highly pleomorphic (variable shape and size) and often resemble cells from other high-grade sarcomas, making them challenging to definitively identify with cytology alone.

The most useful distinguishing features of the cells (compared to many other sarcomas) is that they are often much larger than other sarcoma cells, with a somewhat angular appearance, and often have deeply basophilic (dark blue) cytoplasm. Most cells are found individually scattered throughout the preparations but occasional small aggregates may also be found. In those rarer tumours which exfoliate well, some large aggregates may also be found.

Cutaneous haemangiosarcomas often have a better prognosis than ether subcutaneous or visceral versions – as a general rule, the deeper the haemangiosarcoma, the worse the prognosis. Complete excision can be curative of cutaneous haemangiosarcomas, as metastasis is less common than other variants.

In some cases, vasoformative features may be seen – this is most often recognised as mesenchymal cells that appear to be forming a channel around red blood cells, indicating formation of aberrant vessels.

Metastatic neoplasms (FIG 6.32)
Neoplasm type: can be any
Age: variable but older
Location: any cutaneous
Gross appearance: variable, often multiple masses
Species/breed predispositions: varies
Cytological appearance/further comments: metastasis to the skin from internal masses is uncommon but can occur, most commonly with carcinomas (such as renal carcinomas or urothelial carcinomas) but any neoplasm can implant within the skin. Such tumours are likely to display multiple features of malignancy, so much so that their origin may be challenging to discern – in some poorly-differentiated tumours, even the type of tumour (epithelial, mesenchymal etc) can be hard to assess.

Lung-digit syndrome is an uncommon and unusual syndrome in cats, where a pulmonary carcinoma (often a primary bronchial carcinoma) metastasises to the digits (single or multiple). There, the neoplasms often undergo differentiation to columnar epithelial cells, occasionally ciliated, and can appear quite well-differentiated. The original tumour may be clinically silent. The presence of columnar epithelial cells, especially ciliated, in aspirates from a mass on a cat's digit should precipitate a search for a primary lung lesion (although note that columnar metaplasia (squamous epithelium transforming into columnar epithelium) is a common sequel of self-trauma, most often seen in dogs but occasionally cats). Other unusual sites of metastasis of primary lung neoplasia have also been reported in cats, including other parts of the skin, eyes, skeletal muscle, bone, aorta and other organs.

Transmissible venereal tumour (FIG 6.33)
Neoplasm type: round cell
Age: any age (implanted tumour, see below)
Location: usually external genitalia (implanted during coitus), but occasionally on the face or head
Gross appearance: usually multiple raised nodules, sometimes ulcerated; can be large (10cm not unusual for the primary site of implantation)
Species/breed predispositions: dogs only, rare in the UK, usually only in imported animals
Cytological appearance/further comments: this remarkable neoplasm appears to have developed in a canid some eleven thousand years ago – all current versions of this tumour share this common origin from a single individual, and are implanted into the host, usually during coitus.

Cytologically, the tumour appears somewhat similar to a histiocytoma, but the cells contain rounder nuclei and often have high numbers of cytoplasmic vacuoles (see page 40). The masses can occasionally spontaneously regress but, if not, are locally invasive.

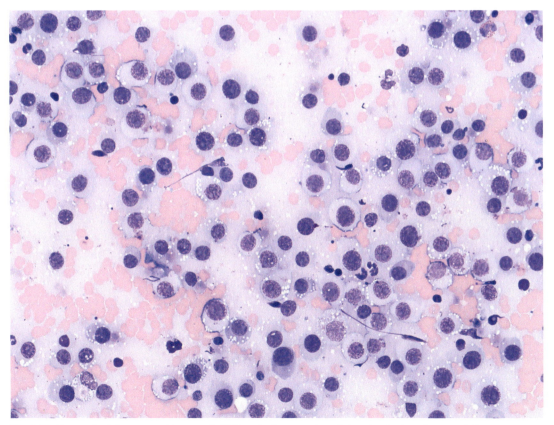

Fig 6.33 Transmissible venereal tumour (×500); note the round nuclei and cytoplasmic vacuolation

> **Key points**
>
> **Cutaneous neoplasia**
> - Mast cell granules often stain poorly with aqueous Romanowsky stains such as Diff-Quik
> - Histiocytomas have not been reported in cats
> - Finding keratin mixed with a non-staining waxy substance suggests aspiration of a sebaceous lesion
> - Dermal melanomas are often less malignant than oral
> - Large amounts of blood, platelet clumps and low numbers of macrophages containing red blood cells/haemosiderin is suggestive of aspiration of a vascular hamartoma or haemangioma

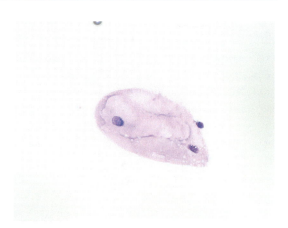

Fig 6.34a Individual adipocyte (×500)

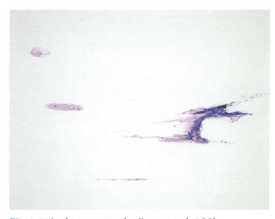

Fig 6.34b Aggregate of adipocytes (×100)

Neoplastic lesions – subcutaneous

The following section contains a list of commonly sampled subcutaneous neoplastic lesions (that is, lesions which do not usually have an obvious dermal component – as ever in medicine, exceptions will occur – histiocytic sarcomas in particular can be cutaneous but mostly appear subcutaneous, so are found here rather than the cutaneous section). They are presented in rough order of commonality (so the further down this list you travel, the less common the lesion and the less likely the diagnosis).

The sections include a brief description of the most relevant non-cytological signalment factors which may aid diagnosis (such as common locations, age and breed) and the typical cytological features present on sampling. The focus of this book is on diagnosis; for up-to-date information on treatment, other sources should be consulted.

Lipoma (FIG 6.34)
Neoplasm type: mesenchymal
Age: usually middle-aged to older
Location: any fatty tissue

Gross Appearance: smooth and often mobile mass, but can be firm/attached if between fascial planes or muscles, or if infiltrative (see below)
Species/breed predispositions: very common in dogs, uncommon in cats; female dogs and castrated male Siamese cats predisposed
Cytological appearance/further comments: lipomas are the most common canine neoplasm aspirated, and cytologically the cells appear as well-differentiated adipocytes (see page 133). Exfoliation is variable, with some aspirates containing large sheets of cells and others containing only a few individual cells. The methanol in staining solutions dissolves extracellular fat (which is only then apparent as a non-staining circular space), so it is worth noting prior to

staining whether a preparation appears greasy or not (as this can help interpretation in very poorly cellular samples).

As the fat cells are well-differentiated, they appear identical to aspirates from non-neoplastic adipose tissue, which is why it is important to be clear whether a lesion is cutaneous or subcutaneous. Cutaneous lipomas are very rare, even in dogs, so fat cells found on aspirates from subcutaneous lesions probably represent inadvertent sampling of the subcutaneous fat layer.

It is always worth assessing suspected lipomas closely, as occasionally other tumours (particularly mast cells tumours) are embedded deep within fat, and aspirates from these can contain high numbers of adipocytes.

An infiltrative lipoma is a benign lipoma variant which is locally invasive – these lesions can feel firm and adhered to underlying tissue, and less obviously discrete than typical lipomas. Aspirates from them can also include small aggregates of skeletal muscle (see page 134). (Fig 6.35)

Soft tissue sarcoma (FIG 6.36)
Neoplasm type: mesenchymal
Age: middle-aged to older
Location: often limbs or joints, trunk, head (cats)
Gross Appearance: solitary firm masses, sometimes multilobulated, sometimes firmly attached
Species/breed predispositions: very common in dogs, uncommon in cats; large breed dogs predisposed
Cytological appearance/further comments: soft tissue sarcomas have traditionally been divided into haemangiopericytomas, peripheral nerve sheath tumours and others, but the classification is used less commonly now as there is little clinical benefit from doing so – cytologically the lesions appear identical, and biologically the lesions behave in a very similar manner, in that they are locally invasive but usually have low metastatic potential.

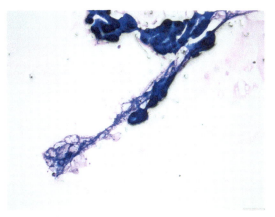

Fig 6.35 Adipocytes and skeletal muscle in an infiltrative lipoma (×100)

On cytology, the lesions consistent of variable numbers of mesenchymal cells – variable because soft tissue sarcomas can frequently exfoliate very poorly (presumably because the cells are tightly adhered to basement membrane).

When aspirates are highly cellular, they are not a diagnostic challenge – they contain high numbers of mostly fusiform (spindle-shaped), occasionally stellate (star-shaped), mesenchymal cells found individually in large aggregates, often with a 'storiform' pattern (see page 80, Fig 4.4). The cells are often binucleate (sometimes resembling alien heads or insect heads) and some sarcomas contain 'crown cells' – large multinucleate cells, with the nuclei arranged around the periphery of the cell (Fig 6.37) (the presence of crown cells raises strong suspicion for soft tissue sarcoma even in poorly cellular specimens).

These tumours are much more difficult to diagnose, however, when cellularity is low. The problem is that mesenchymal cell proliferation from fibrosis can appear identical cytologically to neoplastic mesenchymal cells from a soft tissue sarcoma (Fig 6.38). With lower cellularity specimens, it is often impossible to distinguish between fibrosis and a soft tissue sarcoma. The history becomes very important here – if a lesion appeared suddenly or there is a history of trauma, then fibrosis is

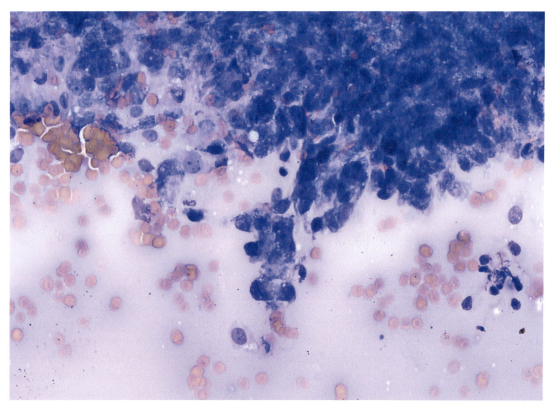

Fig 6.36a Mesenchymal aggregate from a soft tissue sarcoma (×500)

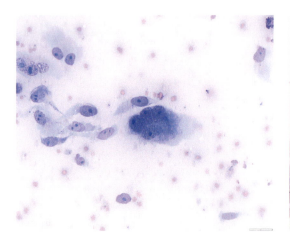

Fig 6.36b Atypical mesenchymal cells from a high-grade sarcoma (×1000)

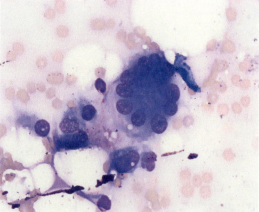

Fig 6.37 Crown cell with multiple peripheral nuclei (×1000)

a significant consideration. If the lesion has already been present for several weeks without any known trauma, then soft tissue sarcoma becomes more likely.

The take-home message: always consider fibrosis as an alternative explanation for mesenchymal cells on cytological specimens, particularly when cellularity is low, there is concurrent

Skin and subcutaneous lesions | Chapter 6   153

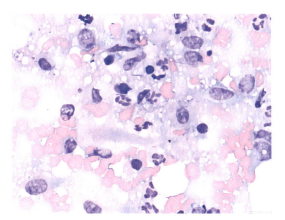

Fig 6.38 Mesenchymal cells and neutrophilic inflammation in reactive fibrosis (×1000)

inflammation, or when the lesion arose suddenly or after trauma.

Cytologists are sometimes called upon to distinguish between regrowth of a sarcoma at a surgical site, or proliferating scar tissue. As you may imagine given the above information, this can be something of a cytological challenge. Histopathology is sometimes required for more definitive information.

Mast cell tumour (FIG 6.39)

Neoplasm type: round cell
Age: any, usually middle-aged to older; more common in dogs
Location: any area but legs, back and thorax most common

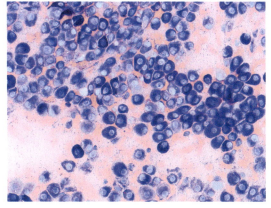

Fig 6.39 Subcutaneous mast cell tumour (×500)

Gross Appearance: often poorly circumscribed mass, mostly single (95%) but occasionally multiple
Species/breed predispositions: boxers, pugs (on average, slightly lower grade neoplasms), Shar Peis (on average higher grade), Staffordshire bull terriers, golden retrievers and Labradors, as well as Persian cats
Cytological appearance/further comments: cytologically identical to cutaneous mast cell tumours except that sometimes the lesions are deeply embedded in fat and can contain significant numbers of adipocytes; at first glance these lesions can appear very similar to lipomas so checking for mast cells is always prudent when lesions appear predominantly fatty (Fig 6.42).

Fibroma/fibrosarcoma (FIGS 6.40–6.43)

Neoplasm type: mesenchymal
Age: usually middle-aged to older (9+), can be as young as 3 years in feline injection-site sarcoma
Location: limbs/head most commonly, injection sites for injection-site sarcoma
Gross Appearance: varies from small and well circumscribed to large and diffuse
Species/breed predispositions: common in cats, rare in dogs; Rhodesian ridgeback and boxers predisposed to fibromas
Cytological appearance/further comments: fibromas/fibrosarcomas appear similar to many other mesenchymal tumours. They may exfoliate poorly, as the cells are often firmly attached to underlying matrix. They contain mostly fusiform (spindle-shaped) mesenchymal cells, individually or in small aggregates – see page 78 for a more detailed description of mesenchymal tumours.

They may contain variable amounts of reddish fibrillar (containing faint striations resembling fibrils) matrix. The appearance of the mesenchymal cells is often correlated with their biological behaviour (i.e. the more malignant features, the more aggressive the neoplasm – see page 92 for malignant features). Many fibromas and fibrosarcomas are low-grade neoplasms – they

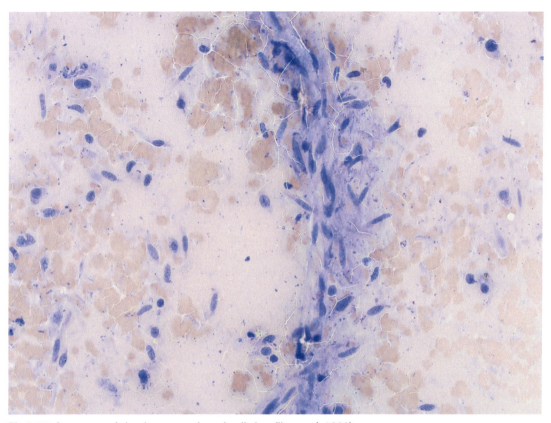

Fig 6.40 Aggregate of slender mesenchymal cells in a fibroma (×1000)

may be locally invasive (fibrosarcomas) but have limited metastatic potential.

Keloidal fibromas (Figs 6.41 and 6.42) and fibrosarcomas are rare variants – these appear similar to other mesenchymal tumours but also contain large amounts of collagen, often with a chaotic tangled appearance (see below). These lesions may have a significant dermal component (usually appearing as a small smooth well-circumscribed and often hairless mass).

Injection site sarcomas are seen in cats relatively commonly – these are often highly aggressive, invasive and frequently recur following surgery. They often display marked atypical features – it can be challenging, however, to distinguish between inflammation following injection (which often contains fibrosis, resembling atypical mesenchymal cells) and sarcomas – here, the history is most useful, as a recent history of injection (within a few weeks) is more likely to be associated with inflammation, whereas injection-site sarcomas will persist for much longer or may appear well after the initial injection.

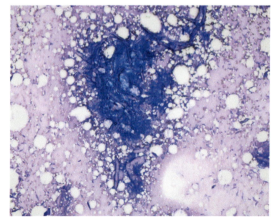

Fig 6.41 Keloidal fibroma showing tangled ribbons of collagen (×100)

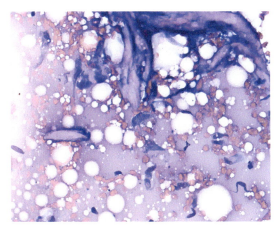

Fig 6.42 Keloidal fibroma (×500)

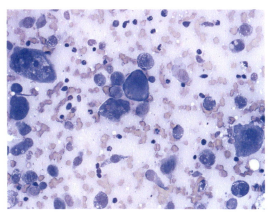

Fig 6.44 Markedly pleomorphic cells from a subcutaneous histiocytic sarcoma (×500)

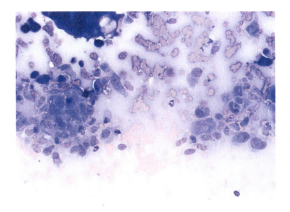

Fig 6.43 Highly pleomorphic cells in an injection site sarcoma (×500)

It is worth bearing in mind that cats which have had a history of significant inflammation following injection may be predisposed to injection site sarcomas and using an alternate injection site (such as the forelimb) may be prudent in these patients (see page 174 for a description of vaccine-site reactions).

Histiocytic sarcoma (FIG 6.44)
Neoplasm type: round cell
Age: middle-aged to older
Location: any location (including cutaneous, although grossly most appear subcutaneous without obvious dermal component), synovial tumours are commonly histiocytic sarcomas *Gross Appearance:* usually soft subcutaneous mass, firm joint masses
Species/breed predispositions: Bernese mountain dog, flat coat retriever, miniature schnauzer, Rottweiler, golden retriever all predisposed
Cytological appearance/further comments: despite the name 'sarcoma', these lesions are tumours of histiocytic cells (dendritic cells and macrophages). Subcutaneous (and cutaneous) histiocytic sarcomas are usually dendritic.

These lesions often contain highly pleomorphic and frequently bizarre cells, often with high numbers of atypical mitotic figures. They often contain multiple features of malignancy – see page 92 for a fuller description.

Myxoma/myxosarcoma (FIG 6.45)
Neoplasm type: mesenchymal
Age: middle-aged to older
Location: usually trunk or limbs
Gross Appearance: soft often poorly-delineated masses, often produce a viscous or jelly-like substance on sampling (can appear very similar to synovial fluid)
Species/breed predispositions: rare in both dogs and cats
Cytological appearance/further comments: the neoplastic cells are similar to other sarcomas – in myxomas (the more benign variant), cells are relatively monomorphic unremarkable fusiform

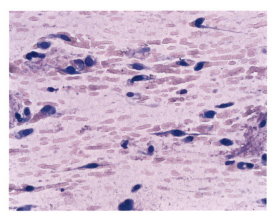

Fig 6.45 Myxosarcoma – the mesenchymal cells and red blood cells are embedded in a thick pink matrix; note the 'windrowing' of the cells (lining up in straight rows), indicating viscosity (×500)

(spindle-shaped) cells, usually found individually or in small aggregates. Cells from myxosarcomas usually display more overtly atypical features (see page 92), such as pleomorphism, multinucleation and multiple nucleoli.

The most striking cytological feature of these neoplasms, however, is the large amount of background material. 'Myxoid' means 'relating to mucous', and these tumours often produce large amounts of the stuff. Cytologically, it appears as variably-dense and often fibrillar (i.e. having the appearance of containing tiny strands or fibrils) pink to purple matrix, often dominating the aspirates, with the cells scattered throughout this background material. The viscous nature of the mucoid material means that cells, particularly red blood cells, are often seen 'windrowing' (lined up in neat rows – see page 52), in contrast with other matrix-rich sarcomas (such as chondrosarcomas).

The biggest diagnostic challenge with these lesions is that cytologically they often resemble joint fluid, and whilst most synovial fluid samples tend to be less cellular and mostly contain mononuclear cells (macrophages) (see page 62), it can be very challenging to distinguish between myxoma/sarcoma and synovial fluid in less-cellular and less well-preserved samples, especially in lesions on or near joints.

Myxomas and myxosarcomas often behave in a similar fashion to soft tissue sarcomas – locally invasive but with low metastatic potential. It should also be borne in mind, however, that some other tumours can also produce significant amounts of mucoid-material (usually other sarcomas such as myxoid liposarcomas, but occasionally epithelial tumours can exude similar goop), further complicating the diagnostic picture. Histopathology is often required for these more cytologically complex cases.

Haemangiosarcoma (FIG 6.46)
Neoplasm type: mesenchymal
Age: usually older
Location: any subcutaneous
Gross Appearance: often larger and more diffuse than cutaneous haemangiosarcomas
Species/breed predispositions: none known (not associated with coat length/skin pigmentation, unlike cutaneous form)
Cytological appearance/further comments: the cytological appearance of subcutaneous haemangiosarcomas is similar to elsewhere (see page 147 for a description). Subcutaneous haemangiosarcoma carries a worse prognosis than its cutaneous counterpart, and they

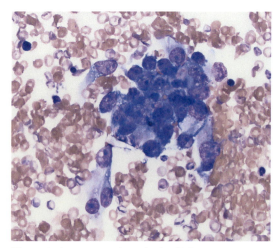

Fig 6.46 Aggregate of atypical cells in subcutaneous haemangiosarcoma (×500)

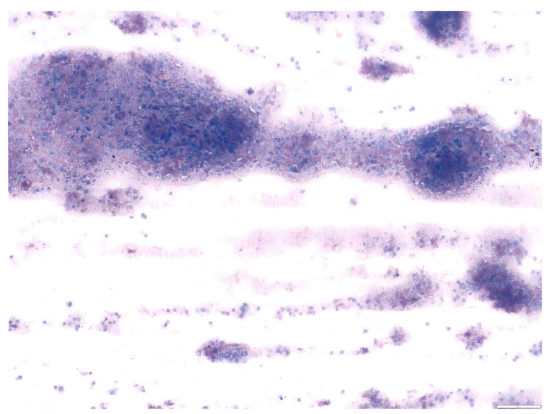

Fig 6.47 Chondrosarcoma – low power; the cells are embedded in abundant extracellular matrix (×100)

often behave more aggressively – further staging is recommended when this tumour is diagnosed or suspected. They can be challenging to remove or even identify surgically as they are often surrounded by extensive subcutaneous bruising.

Chondroma/chondrosarcoma (FIGS 6.47–6.49)

Neoplasm type: mesenchymal
Age: middle-aged to older
Location: usually around flat bones rather than long bones, mostly ribs (costochondral junction), nose or pelvis in dogs, scapula and digits in cats; mostly osseous or periosteal but often feel subcutaneous; very rarely occur extraskeletally (i.e. not over underlying bone)
Gross Appearance: very firm masses, can get very large, usually overlying bone; often fixed in place and feel very firm on sampling

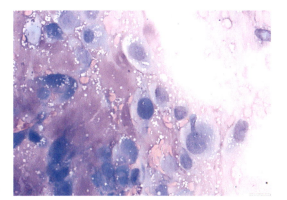

Fig 6.48 On higher power, the atypical features of the mesenchymal cells are more apparent (pleomorphism, anisocytosis, anisokaryosis) ×1000

Species/breed predispositions: usually medium to large dogs; rare in small and giant breeds, rare in cats (possibly more common in male cats)

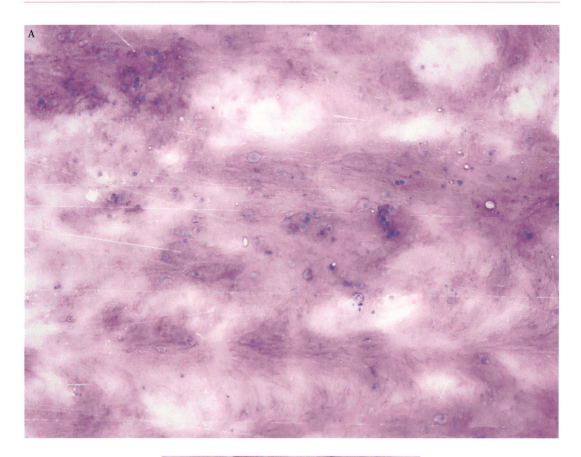

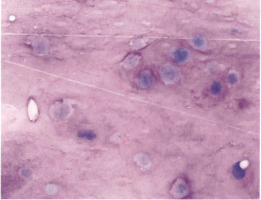

Fig 6.49a and b Low (×100) and high (×500) power appearance of lacunae

Cytological appearance/further comments: the neoplastic cells appear similar to other sarcomas (see page 78), although as with myxomas/myxosarcomas, overall cellularity can be quite low and aspirates are often dominated by matrix. In chondromas/chondrosarcomas, the matrix is not usually viscous and therefore windrowing is not seen. Chondroid is often fibrillar (striated, with the appearance of containing fibrils) and often deeply purple. The cells are sometimes observed on small islands ('lacunae') embedded within the matrix (Fig 6.49), and the rounded shape of these cells within the lacunae can give the more imaginative cytologist the impression of an owl's eye peering back at them from the specimen.

Liposarcoma (FIG 6.50)
Neoplasm type: mesenchymal
Age: middle-aged to older
Location: any subcutaneous
Gross Appearance: can appear similar to lipomas but are often infiltrative and therefore firmer and more attached
Species/breed predispositions: rare in both dogs and cats, but dogs slightly more commonly affected; Shetland sheepdogs slightly predisposed
Cytological appearance/further comments: usually have a very fatty background with high numbers of non-staining fat droplets. The neoplastic cells appear as highly atypical mesenchymal cells, and can be fusiform, stellate, caudate or sometimes rounded. The cells usually contain variable numbers of irregularly-sized clear vacuoles. These lesions can be cytologically challenging because the appearance of irregular pleomorphic (variably-shaped) cells containing clear vacuoles is similar to the cytological appearance of both marked macrophagic inflammation within fat and sebaceous carcinomas. In general, macrophages do not display nearly as much nuclear variation as either of the neoplastic lesions, and sebaceous carcinomas are usually cutaneous, but there are exceptions. Additionally, both mammary lesions and salivary lesions can contain vacuolated and atypical-appearing cells, and both are usually subcutaneous.

Liposarcomas are locally invasive, often markedly so, although reports of metastasis are rare.

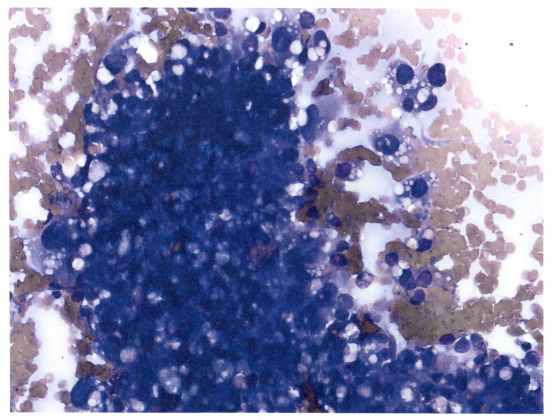

Fig 6.50 Liposarcoma; note fat droplets and irregular clear vacuoles within mesenchymal cells (×500)

Lymphoma (FIG 6.51)
Neoplasm type: round cell
Age: any, usually middle-aged to older
Location: any subcutaneous
Gross Appearance: often discrete subcutaneous mass
Species/breed predispositions: see below
Cytological appearance/further comments: true subcutaneous lymphomas – that is, lymphoma with a predilection for subcutaneous tissue – is very rare in dogs and cats. Subcutaneous aspirates which appear to contain lymphoma probably actually reflect sampling of a neoplastic infiltrate within a subcutaneous lymph node or lymphoid nodule. Regardless, lymphoma here resembles lymphoma in other locations (see page 86) – a monomorphic, rather than mixed, population of lymphocytes. Large cell lymphoma is much less challenging to diagnose cytologically than small cell (as reactive lymphoid populations usually contain 70–80% small lymphocytes).

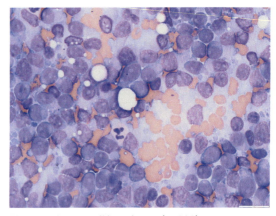

Fig 6.51 Large cell lymphoma (×1000)

Leiomyoma/leiomyosarcoma (FIG 6.52)
Neoplasm type: mesenchymal
Age: variable
Location: mostly on the dorsum, occasionally limbs and muzzle
Gross Appearance: solitary firm dermal or subcutaneous nodules
Species/breed predispositions: none known; rare in both dogs and cats
Cytological appearance/further comments: these are very rare lesions in both the skin and subcutis. They often exfoliate poorly and usually contain scattered fusiform (spindle cells) with an appearance resembling smooth muscle (a haphazard arrangement of oval nuclei within a background of pale pink cytoplasm or matrix). Because of their rarity and poor exfoliation, they are challenging to diagnose cytologically, but the presence of even small amounts of material resembling smooth muscle should raise the cytologist's suspicions. These lesions usually follow a benign clinical course.

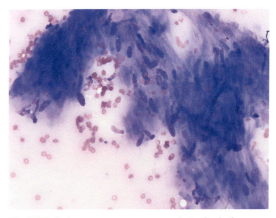

Fig 6.52 Leiomyoma; appearance is typical of smooth muscle but the location and abundance of cells are more suggestive of neoplasia (×500)

Rhabdomyosarcoma
Neoplasm type: mesenchymal
Age: can occur in very young patients, especially the more aggressive neoplasms
Location: often head/neck, mostly commonly larynx, occasionally tongue
Gross Appearance: variable but most often irregular firm masses
Species/breed predispositions: too few reported
Cytological appearance/further comments: these are thankfully very rare but sometimes highly aggressive tumours of skeletal muscle, which can occur in patients as young as a year old. They have a very variable cytological appearance, often containing highly pleomorphic cells. Due

to their often poorly-differentiated nature, the cells can be hard to identify, but there are two features which can raise a cytologist's suspicion of the presence of this lesion. Some cells may contain faint striations within their cytoplasm, reminiscent of those observed within well-differentiated skeletal muscle, and 'strap cells' may be identified – these are atypical mesenchymal cells with multiple nucleoli lined up in a row, somewhat resembling peas in a pod.

> **Key points**
>
> **Subcutaneous neoplasia**
> - Fat cells from a lipoma appear identical to aspirates from non-neoplastic adipose tissue
> - Some tumours (particularly mast cells tumours) are embedded deep within fat, and aspirates from these can contain high numbers of adipocytes
> - Mesenchymal cell proliferation from fibrosis can appear identical cytologically to neoplastic mesenchymal cells from a soft tissue sarcoma

Specific location: perianal region

Although any tumour can occur in the perianal region, the two most common neoplasms in dogs are hepatoid gland tumours and anal sac apocrine gland adenocarcinomas (sometimes called AGASACA) (both tumours are rare in cats). Distinguishing between these lesions cytologically is very useful given the very different prognoses for these two lesions.

Hepatoid gland (perianal) tumour (FIGS 6.53, 6.54)

Neoplasm type: epithelial
Age: can be any but 8–13 most common (dogs)
Location: usually perianal, can also appear around tail base, around the prepuce or rarely on the hindlimbs
Gross appearance: raised masses with sparse hair, often ulcerated
Species/breed predispositions: very common in dogs, especially entire males, but can occur in neutered males and females – breeds more commonly affected include Siberian huskies, Samoyeds and German wirehaired pointers
Cytological appearance/further comments: 'hepatoid' epithelial cells are so called because of their similar appearance to liver cells. They have round central nuclei, usually dense and generally with a single nucleolus, and moderate to abundant pale pinkish-red (eosinophilic) cytoplasm containing fine granules – it is the granules which give the cells their similar appearance to hepatocytes. The clusters often contain variable numbers of smaller denser nuclei, known as 'reserve cells' and thought to represent basal epithelium.

They are often ulcerated and frequently accompanied by inflammation, often predominantly macrophagic, and there may be evidence of prior haemorrhage (see page 98). The great majority of these tumours are benign perianal adenomas, but occasional malignant versions can occur which can be difficult to distinguish from their benign counterparts cytologically. Excision and submission for histopathology is usually recommended for this reason, although castration or anti-androgenic therapy is often used as adjunctive therapy to reduce the size of the masses and prevent further lesions occurring.

The number of reserve cells within these lesions does not appear to be predictive of malignancy, but any of the typical features of malignancy (see page 92) should raise the cytologist's suspicion of a more malignant process (as with any neoplasm).

Apocrine gland anal sac adenocarcinoma (AGASACA) (FIG 6.55)

Neoplasm type: epithelial but neuroendocrine-appearing (see below)
Age: 5+

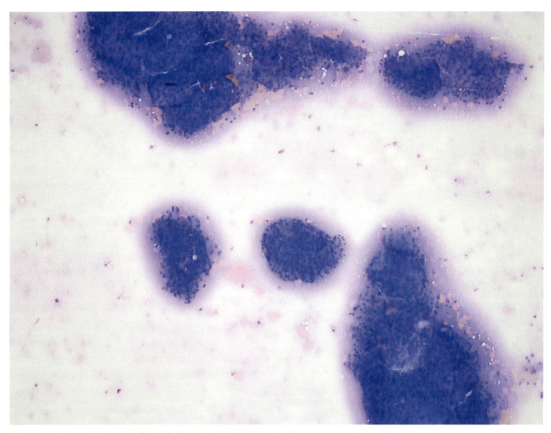

Fig 6.53 Hepatoid tumour (×100): Rounded clusters of uniform-appearing cells

Location: perianal, metastasis often to sublumbar lymph nodes

Gross appearance: variably-sized masses in the wall of the anal sac, about half are visible at presentation (remainder found via palpation)

Species/breed predispositions: common in dogs, rare in cats (but less rare than hepatoid epithelial tumours); breeds affected include English cocker spaniels, Dandy Dinmonts, German shepherds, English springer spaniels

Cytological appearance/further comments: although these are not 'true' neuroendocrine tumours (they are formed from sweat glands, which are eccrine, not apocrine) this is largely academic from a cytological perspective. The salient diagnostic point is that these lesions appear as classic neuroendocrine tumours (see page 76). Aspirates often have high numbers of

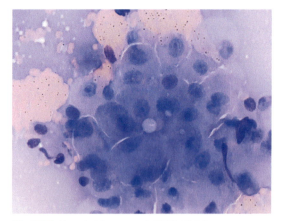

Fig 6.54 Hepatoid tumour (×500): At this magnification the granular appearance of the cytoplasm, similar to hepatocytes, can be appreciated

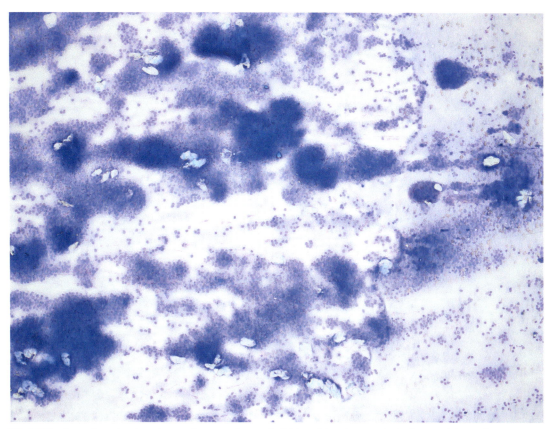

Fig 6.55a Apocrine gland anal sac adenocarcinoma (×100); cell borders are indistinct and the cells appear to be free nuclei in a sea of cytoplasm

bare nuclei. Where intact, the cells have indistinct borders and appear as free nuclei within a lake of pale pink cytoplasm. Anisokaryosis (nuclei size variation) is minimal but amongst the otherwise uniform nuclei, occasional nuclei up to twice as large are sometimes seen. Acinar structures are often commonly found and, again where intact, the clusters of cells are often more cohesive than other neuroendocrine tumours (with the possible exception of thyroid tumours).

As with other neuroendocrine-appearing tumours, their bland cytological appearance often masks aggressive clinical behaviour. Up to 90% of these lesions have metastasised at the time of diagnosis (usually initially to the sublumbar lymph nodes, then on into the liver or spleen). Hypercalcaemia (humoral hypercalcaemia of malignancy – HHM) is a common neoplastic side effect of these tumours, and assessment of a patient's serum calcium as well as further staging is strongly recommended.

Non-neoplastic lesion: Anal sac inflammation/impaction (FIG 6.56)

In addition to neoplasia in this region, impaction of the anal gland with consequent inflammation and possible secondary infection can also produce a firm mass, which can be large and often persists for a long time – it can be very difficult to distinguish impacted anal glands from tumours via palpation.

Cytologically, the principal finding of an impacted anal gland is a large amount of keratin, usually present in large clumps. There is generally (although not always) concurrent

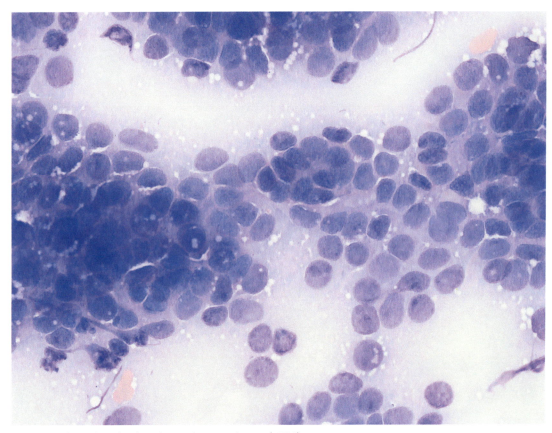

Fig 6.55b Apocrine gland anal sac adenocarcinoma (×500)

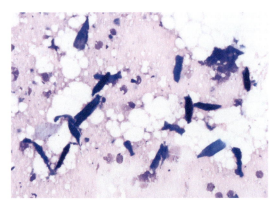

Fig 6.56 Impacted anal gland; keratin, fat and poorly preserved leukocytes (probably neutrophils) (×1000)

inflammation, often neutrophilic, macrophagic, or both (pyogranulomatous). Bacteria are also likely to be present, either as contaminants from faeces or as secondary infection.

The picture can be further complicated because neoplasia in or near the anal sac can cause impaction; careful assessment of slides that appear initially to contain impaction is recommended to avoid missing neoplastic cells interspersed with the keratin and inflammation.

Specific location: mammary lesions

Dogs
Unfortunately, examining aspirates from canine mammary masses can be a frustrating cytological exercise. The diagnosis of lesions of non-mammary tissue is relatively straightforward – or, at least, as straightforward as cytology gets (see above for cutaneous and subcutaneous masses). Masses comprised of mammary tissue,

however, are extremely challenging to assess. This is because these lesions are extremely heterogeneous, even when inflammatory or hyperplastic.

Canine mammary lesions are complex three-dimensional structures which can contain pockets of different cell types (epithelial, mesenchymal) and tissue types – three different aspirates from the same mammary mass in a dog can appear as three separate entities cytologically. Bluntly, the cytological appearance of mammary masses is often poorly correlated with their histological appearance, as well as their biological behaviour.

Further complicating cytology, mammary epithelium is often *myoepithelium* – it shows some characteristics of muscle, in that it is contractile, and the cytological upshot of this is that epithelial cells aspirated from the mammary glands have a somewhat mesenchymal appearance. Mammary epithelium often appears similar to basal epithelium in the centre of clusters (see page 132 for a more detailed description), containing small rounded cells with dense nuclei and little cytoplasm, but at the periphery the cells start to take on a more spindloid appearance and 'fray' away from the clusters in a similar way to mesenchymal aggregates (Fig 6.57). It can be challenging, if not impossible, to distinguish between individual spindloid myoepithelial cells and mesenchymal cells on mammary preparations.

Mammary tissue can also differentiate into other tissue types, including cartilage and bone – this usually occurs in mixed mammary tumours.

Mammary aspirates are also often full of secretory product (appearance as a smooth pale blue substance) as well as substantial numbers of 'foam cells' – these may actually be epithelial cells, despite their strong resemblance to activate macrophages (again, telling the difference between these possibilities is effectively impossible on standard stains).

The overall effect of all of the above is that mammary aspirates are often quite mixed, with

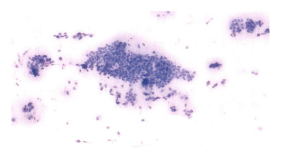

Fig 6.57 Myoepithelium; the cells are present in a dense cluster but the edges are less rounded and have a more mesenchymal appearance

epithelial cells, mesenchymal cells, large foamy cells, secretory material, and frequently some degree of neutrophilic and/or macrophagic inflammation (Fig 6.58), and this cytological appearance can be seen with inflammation, hyperplasia or neoplasia.

The author finds the easiest way to make sense of mammary aspirates is to concentrate on the epithelial cells – well-differentiated epithelium with few signs of malignancy (see page 92) are more likely to reflect hyperplasia, adenoma or well-differentiated (and likely lower grade) carcinoma, whereas atypical features are more likely to be associated with higher-grade carcinomas. This is a less reliable feature than in other locations, however – very malignant-appearing

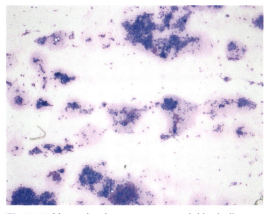

Fig 6.58 Very mixed mammary material including extracellular matrix, clusters of epithelium and scattered bare oval nuclei, more mesenchymal appearing cells and macrophages

epithelium is sometimes associated with hyperplasia, whereas more innocuous-looking epithelium is sometimes found within malignant mammary tumours.

The concurrent presence of significant numbers of mesenchymal cells, and/or fibrillar matrix material resembling chondroid (often an intense purple colour) or osteoid (usually pinker), especially when accompanied with mesenchymal cells resembling chondroblasts or osteoblasts (see pages 266) is most suggestive of sampling a complex or mixed mammary tumour – these are often lower-grade mammary neoplasms.

Given the above challenges, cytology of mammary lesions in dogs is often restricted to confirmation of whether the mass is mammary or non-mammary in origin, and histopathology is often required for more definitive information.

Cats

Thankfully, and atypically for the species, feline cytology is usually more straightforward and more diagnostically rewarding. Mammary tumours are relatively common in cats, mostly occurring in intact females. The majority of mammary masses in older cats (approximately 80%) are carcinomas (mostly adenocarcinomas; myoepithelial involvement is relatively rare), and cytologically they usually have an appearance more consistent with their biological behaviour – that is, aspirates generally contain crowded and disorganised epithelial cells displaying multiple atypical features (Fig 6.59), often including signet ring cells (see page 95, Fig 4.72).

Given the high rate of malignancy in feline mammary tumours, however, even harvests of more uniform-appearing epithelium should be treated carefully. Further staging via aspiration of enlarged lymph nodes and imaging of the chest and abdomen is recommended.

An exception to the general rule that mammary masses are often malignant neoplasms occurs in young intact females, typically less than two

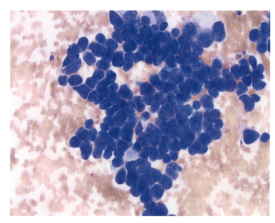

Fig 6.59 Feline mammary carcinoma; cells display variations in nuclear size and cell size (anisokaryosis and anisocytosis), multiple nucleoli and nuclear moulding (×500)

years old. These patients are prone to a form of hyperplasia known as *fibroepithelial hyperplasia*. This is a benign condition which often responds to neutering. Cytologically, aspirates from these lesions often contain dense clusters of cuboidal epithelium, resembling basal epithelium (see page 132), interspersed with frequently large amounts of pink fibrillar (containing striations resembling fibrils) matrix, and fusiform (spindle-shaped) mesenchymal cells (Fig 6.60).

Just as care should be taken with even relatively bland-appearing epithelium in the

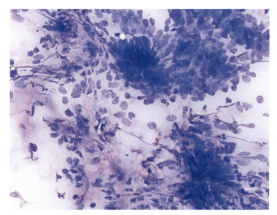

Fig 6.60 Feline fibroepithelial hyperplasia: A mixture of epithelial cells, mesenchymal cells and pink extracellular matrix (×500)

mammary masses of older feline patients, caution is advised when diagnosing mammary tumours in young entire females. As with much of cytology, context is of high importance.

Specific location: salivary lesions

The proximity of the submandibular salivary gland to the lymph node has frustrated many veterinary surgeons over time; the time a cytologist is most likely to inspect salivary material under their microscope is when an attempt at aspirating the submandibular lymph node has been made. It is almost impossible to distinguish between the structures cytologically. Salivary material is cytologically distinctive – the material aspirated is often viscous, so cells are frequently windrowing (lined up in discrete rows – see page 52).

Embedded within this viscous material there are likely to be salivary epithelial cells, most of which are secretory, and have a cytological appearance to match: they have small round nuclei and abundant pale cytoplasm filled with clear vacuoles. The overall appearance is similar to sebaceous epithelium (see page 132), although the vacuoles are less regular and the general impression is somewhat less uniform. There are also sometimes present smaller denser clusters of non-secretory epithelial cells – these appear very similar to basal epithelium (see page 132) in that they have much less cytoplasm, often mid- to dark-blue in colour, although they are often surrounded by a pale reddish-pink halo, which may represent basement membrane (Figs 6.61, 6.62).

Salivary adenoma/adenocarcinoma

Neoplasm type: epithelial
Age: usually older
Gross Appearance: firm subcutaneous swellings or discrete masses
Species/breed predispositions: uncommon in both dogs and cats
Cytological appearance/further comments: well-differentiated salivary adenomas appear similar to normal salivary tissue; as with many

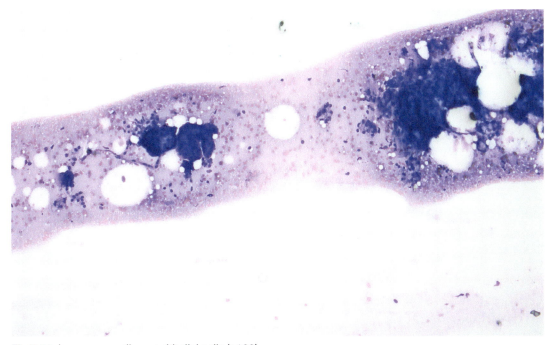

Fig 6.61 Low power salivary epithelial cells (×100)

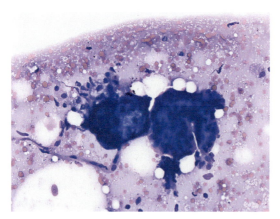

Fig 6.62 High power salivary epithelium; vacuolated secretory cells are in a cluster on the left, with denser non-secretory cells with an eosinophilic halo on the right (×500)

cytological specimens, it can be very challenging to distinguish between low-grade neoplasia and normal tissue or hyperplasia, and the clinical context usually greatly augments the diagnosis in these cases (for instance: 'How long has the mass been present?' 'How quickly is it growing?' 'Has it continued to grow?' – low-grade adenomas are slow growing expansile masses). Note that low-grade salivary neoplasia is less common than malignant salivary tumours, however.

More malignant salivary tumours can have a more confusing cytological appearance – poorly differentiated salivary secretory epithelium can appear similar to activated macrophages, sebaceous carcinomas or liposarcomas. In this context it is extremely helpful to be clear whether the lesion is cutaneous (and more likely to be sebaceous in origin) or subcutaneous (and more likely to be salivary). Salivary tumours can also contain areas of mesenchymal differentiation – in fact, the overall appearance of salivary tumours cytologically can be quite similar to aspirates from mammary tissue.

Non-neoplastic lesion – salivary mucocoele (sialocoele) (FIG 6.63)

These lesions are a consequence of rupture of the salivary gland or salivary ducts, and are relatively common in dogs, slightly less so in cats. Common sites are along the jawline or under the tongue (more common in cats than dogs).

Cytologically, the appearance is predominantly inflammatory – aspirates usually contain mostly macrophages, highly activated. Salivary epithelium (see above) may also be present but this is uncommon. The most distinctive cytological appearance is the presence of variable amounts of wispy flocculent (cloud-like) pale blue material interspersed with the macrophages; this represents the mucous portion of saliva, and it is strongly suggestive of aspiration of a salivary mucocoele (although the absence of it does not exclude the possibility – some mucocoeles secrete altered and more watery saliva which contains very little mucous).

PAS stain (specific for mucopolysaccharides) can help confirm mucocoele (Fig 6.64) but is rarely necessary in the author's experience – the mucous is clearly visible without highlighting, and in the case of more watery mucocoeles, there is very little for the PAS stain to highlight.

Specific location: Thyroid Tumour

Thyroid tissue has a neuroendocrine appearance cytologically. Most neuroendocrine tissue appears similar – the cells are fragile and frequently rupture, so high numbers of bare nuclei are often evidence. The cells are usually found in clusters with indistinct borders – the impression is of small regular nuclei floating in a lake of pale pink cytoplasm (see page 76 for a fuller description of neuroendocrine tissue cytologically). (Fig 6.65)

Given the similar appearance of neuroendocrine tissues, it can be difficult to distinguish thyroid material from metastatic neuroendocrine tumours, although there may be some clues present – thyroid epithelium is sometimes associated with small amorphous blobs of pale pink colloid (Fig 6.66), and the cells sometimes contain dark pigment granules (somewhat resembling lipofuscin within the liver), thought to be tyrosine granules (Fig 6.65). Thyroid epithelium is also

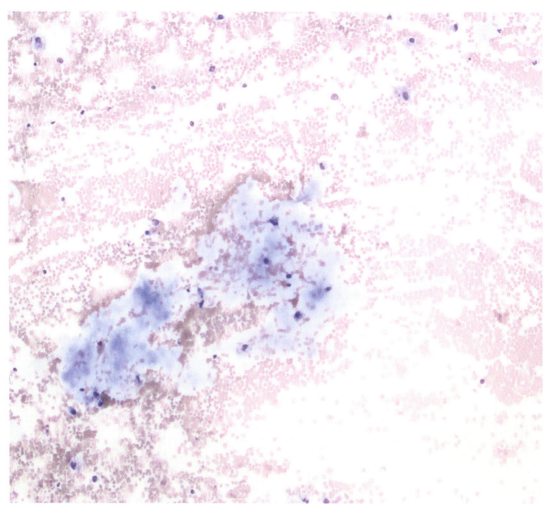

Fig 6.63a Low power sialocoele; note the large cloudy blue blobs of mucous, characteristic of these lesions (×100)

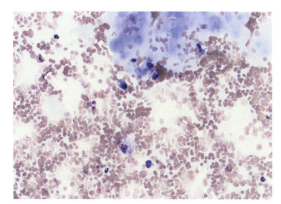

Fig 6.63b Higher power sialocoele, showing mucous and macrophagic inflammation (×500)

slightly more cohesive than other neuroendocrine tissues (though often not quite as cohesive as anal sac apocrine gland adenocarcinomas).

If any of these features are present, it is likely that thyroid tissue has been aspirated. Without these clues, other neuroendocrine lesions remain possible (for instance, carotid body tumours – tumours of the chemoreceptor cells associated with the carotid artery, also known as chemodectomas – can appear in a similar location with a similar appearance).

The text above has coyly referred to the thyroid lesions above as 'thyroid tissue' – this is because

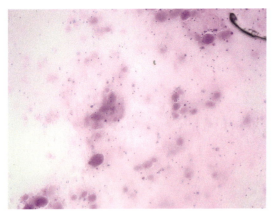

Fig 6.64 Mucous highlighted with PAS stain (×100)

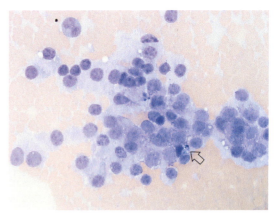

Fig 6.65 Thyroid tissue from a canine thyroid carcinoma; note the dark blue-green pigment (open arrow) (×1000)

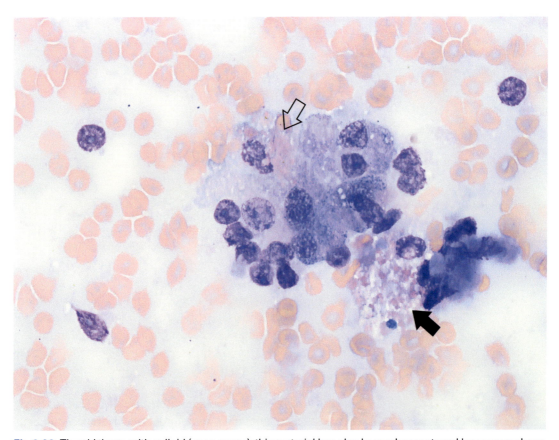

Fig 6.66 Thyroid tissue with colloid (open arrow); this material has also been phagocytosed by a macrophage (black arrow) (×1000)

the interpretation of samples from the thyroid lesion is highly contextual. Whilst some thyroid carcinomas can appear markedly atypical (Fig 6.67), the majority have a very bland cytological appearance, in keeping with many neuroendocrine tumours. This makes it hard to distinguish them from samples of normal thyroid tissue, and here the context becomes important: most thyroid masses in cats represent hyperplasia or functional adenomas, and there is limited value is aspirating these lesions, especially when hyperthyroidism has already been diagnosed – the chances of a cytological sample being able to distinguish the rare feline thyroid carcinoma from hyperplasia/adenoma are slim.

In contrast, most thyroid epithelial masses in dogs are carcinomas (in the region of 90%) – therefore, aspiration is useful because the presence of thyroid tissue in a thyroid mass in dog is strongly suggestive of a thyroid carcinoma (and helps to distinguish from other possible masses in this location). With the advent of better imaging, however, this general rule of thumb has become slightly less useful; finding thyroid epithelium in an aspirate from a small thyroid lesion which is not palpable and only visible using MRI makes a diagnosis of carcinoma (versus adenoma) less clear.

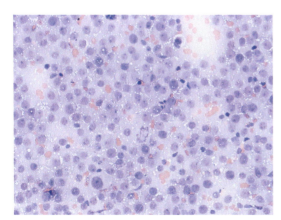

Fig 6.67 Thyroid carcinoma displaying more atypical features including increased mitotic rate, prominent and often multiple nucleoli, increased nuclear size variation (anisokaryosis) (×500)

The parathyroid glands are also in this location, and appear almost identical to thyroid epithelium, although some sources suggest the cytoplasm of parathyroid cells sometimes contains small pale eosinophilic linear structures.

Inflammatory lesions of the skin and subcutis

The skin being the major barrier to the outside world, it is a common site of inflammatory skin lesions, which can sometimes strongly resemble tumours; one of the key uses of cytology is to distinguish inflammation from neoplasia. Difficulties can arise when inflammation and neoplasia occur concurrently – not uncommon given the reach of a dog's tongue and the personality it is attached to, and cytologists should bear in mind that any of the tumours above can be accompanied by significant inflammation, particularly neutrophilic. Some neoplasms are particularly prone to certain types of inflammation (Fig 6.68), however – below follows a brief list of the most commonly found:

- squamous cell carcinoma – neutrophilic inflammation
- mast cell tumour – eosinophilic inflammation
- histiocytoma – lymphocytic inflammation.

Inflammation types

The broad types of inflammation, and the causes of them, are similar to those found elsewhere in the body. See the section starting page 59 for a discussion of these broad categories of inflammation.

Neutrophilic inflammation (FIG 6.69)

This is the most commonly found inflammatory pattern, often associated with infection or trauma. The neutrophils are often accompanied by low numbers of macrophages in more intense inflammatory conditions – the macrophages here are often activated and frequently contain

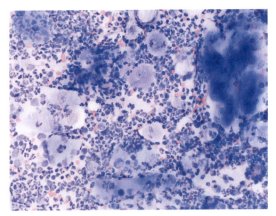

Fig 6.68a Squamous cell carcinoma with neutrophilic inflammation (×500)

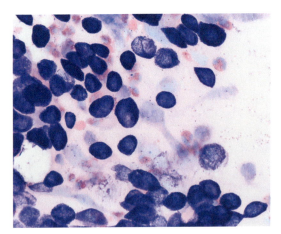

Fig 6.68b Mast cell tumour with eosinophilic inflammation (×500)

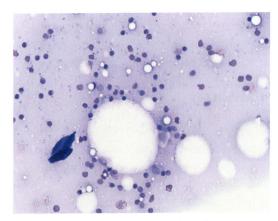

Fig 6.68c Histiocytoma with lymphocytic inflammation (×500)

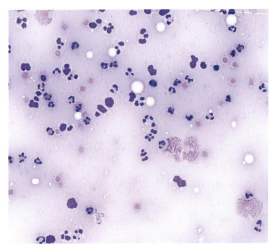

Fig 6.69 Neutrophilic inflammation in the skin (×100)

phagocytosed neutrophils (a finding that confirms inflammation). Squamous cell carcinomas often contain significant neutrophilic inflammation.

Macrophagic inflammation (FIG 6.70)

Predominantly macrophagic inflammation is generally associated with more chronic conditions, or with invading organisms more challenging to neutralise (such as fungi). The most common conditions which produce macrophagic inflammation in the skin and subcutis are ruptured epidermal inclusion cysts and steatitis, summarised below. All lesions with significant macrophagic inflammation can sometimes be mistaken for neoplasia due to the highly plastic appearance of activated macrophages and the reactive fibroblasts that often accompany them.

Ruptured epidermal inclusion cysts (FIG 6.71)

'Epidermal inclusion cyst' is a generic term for a multitude of adnexal lesions (see page 179), all of which contain significant amounts of keratin. When these lesions rupture, keratin is exposed to the subcutaneous tissue, and this elicits a strong foreign body-type reaction. Longstanding lesions of this nature can contain highly activated macrophages, as well as multinucleate macrophages and epithelioid macrophages (macrophages present in clusters

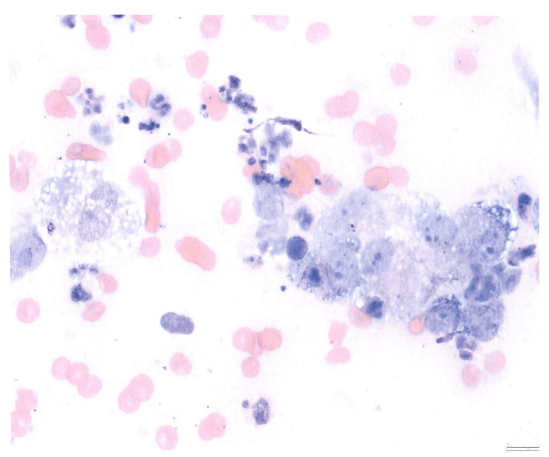

Fig 6.70 Macrophagic inflammation in the skin; note the phagocytosis of neutrophils in the cells on the right, as well as the multiple nucleoli present in these cells, slightly mimicking malignancy (×500)

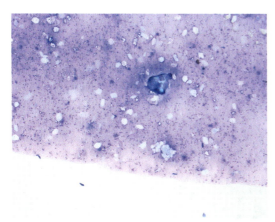

Fig 6.71 Ruptured epidermal inclusion cyst (low power); keratin and high numbers of leukocytes are visible (×100)

resembling epithelium). To the unwary, these busy macrophages can mimic malignant cells.

This type of inflammation takes a long time to settle, as the keratin must be cleared before it subsides – occasionally excision of these lesions is the fastest way of resolving them.

Steatitis (inflamed adipose tissue) (FIGS 6.72, 6.73)
Fat is prone to inflammation following trauma – the presence of even a few macrophages alongside adipocytes indicates inflammation and possible blunt trauma (not uncommon in large lipomas). With more severe inflammation, the adipocytes often collapse into denser basophilic structures, hard to identify. The combination of these collapsed aggregates of adipocytes and highly

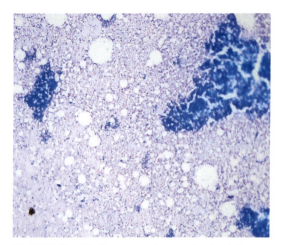

Fig 6.72 Steatitis (low power); many fat droplets in the background and collapsed aggregates of adipocytes (now blue-coloured) can be seen (×100)

activated macrophages can be confusing and may appear similar to malignancy in some cases.

When multiple area of steatitis are present, underlying conditions such as pancreatitis (causing fat digestion due to release of lipase) should be considered.

Vaccine reactions (FIG 6.74)

Injection site reactions generally produce significant macrophagic inflammation as well as fibrosis, and, as ever with fibroplasia, it can be difficult to distinguish between reactive mesenchymal cells and neoplastic ones. Context is very useful here (is there a history of injection within a few weeks?).

Vaccine reactions sometimes have a distinctive appearance cytologically; vaccines often contain

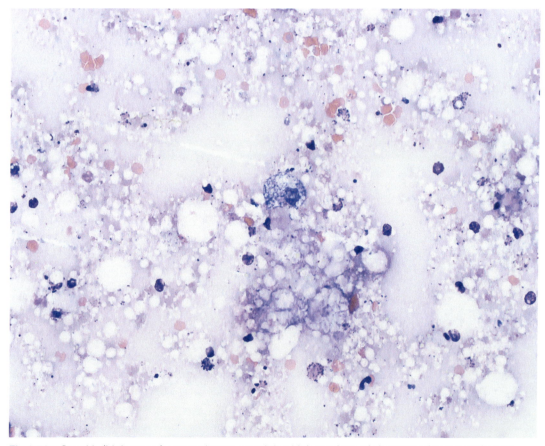

Fig 6.73a Steatitis (high power); macrophages containing high numbers of clear vacuoles resembling fat droplets are embedded (×500)

Skin and subcutaneous lesions | Chapter 6   175

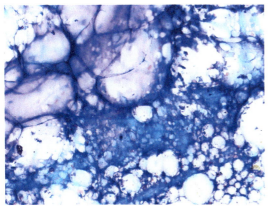

Fig 6.73b Steatitis: a collapsed aggregate of adipocytes adjacent to more typical-appearing fat cells (×500)

adjuvant to prolong the effect of the immune stimulation, and this material is sometimes visible phagocytosed within macrophages. Sources vary on the description of this material, probably because of different staining techniques or, more likely, different adjuvant. In the author's experience of working in the UK, vaccine adjuvant usually appears as a slightly cloudy bluish-grey material, often present in the background and phagocytosed within macrophages.

It is worth noting that cats which have significant vaccine reactions are reported to be more prone to injection-site sarcomas, and it may be prudent to consider different locations for vaccination in these patients.

Eosinophilic inflammation (FIG 6.75)
Eosinophils are both distinctive and useful cytologically, as they tend to narrow the differential list significantly. They are associated with hypersensitivity or parasitism – insect bites are a relatively common cause. Eosinophilic plaques and granulomas ('rodent ulcers') occur relatively commonly in cats, and rarely in dogs (huskies

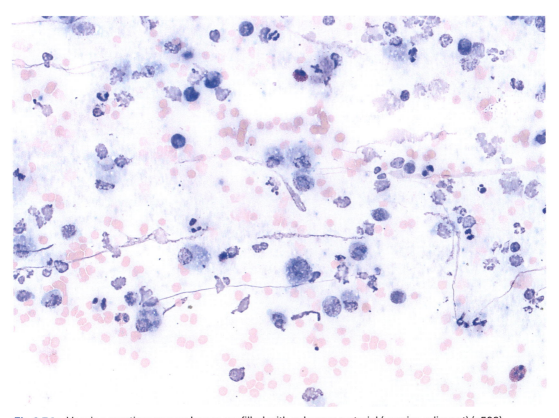

Fig 6.74a Vaccine reaction; macrophages are filled with pale grey material (vaccine adjuvant) (×500)

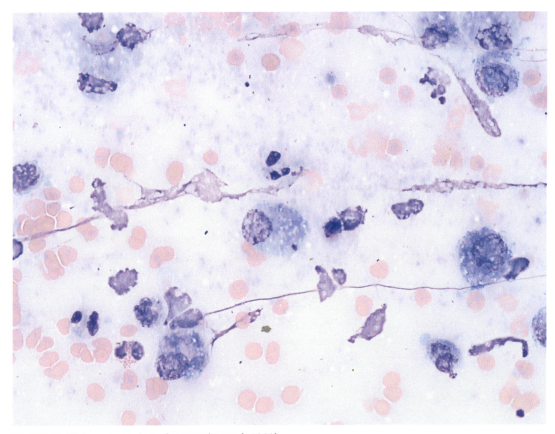

Fig 6.74b Higher power view of macrophages (×1000)

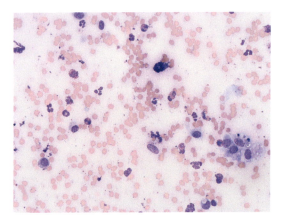

Fig 6.75 Mixed, mostly eosinophilic inflammation, in the skin; the cells on the right are harder to identify; they are probably a mixture of mesenchymal cells and macrophages (×500)

and other Arctic circle breeds are reported to be predisposed) – the cause is unclear but likely to be immune-mediated.

Eosinophilic inflammation is also common in mast cell tumours – some difficulties can occur as mast cells are often present in low numbers with marked eosinophilic inflammation. As ever, the context and proportion of cells becomes important – if mast cells are significantly in the minority compared with eosinophils, then mast cell neoplasia is unlikely, but there will be edge cases or grey areas where the distinction is challenging to make.

Lymphocytic inflammation

True lymphocytic inflammation is uncommon in the skin and subcutis except in young patients (less than a year old), and even then, the inflammatory pattern tends to be mixed rather than predominantly lymphocytic. In most cases, high numbers of lymphocytes on aspirates from the skin indicate sampling of a lymph node/nodule, or cutaneous lymphoma, but lymphocytic inflammation occasionally occurs in some infections (although again the pattern is usually mixed) and small lymphocytes can also be present in high numbers in regressing histiocytomas. An aspirate containing small lymphocytes and rare large cells resembling histiocytes, especially in a young animal with a 'button' tumour, is likely to reflect sampling of a histiocytoma (Fig 6.76).

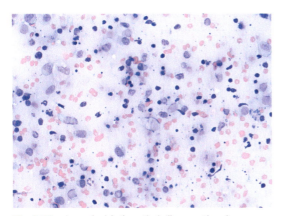

Fig 6.76a Lymphohistiocytic inflammation from a histiocytoma (×500)

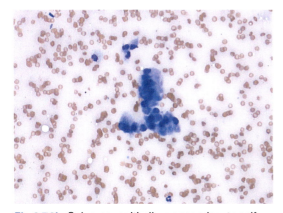

Fig 6.76b Columnar epithelium secondary to self-trauma (×500)

Plasmacytic inflammation

Again, this is a relatively uncommon finding – high numbers of plasma cells can indicate antigenic stimulation or unusual infections (such as Leishmania) – a close search for infectious agents should be made if plasma cells are present in high quantities. Plasma cell pododermatitis is a significant consideration in plasma-cell rich aspirates from puffy or spongy pads in cats (dogs are very rarely affected).

Aspirates from plasmacytomas usually contain atypical plasma cells, frequently multinucleate, which are usually easily distinguishable from their non-neoplastic counterparts, although they may look so different from normal plasma cells that the diagnosis may be challenging (see page 86 for description).

Mixed inflammation

Many skin aspirates contain mild mixed inflammation, in particular neutrophils, macrophages and occasional lymphocytes or plasma cells. Mixed inflammatory patterns are very non-specific and can be associated with many inflammatory or neoplastic conditions – finding mild mixed inflammation alone is unlikely to help in achieving a diagnosis.

Epithelial dysplasia/metaplasia

Dysplasia is a morphological change within cells, most commonly seen with epithelium, usually secondary to inflammation. The change varies from case to case, often dependent on the degree and duration of inflammation, but the changes often resemble malignancy. Changes include pleomorphism (variable size and shape of cells), binucleation and increased mitotic rate; a diagnosis of neoplasia should be made with caution where inflammation is present. In the author's experience, however, even with marked prolonged inflammation, the dysplastic changes are often relatively mild, and therefore with marked features of malignancy, a diagnosis of neoplasia can be made with more confidence (an exception to this rule is dysplastic changes within epithelium in tightly enclosed spaces, such as the nasal cavity or the retro bulbar space; here, dysplasia can be marked and strongly mimic malignancy).

Metaplasia is a change from one cell type to another (i.e. cuboidal epithelium to squamous epithelium). In skin masses, the most common type observed is from cutaneous squamous epithelium to cuboidal, usually secondary to self-trauma; finding small clusters of cuboidal epithelium in skin aspirates is often an indication of self-trauma (although care should be taken with this finding in aspirates from cat's feet, as lung digit syndrome is a significant differential (metastasis of pulmonary neoplasia to the digits).

> **Key points**
>
> **Skin inflammation**
> - Lesions with marked macrophagic inflammation can be mistaken for neoplasia due to the highly plastic appearance of activated macrophages and pleomorphic fibroblasts
> - Multiple areas of steatitis can be a sequel to severe pancreatitis
> - An aspirate containing small lymphocytes and rare large cells resembling histiocytes, especially in a young animal with a 'button' tumour, is likely to reflect sampling of a histiocytoma
> - Squamous epithelial cells can transform to cuboidal epithelium with self-trauma

Infectious diseases

Bacterial

Most cutaneous infections are bacterial. The skin is populated by many commensal organisms, and most of the pathogens or potential pathogens are cocci. *Staphylococcus* and *Streptococcus* are the most commonly isolated, but there are many different possibilities. When a foreign body has penetrated the skin, or when there has been significant licking, the infection present is often mixed (containing both bacilli and cocci), and where spirochaetes (spiral-shaped rods) are observed, then licking is likely to have occurred.

Mycobacterium can also be present in cutaneous lesions – this often provokes macrophagic inflammation; the organisms themselves are hard to see without special stains (see page 114).

Fungal

The most common cutaneous fungal infections are *Malassezia* and dermatophytosis (ringworm). These are usually superficial infections, although occasional raised dermal lesions known as *kerion* are present. Other cutaneous fungal infections are uncommon in the UK but are always worth considering when extensive macrophagic inflammation is present. They are discussed in more detail on page 116.

When intra-dermal fungal infections are found in cats, they are often a lone lesion (frequently by opportunistic pathogens – *mycetoma* – see page 179) (Fig 6.77), but in dogs, dermal fungal infections (other than ringworm or *Malassezia*) are often a manifestation of a deeper or systemic infection.

Parasitic

Dermal parasitic lesions are very rarely seen on cytology specimens – possibilities include (but are not limited to) the worm-like microfilariae (larval stages of *Dirofilaria repens* (cytologically almost indistinguishable from those of *Dirofilaria immitis* – canine heartworm (see page 125, Fig 5.22)) and larvae of *Dracunculus insignis* (related to the human Guinea worm).

Skin and subcutaneous lesions | Chapter 6

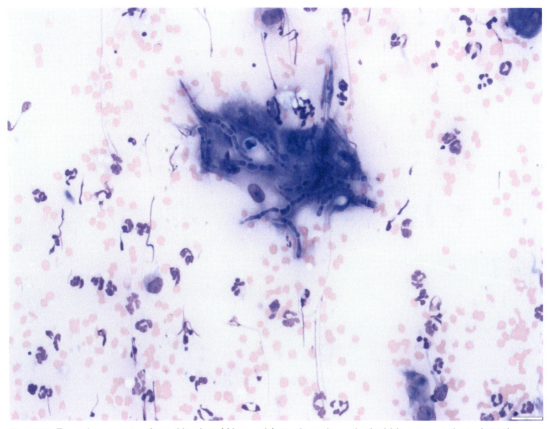

Fig 6.77 Fungal mycetoma; fungal hyphae (*Alternaria*) are densely packed within a macrophage (×500)

Non-inflammatory/non-neoplastic lesions

Epidermal inclusion cyst (FIG 6.78)

There are a number of adnexal lesions which all yield large amounts of keratin and very little else cytologically. These range from non-neoplastic lesions such as follicular cysts to benign hair follicle tumours such as pilomatricoma. Cytologically, it is very difficult to distinguish between these lesions – although very rare malignant tumours yield mostly keratin, the majority of lesions with a harvest of pure keratin are benign. See page 179 for a fuller description.

When these lesions rupture, the keratin within them elicits a strong foreign body response (mostly granulomatous/pyogranulomatous (macrophagic/neutrophilic-macrophagic)) – see page 328 for more detail.

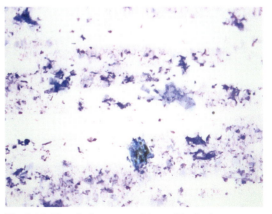

Fig 6.78 Keratin from an epidermal inclusion cyst (×100)

Apocrine cyst

These are benign fluid-filled lesions which yield acellular pale fluid. When a fluid-filled lesion deflates on sampling and no cells are found on cytology, then these lesions may be suspected.

Seroma/haematoma

These lesions are discussed in more detail on page 59 – the main difference between them is that seromas generally contain high-protein fluid (pinkish stippled background with crescent shapes known as 'protein clefts') and macrophages, whereas haematomas contain more blood, and macrophages containing red-cell breakdown products (hematoidin and haemosiderin – see page 98).

Necrosis

This is described in more detail on page 96. It is not a specific finding, as necrosis can occur with intense inflammation and ischaemia, but the presence of swathes of necrosis in a cutaneous lesion raise concern for the presence of a malignant neoplasm. Resampling from the periphery of a lesion may help to avoid any areas of central necrosis.

Mucinosis (Shar Pei)

This condition is characterised by the presence of viscous mucin under the skin, forming small blisters and vesicles. Cytologically, mucin appears as a cloudy blue to bluish-pink material and is not usually accompanied by inflammation. The condition is almost exclusive to Shar Pei, and its presence should alert clinicians to an increased risk of amyloidosis and Shar Pei fever (although it is does not mean these conditions will definitely occur).

Ear Swab Cytology

Rolled swab preparations are a quick and effective technique for screening for bacterial or fungal infection (see page 26 for the procedure). Swab preparations from ears contain very superficial material, mostly keratinised squames and waxy material that does not stain. As the material is so superficial, leukocytes are relatively uncommon – a lack of them does not exclude infection or inflammation, although grossly purulent ears will probably have neutrophils on cytology swabs.

With rolled ear preparations, the cytologist should confirm and quantify the presence of acellular material, squames, leukocytes, bacteria and yeasts (usually *Malassezia*). Low numbers of bacteria and yeasts could potentially represent commensals, but high numbers are more likely to reflect infection (bacteria phagocytosed within neutrophils confirms this). The bacterial morphology is a guide (but not a definitive identification) to the organisms present; bacterial cocci are often *staphylococcus* or *streptococcus*, whereas short bacterial rods raise concern for *pseudomonas*. Again, the context of the clinical appearance should be considered, and culture is needed for definitive examination, but in-house ear swabs can be a guide to treatment whilst awaiting culture results.

Chapter 6 – take home messages

- Samples from 'normal' skin and subcutis often exfoliate poorly and have relatively low cellularity.
- Adipocytes aspirated from lipomas are cytologically identical to those from normal fat – context is needed to definitively identify lipomas.
- It is important, where possible, to identify whether a lesion is cutaneous, subcutaneous, or both.
- Mast cell granules often stain poorly with many in-house stains (aqueous Romanowsky).
- Some mast cell tumours can be nestled within fat and so aspirates may contain primarily adipocytes.
- It can be challenging cytologically to distinguish between reactive mesenchymal cells (fibrosis) from neoplastic cells (sarcoma), especially when cellularity is low; context (such as how long the lesion has been present, history of trauma) is very useful to distinguish between them.
- Cytology of mammary tumours in dogs is challenging due to their complex structure; the biological behaviour is often not well correlated with their appearance cytologically.
- Macrophages (particularly those in ruptured keratin cysts) can display multiple atypical features (such as marked pleomorphism and multinucleation) and mimic malignancy.

Chapter 7

Gastrointestinal system

As with many of the non-cutaneous locations in this textbook, the emphasis here is on the locations most easily (and therefore most commonly) sampled – in this case, the oral cavity and the liver. For the other parts of the gastrointestinal tract (the oesophagus, stomach, intestines and pancreas), this book is limited to a brief description of the normal cytological appearance, although the bibliography contains many sources with more detailed descriptions of these locations.

Oral cavity

Normal cytological appearance (FIG 7.1)

The oral cavity is lined with squamous epithelial cells and filled with non-pathogenic commensal bacterial organisms. Distinguishing between infectious organisms and commensals can be challenging, but there are several clues. *Conchiformibius* (previously known as *Simonsiella*) is a highly distinctive commensal organism. The bacilli line up in parallel so that the colonies often resemble a single large tablet-shaped organism ((Fig 7.2). The presence of *Conchiformibius* colonies indicates that commensals have been harvested.

Neutrophils are a normal finding in samples from the oral cavity, but degenerate neutrophils (see page 60) are a clue to the presence of pathogens, and when neutrophils are seen containing

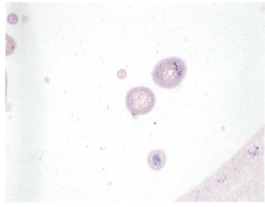

Fig 7.1 Low power view of normal oral material; poorly cellular with scattered squamous epithelium, blood and neutrophils (×100)

phagocytosed bacteria (as elsewhere in the body), infection is confirmed.

Normal oral epithelium generally exfoliates relatively poorly, from both the gums and the tongue. Most cells harvested will be individual, but rare small clusters may also be present. Small amounts of melanin pigment can also be a normal finding. The epithelial cells will often contain embedded bacteria (Fig 7.2).

Most aspirates from a 'normal' oral cavity will contain scattered squamous epithelial cells, mixed bacteria and occasional neutrophils, as well as a small amount of blood.

The tonsils, present at the back of the mouth, contain a mixed lymphoid harvest, similar to lymph nodes, although small amounts

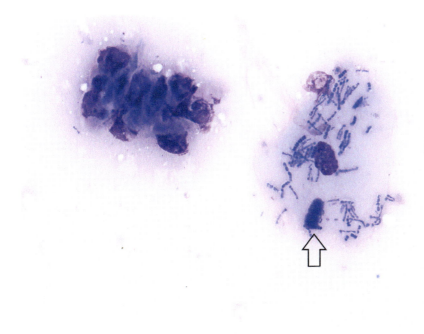

Fig 7.2 Squamous epithelial cell with embedded bacteria including *Conchiformibius* (open arrow) (×1000)

of contaminants (bacteria and squamous epithelium) are sometimes present.

Neoplastic lesions of the oral cavity

As elsewhere, these lesions are listed in rough order of commonality, which is to say the lower down the list, the less likely the diagnosis is.

Epulis
Neoplasm type: mesenchymal/epithelial
Age: usually older
Location: usually rostral mandible, most commonly around canines
Gross Appearance: thickened hyperplastic gum margins and masses
Species/breed predispositions: common in dogs; golden retrievers, cocker spaniels, akitas, Shetland sheepdogs overrepresented

Cytological appearance/further comments: Epulis is a largely outdated term for gum mass but is usually applied to two main lesions that appear grossly identical. The most common is the *peripheral odontogenic fibroma (formerly fibromatous* or *ossifying epulis)*, a slow-growing and usually benign lesion. Unfortunately, although these masses are very common in dogs, they exfoliate extremely poorly cytologically, and the diagnosis is challenging. Aspirates contain scattered oral epithelial cells and, sometimes, low numbers of fusiform (spindle) mesenchymal cells; most often, they appear very similar to 'normal' oral cavity. Diagnosis of these lesions is unlikely to be made cytologically – the use of cytology in these cases is more helpful to exclude other lesions such as melanomas or squamous cell carcinomas.

The second type is the *acanthomatous ameloblastoma*, a less common lesion of odontogenic epithelium. These lesions are more locally aggressive and invasive than the fibroma described above. They do not metastasise but can loosen teeth and occasionally cause pathological fractures. Cytologically, these lesions contain a mixture of both densely packed epithelial cells with small amounts of pale blue cytoplasm and low numbers of individual and largely unremarkable fusiform mesenchymal cells.

Lymphoma
Neoplasm type: round cell
Age: usually middle-aged to older
Location: usually tonsilar but can occur anywhere
Gross Appearance: swollen tonsils or firm swollen lesion elsewhere
Species/breed predispositions: more common in cats
Cytological appearance/further comments: lymphoma can occur anywhere in the oral cavity but usually arises in the tonsils; the appearance is similar to elsewhere (see page 86 for a more detailed description of lymphoma).

Squamous cell carcinoma (FIG 7.3)
Neoplasm type: epithelial
Age: middle-aged to older
Location: any oral
Gross Appearance: pale erosive plaques, often ulcerated, sometimes with proliferative irregular pink tissue
Species/breed predispositions: more common in cats but common in both
Cytological appearance/further comments: although it may be tempting to attempt to

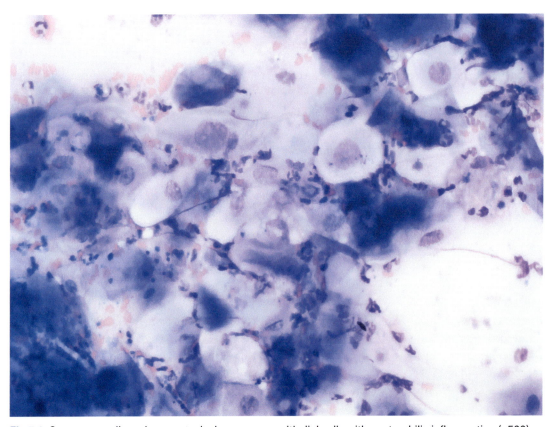

Fig 7.3 Squamous cell carcinoma; atypical squamous epithelial cells with neutrophilic inflammation (×500)

sample ulcerated lesions with impression smears, this approach often harvests superficial inflammation only; needle aspirates are usually superior for diagnosis.

The cytological appearance is similar to elsewhere (see page 138); aspiration of the tonsils and submandibular lymph nodes is usually prudent to check for metastasis. Care must be taken not to confuse normal oral squamous epithelial cells with atypical squamous cells from a squamous cell carcinoma. Epithelial cells from the oral cavity do not normally display nuclear atypia.

Malignant melanoma
Neoplasm type: round cell
Age: middle-aged to older (usually older than 6)
Location: any oral
Gross Appearance: raised sometimes pigmented plaque, can be ulcerated
Species/breed predispositions: common in dogs, rare in cats. Breeds at risk include vislas, schnauzers, chow chow, Shar Pei, cocker spaniel and Irish setters.
Cytological appearance/further comments: see page 87 for more detailed descriptions. Oral lesions are more common in dogs and are usually more aggressive than dermal masses. When metastasis occurs (in approximately 80% of cases), it is commonly to the mandibular or retropharyngeal lymph nodes, and often from there to the lungs.

Mast cell tumour (FIG 7.4)
Neoplasm type: round cell
Age: variable, usually older
Location: only rarely found in oral cavity
Gross appearance: raised mass, occasionally ulcerated
Cytological appearance/further comments: see pages 52 and 135 for more detailed descriptions. Oral mucosal mast cell tumours are rare but are reported to have a more aggressive clinical course and around 55% of canine oral mast cell tumours are reported to have

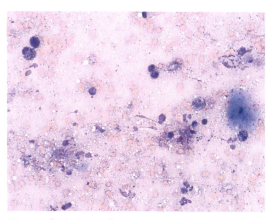

Fig 7.4 Oral mast cell tumour; most cells are ruptured but there are many mast cell granules with occasional intact mast cells; a squamous epithelial cell with embedded bacteria is also seen (×500)

metastasised to local lymph nodes at the time of diagnosis.

Plasmacytoma
Neoplasm type: round cell
Age: 5+ in dogs; rare in cats
Location: only occasionally found in oral cavity
Gross appearance: raised mass, occasional ulcerated
Species/breed predispositions: terriers, cocker spaniels, standard poodle; rare in cats
Cytological appearance/further comments: see page 86 for more detailed descriptions.

Other oral neoplasms include sarcomas (see page 78), metastatic neoplasia, other odontogenic tumours (other than acanthomatous ameloblastoma) and clear cell tumours, but these are all relatively uncommon.

Inflammatory lesions of the oral cavity

The 'normal' oral cavity includes neutrophils, as it contains many bacteria and is often in a state of low-grade inflammation (or not so low grade, in many older dogs and cats). Eosinophilic plaques are sometimes found, more commonly in cats – as with cutaneous eosinophilic plaques and granulomas, they are thought to have an immune-mediated origin. Other types of inflammation are uncommon and the causes for them are similar to other locations (see page 59).

> **Key points**
>
> **Oral cavity**
>
> - The presence of *Conchiformibius* colonies indicates that commensals have been harvested.
> - 'Normal' oral cavity aspirates contain squamous epithelial cells, mixed bacteria and occasional neutrophils, and blood
> - Oral malignant melanomas are more common in dogs than cutaneous, and they are usually more aggressive

Liver

Needle aspirates of the liver are simple and relatively risk-free; the chances of significant haemorrhage are slim, and lower than with large-bore needle biopsies, although assessment of clotting factors may be prudent prior to sampling, especially in more excitable patients.

Normal appearance

Blood: Liver aspirates are usually moderately and often markedly haemodiluted (Fig 7.5); it's a rare aspirate of the liver that doesn't contain a large amount of blood. Using smaller bore needles and less suction can help to reduce the haemodilution of liver samples.

Hepatocytes: Aside from blood, aspirates from 'normal' liver should contain moderate to high numbers of hepatocytes – the liver's resident population of epithelial cells – usually found in variably-sized clusters and sheets. Hepatocytes have a helpfully distinctive appearance. When harvested in high numbers, the sheets of hepatocytes are often found in a trabecular pattern (see page 75, Fig 4.30).

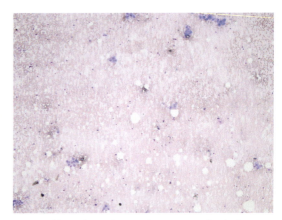

Fig 7.5 Hepatic aspirate at low power, displaying typical amount of blood contamination (×100)

Hepatocytes have a hexagonal shape, although this is often not well-preserved on samples and they usually appear more rounded. Well-differentiated hepatocytes have uniform round to slightly oval central nuclei, roughly 1.5 erythrocytes in diameter, with coarse dense chromatin and usually a single small round nucleolus. They have low nuclear to cytoplasmic ratios and have moderate to abundant amounts of pale eosinophilic cytoplasm, with a characteristic finely granular appearance (Figs 7.6–8) (perianal epithelium also has similar appearing finely granular cytoplasm, hence the term 'hepatoid' epithelium). Binucleation is relatively common.

Some hepatocyte nuclei contain 'brick' inclusions – rectangular crystalline structures of no known clinical significance, but useful to recognise as a normal finding.

Many hepatocytes contain small amounts of blue-green pigment granules, generally thought to be lipofuscin (Fig 7.9). This is a 'wear and tear' pigment which accrues though the lifetime of the hepatocyte – finding very few or no cells with pigment is a cytological clue that the cells observed are likely to be young, although the causes for this are many and varied (inflammation, neoplasia, nodular regeneration – see below).

Neutrophils and small lymphocytes: most aspirates from the liver contain low numbers of neutrophils and small lymphocytes, most likely a

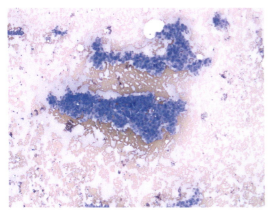

Fig 7.6 Low power hepatocytes (×100)

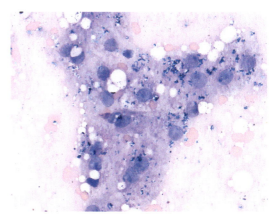

Fig 7.9 Cytoplasmic pigment in hepatocytes (×1000)

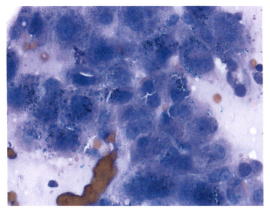

Fig 7.7 Hepatocytes displaying typical granular cytoplasm, also often containing larger blue-green granules of cytoplasmic pigment; frequent binucleate cells are visible (×1000)

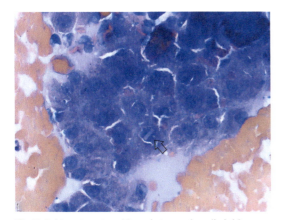

Fig 7.8 Hepatocyte with an intranuclear 'brick' inclusion (open arrow) (×1000)

combination of the large amounts of blood usually present and the fact that the liver receives many antigens directly from the intestinal blood supply. This can make assessment of whether a liver is inflamed cytologically challenging. The presence of inflammatory cells in small pockets rather than evenly distributed throughout the film can be a clue, but overall the assessment of inflammation is subjective, and improves with experience of both liver aspirates and blood films.

Biliary epithelium: although hepatocytes should form the majority of epithelial cells harvested, occasional small clusters of biliary epithelium are not unusual. Biliary epithelium is found in much denser clusters than hepatocytes; the cells have much lower amounts of cytoplasm (Fig 7.10), somewhat resembling basal epithelium (see page 132) although the clusters generally are not found in papillary formations. Biliary epithelium can sometimes be markedly vacuolated. Frequent clusters of biliary epithelium could indicate biliary hyperplasia or potentially neoplasia.

Mesothelial cells: any aspirates of structures within the peritoneal (or pleural) cavities can contain sheets of mesothelium, which form the lining of these cavities. It is worth familiarising oneself with them as a cytologist as they resemble epithelial cells and can raise concern for the presence of a carcinoma. Sheets of mesothelium

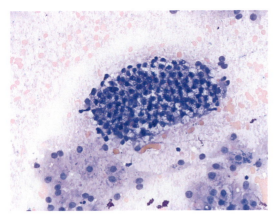

Fig 7.10 Cluster of vacuolated biliary epithelium (×500)

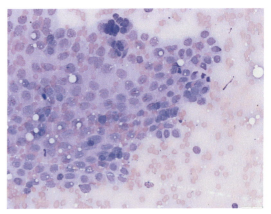

Fig 7.12 Higher magnification sheet of mesothelium; note the prominent clear gaps between cells (×500)

have a somewhat characteristic appearance (Figs 7.11, 7.12) – in samples from the liver, they can be mistaken for biliary epithelium, although they usually have slightly more cytoplasm and often the gap junctions between the cells can be appreciated.

Variations in hepatocytes

Hepatocytes are in the firing line of a steady stream of antigens from the intestine; as well as this, they perform myriad metabolic and homeostatic functions. As a consequence, there are several variations in their normal appearance associated with this which gives some indication of the current state or activity of the liver.

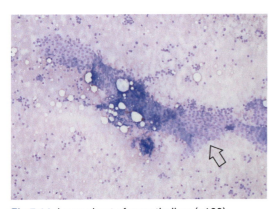

Fig 7.11 Large sheet of mesothelium (×100)

Cytoplasmic vacuolation – indiscrete: vacuoles can appear in hepatocytes for many reasons. The most common form is 'indiscrete' vacuolation. Here, the vacuoles have indistinct borders so that the vacuolation appears more like a patchy thinning or rarefaction of the cytoplasm, more obvious at the periphery of the cells (Fig 7.13).

This form of vacuolation is very non-specific – the cytological equivalent of a moderately elevated ALT – and can be associated with a variety of hepatocellular insults (inflammation, neoplasia, hypoxia, etc.), nodular regeneration (see below) or glycogen deposition (this last usually associated with corticosteroid therapy or Cushing's disease).

Cytoplasmic vacuolation – discrete: this is easier to spot, as the vacuoles here have clear round edges and appear as bubbles within the cytoplasm of the hepatocytes (Fig 7.14). This is a more specific finding than indiscrete vacuolation; it occurs following increased lipid deposition within the cells, although this can be primary or secondary. It is most marked in feline patients with hepatic lipidosis but can also be secondary to diseases such as pancreatitis, cholangiohepatitis or diabetes mellitus.

Reduced pigmentation: as discussed above, reduced amounts of cytoplasmic pigment can

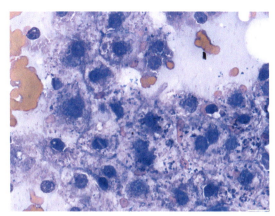

Fig 7.13 Indiscrete vacuolation in hepatocytes; note the patchy moth-eaten appearance of the cytoplasm (×1000)

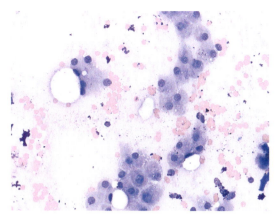

Fig 7.15 Hepatocytes with reduced cytoplasmic pigmentation

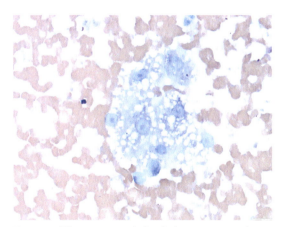

Fig 7.14 Discrete vacuolation in hepatocytes; clear vacuoles can be seen in the cytoplasm (×1000)

be a sign of 'younger' hepatocytes, although the causes of this are varied (Fig 7.15).

Bile casts: bile casts are dark grey to black linear clumps of pigment, found between the hepatocytes. As they represent bile building up in the bile canaliculi, they conform to the hexagonal structure, although often only one or two 'walls' of the hexagon are present (Figs 7.16, 7.17). They indicate cholestasis, although they are not specific (i.e. they can be present in pre-hepatic, intra-hepatic or post-hepatic cholestasis). Rounded clumps of dark bile pigment within the cytoplasm of hepatocytes are sometimes seen; these are less specific than bile casts but can also be an indication of cholestasis.

Copper: build-up of copper within hepatocytes can be challenging to spot, as the appearance is similar to lipofuscin. The pigment is paler, however (similar to copper sulphate, for those who remember their chemistry lessons) and often larger (Fig 7.18). It can be confirmed with special stains (rhodanine or rubeanic acid) and can indicate primary copper toxicosis (usually Bedlington terriers) but can also be seen occasionally secondary to other causes of hepatitis.

Increased basophilia: in general cytological terms, increased basophilia (blueness) of cells is usually associated with build-up of nucleic

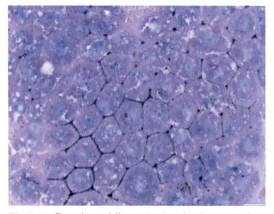

Fig 7.16 Prominent bile casts showing hexagonal shape of canaliculi between hepatocytes (×500)

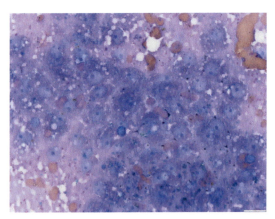

Fig 7.17 More typical appearance of bile casts, mostly only lines of bile present (×1000)

acids (acids are basophilic – that is, they are associated with bases, and stain with basic dyes), which usually means increased metabolic activity (see page 39). Hepatocytes which appear bluer (Fig 7.19) are more active than normal, usually due to inflammation, although neoplasia is also a consideration.

Nodular regeneration/hyperplasia

Nodular regeneration and nodular hyperplasia are hepatic phenomena seen in dogs, where nodular patches of liver (visible ultrasonographically) undergo regeneration or hyperplasia. The lesions are histologically distinct but mostly cytologically identical; the hepatocytes harvested from these regions often display indiscrete vacuolation and may also contain reduced pigmentation, increased basophilia, or other mild dysplastic features (such as increased binucleation or increased nuclear to cytoplasmic ratio) (Fig 7.20, 7.21). Nodular regeneration is one of the reasons why it can be challenging to

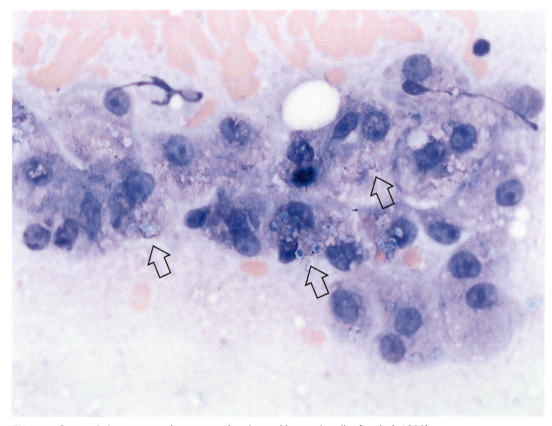

Fig 7.18 Copper in hepatocytes (open arrow); paler and larger than lipofuscin (×1000)

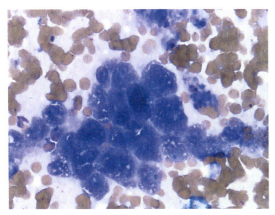

Fig 7.19 Increased basophilia in hepatocytes (mild) (×1000)

confidently diagnose well-differentiated hepatocellular neoplasia in canine patients.

Extra-medullary haematopoiesis

This phenomenon, usually observed in the spleen but occasionally seen in the liver (and less commonly elsewhere) comprises the presence of haemopoietic precursors (nucleated red blood cells and red cell precursors, early neutrophils and neutrophil precursors, megakaryocytes) outside of the bone marrow (Fig 7.22).

It is not associated with any specific disease but must be kept in mind when examining the

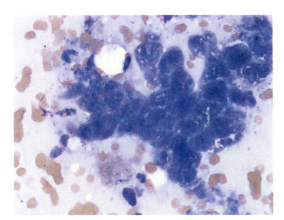

Fig 7.20 Mildly dysplastic hepatocytes (increased basophilia, mild variation in nuclear size (anisokaryosis) (×1000)

liver, as the presence of erythroblasts and myeloblasts can create the impression of a round cell tumour within the liver, and it also makes assessment of inflammation within the liver even more challenging than it normally is (neutrophils observed could be blood derived, part of extra-medullary haematopoiesis, or may be genuinely inflammatory).

Neoplastic lesions of the liver

As elsewhere in the book, the list below is in rough order of commonality; the further down the list, the less common the neoplasm (in general). 'Gross' appearance is of limited use for lesions on the liver, as they are usually found via imaging; instead a brief description of whether they are discrete or diffuse lesions is included.

Metastatic neoplasia (FIG 7.23)

Neoplasm type: varies (see below)
Age: varies (see below)
Distribution: usually discrete masses, but varies
Species/breed predispositions: varies
Cytological appearance/further comments: the liver is a common site of metastasis for many other tumours, which is why it is helpful to become comfortable with the 'normal' appearance of the liver; essentially, any cells which aren't normally present (hepatocytes, biliary epithelium, mesothelium, low numbers of neutrophils and lymphocytes, extra-medullary haematopoiesis) have the potential to be neoplastic. Metastatic neoplasia in the liver is roughly three times more common than primary liver tumours.

The most common metastatic round cell tumour is lymphoma (see below) followed by mast cell tumours – a few mast cells are sometimes seen on liver aspirates, but with increased numbers and particularly when mast cells are found in aggregates (even of two to three cells), or with morphological abnormalities (decreased granules, varied size and shape, binucleation, increased mitotic figures), metastatic mast cell

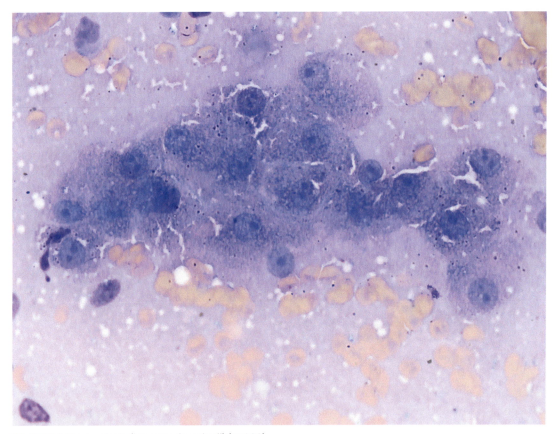

Fig 7.21 Mild dysplasia (increased nucleoli) (×1000)

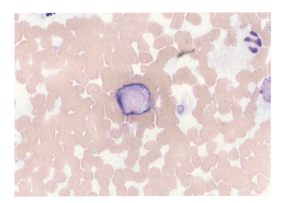

Fig 7.22 Pro-myelocyte within a liver aspirate (granular cell at centre) indicating extra-medullary haematopoesis (×1000)

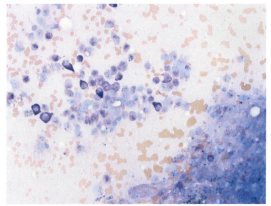

Fig 7.23 Mast cell tumour metastasised to liver; note the reduced granulation of the mast cells; hepatocytes are visible on the right (poorly preserved but the blue-green cytoplasmic pigment gives them away (×500)

disease is a concern. Primary mast cell tumours are rare in dogs, but occasionally occur in cats; primary visceral mast cell tumours are generally more aggressive than cutaneous lesions.

Metastatic carcinomas are also relatively common; the appearance of the cells varies greatly depending on the primary tumour and the degree of malignant change (see page 92 for general notes on the malignant features of epithelial cells). Pancreatic carcinoma is the most commonly observed metastatic carcinoma.

Metastatic sarcomas are occasionally found within the liver, particularly haemangiosarcomas (see page 147), leiomyosarcomas or gastrointestinal stromal tumours (GISTs) – the latter two have a very similar cytological appearance, similar to soft tissue sarcomas (see page 78) although they are sometimes accompanied with large amounts of pinkish fibrillar (stripy, as if it contains fibres) material, presumably extracellular matrix. The cells can appear surprisingly well-differentiated in GISTs and leiomyosarcomas (although they can also be markedly atypical).

Metastatic neuroendocrine tumours often have a typical neuroendocrine appearance (bare nuclei and clusters of cells with indistinct borders; see page 76). They can be very difficult to distinguish from primary hepatic carcinoids (see below) although metastatic neuroendocrine disease is more comon.

Lymphoma (FIG 7.24)
Neoplasm type: round cell
Age: usually middle-aged to older but can be young
Distribution: usually diffuse liver enlargement but occasionally present as discrete mass
Species/breed predispositions: more common in cats than dogs
Cytological appearance/further comments: the liver often contains low numbers of mixed lymphocytes, usually small; the presence of lymphocytes in itself is not especially alarming. When lymphocyte numbers are increased, and when most of the lymphocytes present are intermediate to large, lymphoma is a concern – the appearance of the cells is varied but similar to lymphoma elsewhere in the body (essentially, the presence of a monomorphic (all similar to each other), rather than mixed, population of lymphocytes, raises serious concern for lymphoma, especially when high numbers are present.

Care must be taken when extra-medullary haematopoiesis is also present, as myeloblasts and erythroblasts often appear very similar to large lymphocytes (see page 67, Fig 4.17); the presence of nucleated erythrocytes, increased neutrophils or neutrophilic precursors, megakaryocytes or large cells which appear different to each other are all clues to the presence of extra-medullary haematopoiesis.

Haemangiosarcoma (FIG 7.25)
Neoplasm type: mesenchymal
Age: usually over 10 years
Gross appearance: cavitated mass, sometimes multiple, can be very large
Species/breed predispositions: more common in dogs, often metastatic rather than primary; German shepherds predisposed
Cytological appearance/further comments: the appearance is similar to elsewhere in the body (see page 147); aspirates usually contain mostly blood with relatively few neoplastic cells, often accompanied by macrophages containing haemosiderin (indicative of haemorrhage prior to sampling; see page 98).

Hepatocellular adenoma/carcinoma (FIG 7.26)
Neoplasm type: epithelial
Age: middle-aged to older
Gross appearance: discrete mass, sometime multiple (more common with carcinoma)
Species/breed predispositions: more common in dogs, carcinoma more common than adenoma
Cytological appearance/further comments: with highly malignant hepatic carcinomas, the diagnosis of malignancy is not a challenge (see page 92 for typical features of malignancy),

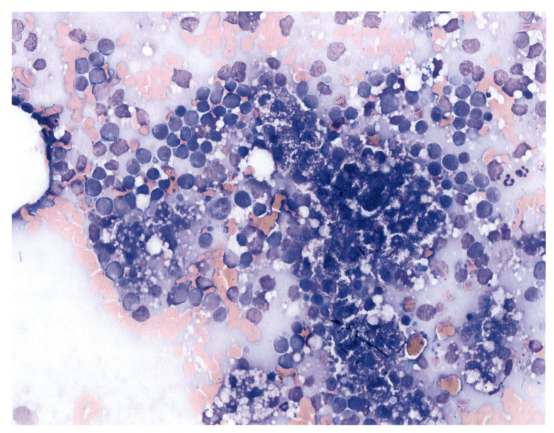

Fig 7.24 Lymphoma infiltration of the liver; note the indiscrete vacuolation of the hepatocytes likely as a result of the neoplasm

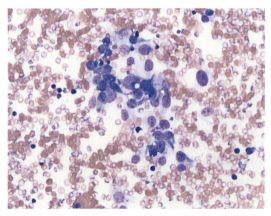

Fig 7.25 Haemangiosarcoma in the liver (×1000)

although sometimes recognising the cells as having hepatic origin (rather than metastatic disease) can be difficult. The main diagnostic challenge is recognising well-differentiated hepatocellular tumours, as distinct from dysplastic cells secondary to inflammation or, in dogs, nodular regeneration or hyperplasia. Features which have been reported to be more associated with neoplasia include multiple nucleoli, single prominent nucleoli, smaller clusters of cells, increased capillaries, increased nuclear: cytoplasmic ratios and reduced pigment. Whilst these features are a guide, in the author's experience all of them can also be seen with nodular regeneration or dysplasia.

As ever with cytology, context is important; **hepatocellular neoplasia is unlikely (not impossible) when there is no obvious discrete mass.** Ultimately, however, it is almost impossible cytologically to either confidently diagnose or completely exclude well-differentiated hepatocellular neoplasia on liver aspirates.

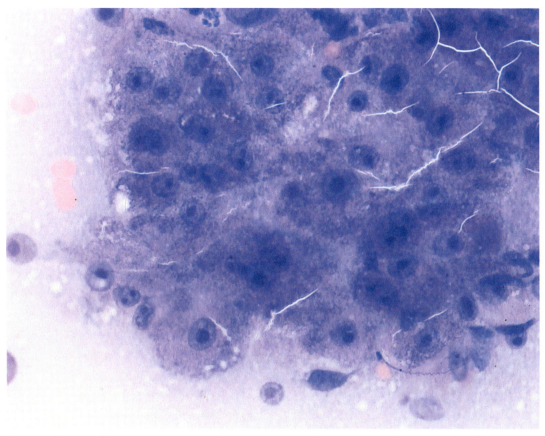

Fig 7.26 Hepatocellular carcinoma; the cells remain recognisably hepatocytes in this case, but display prominent large nucleoli or multiple nucleoli; there is moderate-marked variation in nuclear size (anisokaryosis) and nuclear: cytoplasmic ratio is increased (×1000)

Biliary Carcinoma
Neoplasm type: epithelial
Age: middle-aged to older
Gross appearance: discrete mass/masses
Species/breed predispositions: uncommon/rare in both dogs and cats
Cytological appearance/further comments: biliary epithelial cells are smaller than hepatocytes and found in denser clusters (see page 188, Fig 7.10). As with hepatocellular carcinomas, with cells displaying markedly malignant features, the diagnosis of malignancy is not challenging, but identifying the origin of the cells may be difficult.

With well-differentiated tumours, it can be difficult to distinguish between biliary hyperplasia (uncommon, but occasionally seen especially in cats) and biliary neoplasia, although biliary epithelium outnumbering hepatocytes on a liver aspirate raises significant suspicion of neoplasia (again, in context: neoplasia is unlikely when there is no evidence of a liver mass).

Plasma cell tumour/multiple myeloma
(FIG 7.27)
Neoplasm type: round cell
Age: middle-aged to older
Gross appearance: diffuse swelling, occasionally multiple nodules; likely to also have bone lesions in dogs
Species/breed predispositions: more common in male dogs than female

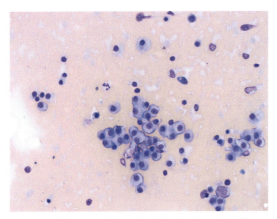

Fig 7.27 Plasma cell neoplasia in the liver (×500)

Cytological appearance/further comments: primary plasma cell tumours of the liver are rare in dogs. Instead, plasma cell neoplasia is usually part of multiple myeloma, a malignant plasma cell neoplasm. It is often accompanied with multiple punched-out lesions in bone, particularly vertebrae and/or marked hyperglobulinaemia (which can lead to hyper viscosity syndrome; nosebleeds and seizures are common symptoms of this). Increased plasma cells in the bone marrow (>20%) and Bence-Jones proteinuria (fragments of immunoglobulins present in the urine; challenging to diagnose in general practice as urinary dipsticks usually only indicate the presence of albumin) lend further support to a diagnosis of multiple myeloma. Hypercalcaemia can also be present.

In contrast to solitary cutaneous plasmacytomas, the plasma cells involved in multiple myeloma are often well-differentiated and cytologically bland. The presence of high numbers of largely unremarkable plasma cells on liver aspirates should raise concern for the presence of multiple myeloma. Increased plasma cells are also seen to a lesser extent with inflammatory conditions of the liver – when mixed with other leukocytes, infection/inflammation may be more likely.

Cats, ever contrary, do not follow the typical pattern above. Plasma cell tumours in the liver in cats are part of a group of conditions known as *myeloma related disorders* (MRD) – they include multiple myeloma, but true multiple myeloma is rare in cats, and other types of MRD predominate. In general MRD in cats is not accompanied by the bone lesions seen in dogs, and hyperglobulinaemia is less common; visceral plasma cell neoplasia may be the only obvious feature (although often multiple organs are affected, most commonly the spleen and liver). Nevertheless, MRD is still an aggressive and often fatal neoplasm.

It can be challenging to distinguish cytologically between well-differentiated plasma cell neoplasm and plasmacytoid lymphoma, a variant of B-cell lymphoma. In general, plasma cells have more cytoplasm and smaller nuclei than plasmacytoid lymphocytes, but the distinction can be difficult in many cases.

Hepatic carcinoid

Neoplasm type: neuroendocrine
Age: in dogs, younger than many other primary hepatic tumours; slightly older in cats
Gross appearance: usually diffuse small nodules in multiple lobes
Species/breed predispositions: very rare in both dogs and cats
Cytological appearance/further comments: these tumours arise from resident neuroendocrine cells within the liver. They have the typical neuroendocrine appearance (see page 76), with many bare nuclei and clusters of cells with indistinct margins. They are very difficult to distinguish from metastatic neuroendocrine tumours (which are actually more common than carcinoids – see above) but should be a differential for neuroendocrine cells observed on liver aspirates.

Inflammatory lesions of the liver

As discussed above, inflammation within the liver can be challenging to identify. Not only are liver specimens usually significantly contaminated with blood they may also contain evidence of extra-medullary haematopoiesis – mild inflammation within the liver is very hard to definitively identify cytologically. The presence of neutrophils in pockets or groups can be an indication that they represent a focal area of inflammation rather than random distribution (Fig 7.28). Other indicators of true hepatic inflammation are neutrophils embedded within hepatocyte clusters, plasma cells (which are very rarely found on 'normal' liver aspirates) and the presence of neutrophils phagocytosed within macrophages (a sure sign of inflammation anywhere in the body).

Macrophagic/granulomatous inflammation can occur in some situations, most notably feline infectious peritonitis, as well as secondary to neoplasia or other infectious diseases (such as toxoplasmosis).

Hepatic splenosis

This is an uncommon non-neoplastic finding within the liver, which occurs after splenic trauma or surgery. Small sections of spleen can find their way to the liver and take root, forming small accessory spleens within the hepatic parenchyma. Their cytological appearance is very similar to normal splenic tissue (see page 249), with aggregates of splenic stroma and often increased lymphocytes. In the author's experience, the stroma in hepatic splenosis can sometimes appear more prominently mesenchymal than within the spleen itself. Therefore, care should be taken in diagnosing mesenchymal tumours or lymphoma in canine patients with a history of splenic trauma.

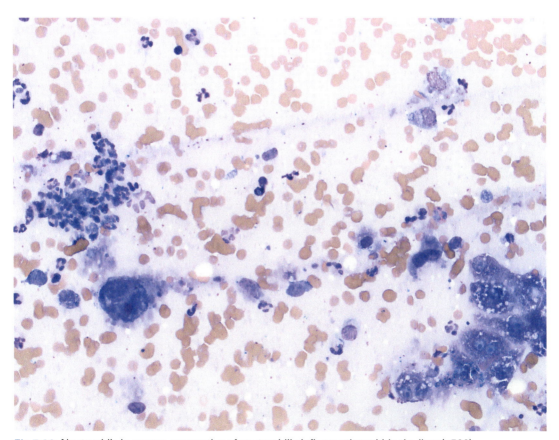

Fig 7.28 Neutrophils in groups, suggestive of neutrophilic inflammation within the liver (×500)

Cystic lesions

A variety of cystic lesions can occur in the liver but, unfortunately, as with other cystic structures, cytology is often unhelpful in diagnosing them, as most cystic structures appear cytologically similar – mildly proteinaceous fluid (pink stippled background with occasional protein clefts – see page 99, Fig 4.81) with low numbers of macrophages. Histopathology of the wall of these structures is usually required, although cytology can be useful to distinguish between a cyst and an abscess. Haematomas or cavitated neoplasia such as haemangiosarcoma can sometimes be identified although the cellular harvest is often low.

> **Key points**
>
> **Liver**
> - Binucleation is relatively common in normal hepatocytes
> - Mesothelial cells can be mistaken for biliary epithelium or other epithelial clusters on liver aspirates
> - Extra-medullary haematopoiesis is a non-specific finding in the liver but it can be mistaken for inflammation or neoplasia
> - Metastatic neoplasia in the liver is roughly three times more common than primary liver tumours
> - Care should be taken in diagnosing mesenchymal tumours or lymphoma in canine patients with a history of splenic trauma due to the possibility of hepatic splenosis

Other gastrointestinal tissues

The other organs/tissues associated with the gastrointestinal tract (stomach, intestines, and pancreas) are not commonly sampled in first opinion practice; they can be challenging to aspirate due to thin walls, small size, mobility etc., and they frequently exfoliate relatively poorly, yielding disappointing harvests mostly containing blood. Consequently, this book does not dwell in any detail on these locations, although a few common cytological findings are outlined below.

Intestinal masses

The most common reason to aspirate an area of gastrointestinal tract is due to the presence of masses within or attached to (or at least suspected of being attached to) the intestinal wall. The most common neoplasm aspirated in this way is lymphoma, and the presence of significant numbers of lymphocytes in aspirates from an intestinal wall should raise concern for lymphoma, although GI-associated lymphoid tissue (such as Peyer's patches) and lymph nodes will also contain increased lymphocytes.

The appearance of lymphoma is similar in other locations (see page 86 for a general description of lymphoma) although the yield of cells is often lower than elsewhere, and the lymphoid population can be more mixed. The typical cytological appearance of large cell lymphoma in cats is of cells with small amounts of cytoplasm which often contains low numbers of small vacuoles (Figs 7.29, 7.30), as well as cytoplasmic fragments also containing vacuoles (see below). Low numbers of these cells can be found in a reactive lymphoid population, but when they comprise a significant proportion of lymphocytes, lymphoma is a concern.

Large granular lymphoma (LGL) is an uncommon but highly aggressive variant of T-cell lymphoma seen mostly in cats. The name is confusing as it is unclear whether the 'large' means large granules or large lymphocytes, but the cytological appearance is distinctive. Aspirates contain high numbers of large lymphocytes containing irregular-sized magenta granules (although the granules may stain less well on in-house aqueous Romanowsky stains – see page 27) (Fig 7.31). This form of lymphoma often responds poorly to chemotherapy and progresses rapidly.

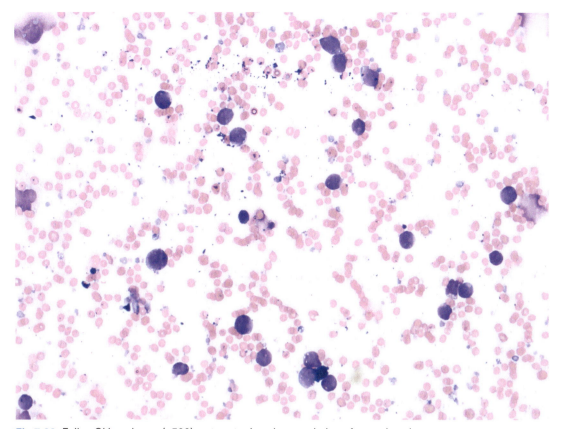

Fig 7.29 Feline GI lymphoma (×500); note cytoplasmic vacuolation of some lymphocytes

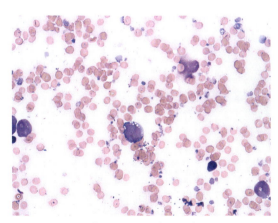

Fig 7.30 Feline GI lymphoma (×1000)

Other less common neoplasms include carcinomas (see page 72, Table 4.2) and mesenchymal tumours such as gastrointestinal stromal tumours (see page 261), as well as occasional mast cell tumours and other less common entities.

A relatively common feature of gastrointestinal neoplasia is the loss of GI integrity. This is not a completely specific finding, as it can also be seen with infarction or necrosis for other reasons, but even if neoplastic cells are not found, evidence of a loss of integrity should raise some concern for underling neoplasia. It is represented cytologically by high numbers of mixed morphology bacteria, usually mixed bacterial rods with rare cocci, accompanied by increased neutrophils containing phagocytosed bacteria.

The bacteria alone can represent inadvertent sampling of the gastrointestinal tract, and neutrophils can be blood derived (there are no neutrophils in the lumen of the GI tract except the stomach in normal circumstances) but the presence of phagocytosed bacteria confirms infection and probable loss of integrity.

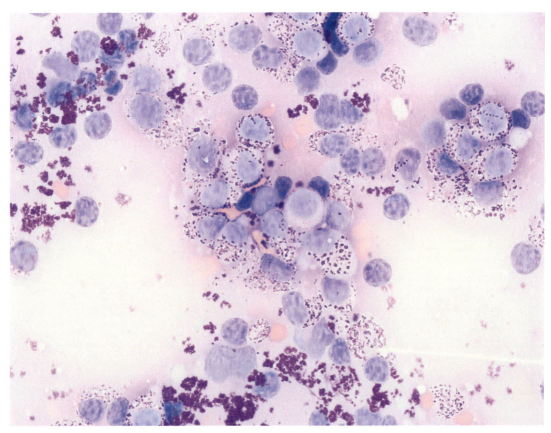

Fig 7.31 Large granular lymphoma, feline intestinal wall (×500)

Pancreas

Pancreatic aspirates most commonly harvest small amounts of exocrine pancreatic epithelium. This has a similar appearance to hepatocytes, containing cells with abundant finely granular cytoplasm, although acinar structures can also often be seen (Figs 7.32, 7.33).

Common findings in pancreatic aspirates include neutrophilic inflammation (pancreatitis) which can be accompanied with necrosis, and pancreatic carcinoma – carcinomas are more common than adenomas, and appear similar to other carcinomas, although their granular cytoplasm can sometimes still be appreciated (see page 92 for general epithelial features of malignancy) (Fig 7.34).

Pancreatic hyperplasia is also sometimes aspirated. This generally yields increased amounts of unremarkable pancreatic epithelium.

Abdominal lymph nodes

Lymph nodes and lymphoid tissue will be discussed in more detail in Chapter 10, but aspiration of enlarged abdominal lymph nodes to distinguish between inflammatory disease and neoplasia is relatively common. Small cell lymphoma can be very challenging to diagnose cytologically (see page 87), but large cell lymphoma has a very similar appearance to elsewhere in the body (see page 86).

Inflammation within abdominal lymph nodes can provide some information about suspected

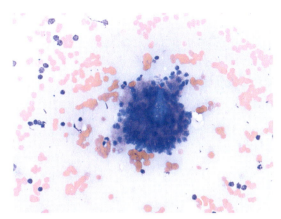

Fig 7.32 Pancreatic epithelium cluster (×500)

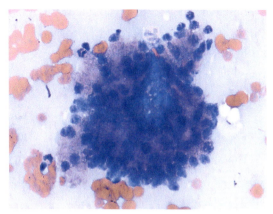

Fig 7.33 Pancreatic epithelium cluster (×1000)

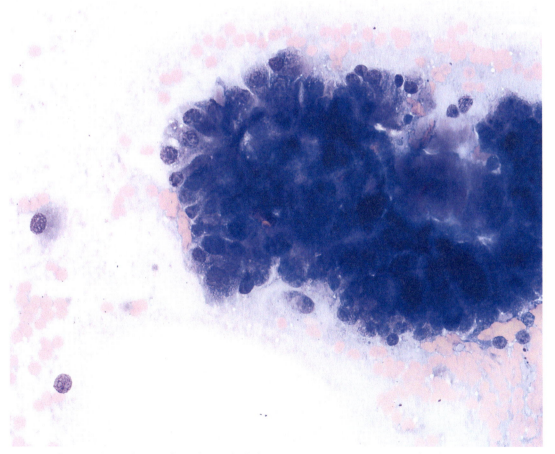

Fig 7.34 Pancreatic carcinoma; the cells retain their granular cytoplasm and so are (just) recognisable as pancreatic, but display marked variation in nuclear size (anisokaryosis) and multiple nucleoli

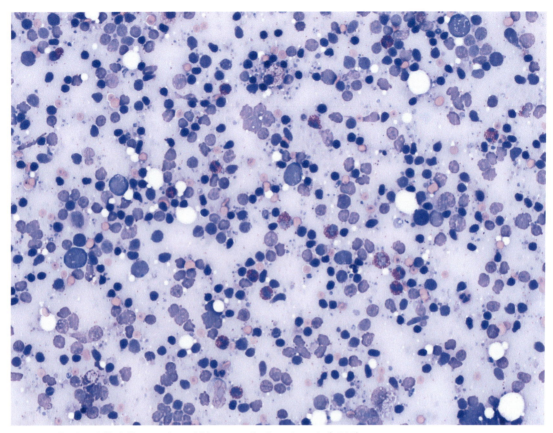

Fig 7.35 Eosinophilic inflammation within a reactive lymph node (×500)

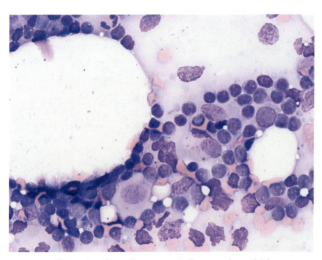

Fig 7.36 Granulomatous inflammation within a lymph node (×1000)

diseases. Eosinophilic inflammation is a relatively common finding (Fig 7.35), usually indicating eosinophilic inflammation in the intestines drained by the node, which could lend support for inflammatory intestinal disease/hypersensitivity, although paraneoplastic increases in eosinophils occur in some neoplasms (particularly mast cell tumours and lymphoma).

Similarly, neutrophilic inflammation is a common finding often indicating a nearby inflammatory process.

Macrophagic (granulomatous) or neutrophilic/macrophagic (pyogranulomatous) inflammation (Fig 7.36) is less common and can indicate a long-standing inflammatory pattern, or can be related to more serious infectious diseases – this pattern in cats raises concern for feline infectious peritonitis or, rarely, Mycobacterial infection (particularly in cats on raw food diets).

Abdominal lymph nodes are also a common site of metastasis for neoplasms of the gastrointestinal tract.

> **Chapter 7 – take home messages**
>
> - The presence of *Conchiformibius* colonies on cytology samples indicates that commensals have been harvested.
> - Oral malignant melanoma is more common in dogs than cats, and oral versions usually behave more aggressively than cutaneous melanoma.
> - Similarly, oral mast cell tumours are reported to be more aggressive than cutaneous.
> - Mesothelium in the liver can be mistaken for biliary epithelium or an atypical epithelial population.
> - It is extremely challenging on liver specimens to distinguish between nodular, hyperplasia, mild dysplasia, and low-grade (well differentiated) hepatic neoplasia
> - Inflammation can be difficult to assess in the liver as samples are often heavily haemodiluted.
> - Extra-medullary haematopoiesis in the liver is non-specific but can be mistaken for round cell neoplasia.
> - Metastatic neoplasia within the liver is roughly three times more common than primary hepatic neoplasia.
> - Lymphoma and mast cell tumour are the most common metastatic neoplasms found within the liver.
> - Loss of gastrointestinal integrity (represented by neutrophils containing phagocytosed mixed bacteria on samples from intestines) is commonly associated with underlying GI neoplasia.

Chapter 8

Genitourinary system

The emphasis of this chapter, as with the other non-cutaneous locations, is on those locations most commonly and most easily sampled of the genitourinary system – in this case, the kidneys, the prostate gland, and the bladder (as well as urine). Other areas – the gonads, uterus, ureters etc. – are relatively rarely sampled, as many veterinary patients are neutered. These locations will receive only brief mentions towards the end of the chapter.

Kidney

Kidneys are easy to sample with relatively low risk. Although the cytological harvest from 'normal' kidneys can be disappointing, the cell harvest increases with inflammation and neoplasia.

'Normal' appearance

Aspirates from normal kidneys often have very low cellularity.

Blood: as with many other internal organs, renal aspirates often contain large amounts of blood, although not usually as much as found in preparations from the liver or spleen. (Fig 8.1)

Renal epithelial cells: the renal epithelial harvest is often very low in aspirates from normal renal tissue, and the cells are often found individually or in very small clusters. Renal epithelial cells are usually round, occasionally cuboidal or slightly columnar. They usually have round central nuclei with coarse chromatin and occasionally a single indistinct nucleolus. The distinctive feature of

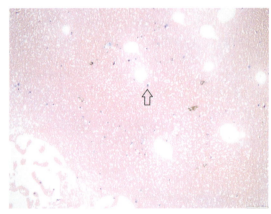

Fig 8.1 Typical low power appearance of renal aspirate with scattered renal epithelium (open arrow and other examples) (×100)

renal epithelial cells is their abundant eosinophilic (reddish-pink) with low numbers of clear vacuoles (droplets of lipid) (Fig 8.2). The vacuoles are more prominent in feline renal epithelium, and often more prominent in males than females.

Renal tubules: as well as individual renal epithelial cells, occasional whole tubules are aspirated, and they look rather like they sound – clusters of epithelial cells compressed into a tubular shape, similar to a cast in urine (see page 206) (Fig 8.3).

Glomeruli: intact glomeruli are occasionally found, and they appear as a tuft of capillaries and vascular endothelium with a cluster of associated renal epithelial cells (Fig 8.4).

Leukocytes: renal aspirates usually have very few leukocytes other than those associated with the accompanying blood, although the author

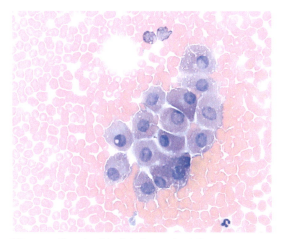

Fig 8.2a Renal epithelial cluster (×500)

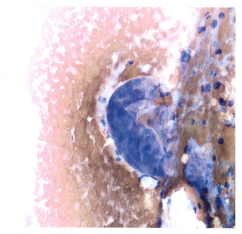

Fig 8.3 Renal epithelial tubule (×500)

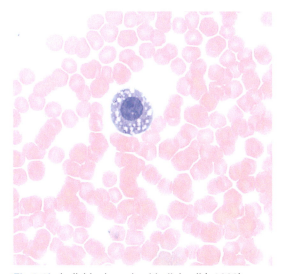

Fig 8.2b Individual renal epithelial cell (×1000)

has occasionally encountered low numbers of mixed lymphocytes on otherwise unremarkable renal aspirates.

Renal cystic structures

As mentioned previously, cytology is an insensitive and often unhelpful tool for cystic structures, as the cytological appearance of cysts is often similar regardless of the cause: mildly proteinaceous fluid (pink stippled background with occasional protein clefts – see page 99, Fig 4.81) with

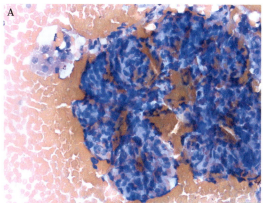
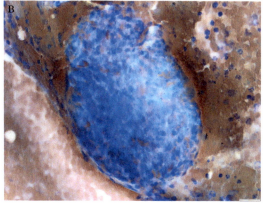

Fig 8.4a and b Glomerular tufts (×500)

low numbers of activated macrophages. Histopathology is usually needed for definitive information. Cytology can be useful to distinguish between cysts, abscesses and neoplasia (although many neoplasms do not exfoliate into fluid).

Renal neoplasia

As elsewhere, these lesions are arranged in rough order of commonality: the further down the list, the less likely the neoplasm. As with the liver, metastatic neoplasia is more common than primary renal neoplasia, which is relatively rare in both dogs and cats.

Renal lymphoma

Neoplasm type: round cell
Age: middle-aged to older
Gross appearance: usually bilateral renal enlargement
Species/breed predispositions: most common in cats
Cytological appearance/further comments: lymphoma usually results in generalised enlargement of both kidneys, and the appearance is similar to elsewhere in the body (see page 86). Lymphoma usually exfoliates much better than 'normal' kidneys, although the fragile neoplastic lymphocytes are often ruptured. Usually a few scattered renal epithelial cells or glomerular tufts confirm the presence of the neoplasm within renal tissue, although occasionally the kidney tissue is completely effaced.

Metastatic neoplasia

Neoplasm type: varies
Age: varies
Gross appearance: varies
Species/breed predispositions: varies
Cytological appearance/further comments: metastatic neoplasia is more common in the kidneys than primary tumours (approximately twice as common). In cats, lymphoma (described above) is the most common; in dogs, lymphoma, haemangiosarcoma (see page 147) and carcinomas (variable origin – see page 71 for general details of epithelial neoplasia) are mostly commonly encountered.

Renal carcinoma (FIG 8.5)

Neoplasm type: epithelial
Age: usually middle-aged to older, occasionally young dogs
Gross appearance: usually unilateral renal mass; occasionally bilateral or multiple masses
Species/breed predispositions: most common in dogs than cats; seen in German shepherds as part of hereditary dermatofibrosis
Cytological appearance/further comments: the most common primary renal neoplasm, primary renal carcinomas can vary in appearance but many display markedly atypical features and they commonly metastasise; often to the lung but can be any location, including cutaneous. It is challenging to distinguish between primary renal carcinoma and metastatic carcinoma, but a common feature of renal carcinoma is the presence of prominent pink smooth secretory material, sometimes in large amounts. It can be found embedded within clusters, often surrounded by acinar structures (see page 75, Fig 4.31), or free in the background. The absence of this does not exclude renal origin, but the presence of this material lends significant support for it.

Hereditary dermatofibrosis is a rare genetic disorder of German shepherds, characterised by the presence of multiple subcutaneous fibrous nodules, uterine leiomyomas and renal epithelial neoplasia (cysts, adenomas or carcinomas).

Urothelial (transitional cell) carcinomas occasionally develop in the renal pelvis. They are described in more detail on page 212.

Renal sarcoma (FIG 8.6)

Neoplasm type: mesenchymal
Age: middle-aged to older
Gross appearance: multiple cavitated masses (haemangiosarcoma); single masses (other sarcomas)

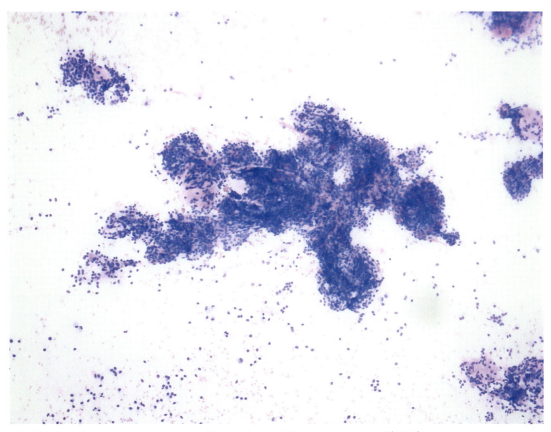

Fig 8.5a Renal carcinoma, low power, with prominent pink secretory material (×100)

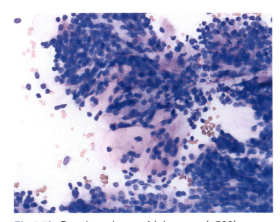

Fig 8.5b Renal carcinoma, high power (×500)

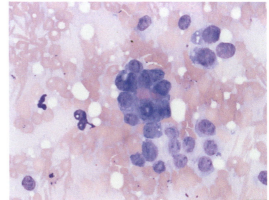

Fig 8.5c Renal carcinoma (×1000)

Species/breed predispositions: more common in dogs

Cytological appearance/further comments: primary renal sarcomas are uncommon to rare, with the exception of haemangiosarcoma, although as with carcinomas it is often challenging to distinguish between primary renal haemangiosarcoma and metastatic disease (which is much more common). The appearance is similar to elsewhere (see page 147 for haemangiosarcoma and 78 for other sarcomas).

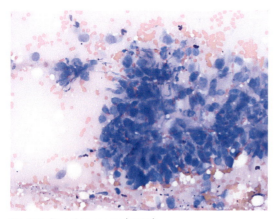

Fig 8.6 Renal sarcoma (×500)

Nephroblastoma (FIG 8.7)
Neoplasm type: embryonal (see below)
Age: usually less than 2 years old
Gross appearance: unilateral solitary mass usually
Species/breed predispositions: possible males predisposed
Cytological appearance/further comments: these tumours develop from common stem cells within the kidney; they are usually congenital although are generally only detected in later life. The cytological appearance varies as the tissue within the lesions can differentiate into epithelial or mesenchymal cells.

A common appearance is that of a 'sticky' lymphoma; i.e. large blastic cells resembling large lymphocytes with prominent nucleoli, but often found in obviously cohesive clusters, more

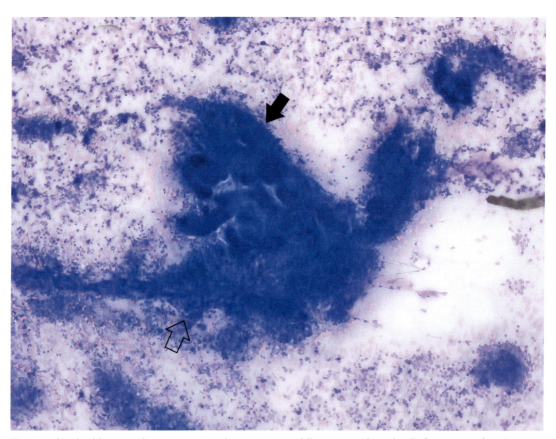

Fig 8.7a Nephroblastoma, low power; note the areas resembling mesenchymal cells (open arrow) and epithelial cells (black arrow) (×100)

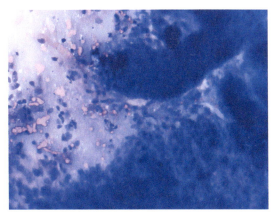

Fig 8.7b Nephroblastoma, high power (×500)

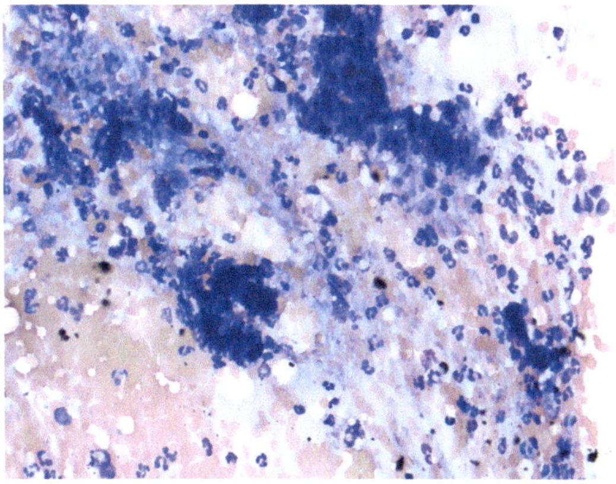

Fig 8.8 Neutrophilic inflammation in the kidney

typical of epithelial cells. Sometimes there are also clusters of epithelial cells and aggregates of mesenchymal cells also present, and these are occasionally the most prominent cells observed. Rare tumours can also contain extracellular matrix representing the presence of cartilage or osteoid.

In cats and dogs, these tumours frequently metastasise, although some reports suggest that those tumours with more differentiated tissues (i.e. more epithelium and mesenchymal cells) may behave in a less aggressive fashion.

Renal inflammation

Inflammatory patterns in the kidneys are similar to inflammation elsewhere; neutrophilic inflammation (Fig 8.8) is most commonly found and, in the case of pyelonephritis, bacteria can sometimes be identified on cytological specimens; the presence of bacteria on renal aspirates is rarely normal, and if they are observed phagocytosed within neutrophils, infection is confirmed. Macrophagic (granulomatous) inflammation is less commonly found, and is associated with more chronic inflammatory conditions, or with other infectious agents such as FIP in cats or fungal organisms.

Low numbers of mixed lymphocytes are sometimes found (see page 68, Fig 4.18), but high numbers of lymphocytes raise concern for lymphoma. Eosinophilic inflammation is rarely seen but can be paraneoplastic (often secondary to lymphoma or mast cell tumours) or, rarely, parasites or hypersensitivity reactions.

> **Key points**
>
> **Kidney**
> - 'Normal' kidney aspirates have low cellularity, with blood, renal epithelial cells, occasional tubules and occasional glomerular tufts
> - Metastatic neoplasia is more common than primary renal neoplasia
> - Lymphoma is generally bilateral; renal carcinoma is more typically unilateral

Urine

Cytological evaluation of urine is distinct from sediment analysis, as the staining highlights some features (bacteria, nucleated cells) but damages or otherwise makes some features such as crystals or casts harder to identify. In general, urine cytology is most useful to assess the morphology of epithelial cells when they are identified on sediment analysis. It can also be helpful to identify types of inflammation

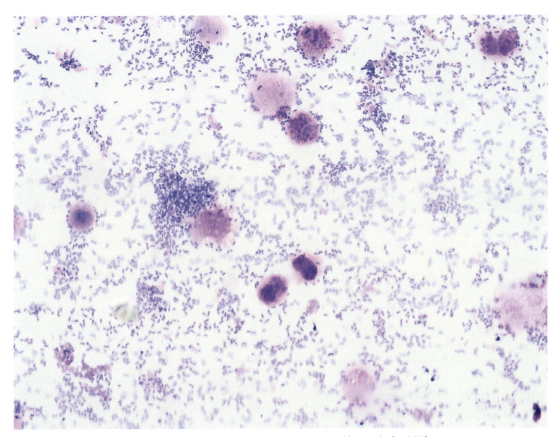

Fig 8.9 Highly degenerate neutrophils in urine with high numbers of bacteria (×1000)

and confirm the presence of infectious agents when sediment examination is unequivocal. Crystal examination and identification is more usefully carried out on fresh in-house samples via sediment analysis (examining concentrated unstained urine).

Urine samples are often poorly cellular, and concentrated cytology preparations are usually required for detailed examination. Cytocentrifuged preparations (see page 13, Fig 1.13b) are most useful.

Urine is not a pleasant substance for a nucleated cell to find itself in; even more so than other fluids, urine has a deleterious effect on the preservation of nucleated cells, which must be borne in mind when examining urine cytology. Degenerate neutrophils are often markedly degenerate within urine, sometimes losing their characteristic nuclear shape altogether, developing round nuclei somewhat reminiscent of lymphocytes. Pale cells with round nuclei containing phagocytosed bacteria on urine cytology samples are likely to be highly degenerate neutrophils (Fig 8.9).

'Normal' appearance

Cytologically normal urine has a smooth clear background and is largely acellular. Variable numbers of erythrocytes may be present, dependent on the sampling method (more prominent in cystocentesis samples). Low numbers of scattered anucleate squames and squamous epithelial cells (see page 97) may also be found, more prominent on free-catch and catheterised samples. Spermatozoa may also be found in intact or very recently castrated male dogs. These stain very pale blue cytologically and are occasionally difficult to visualise.

Bacteriuria

Free catch samples often contain contaminants, including bacteria and occasionally yeasts, but when accompanied by significant inflammation, infection is suspected, and confirmed when organisms are found phagocytosed within neutrophils (see page 107, Fig 5.1b). In contrast, bacteria are not expected to be seen in cystocentesis samples and their presence here should raise significant suspicion of infection, even when not accompanied by inflammatory cells (Fig 8.10).

Inflammation

Neutrophilic inflammation is most common in urine samples, often associated with urinary tract infection, although when highly degenerate, neutrophils can be challenging to identify (see page 210 above). Other inflammatory patterns are rare.

Neoplasia

Neoplastic cells exfoliate relatively uncommonly into urine, but it is occasionally possible to identify neoplastic processes in urine samples. Urothelial (transitional cell) carcinoma is the most common bladder neoplasm in dogs and cats by a large margin (approximately 90% of bladder tumours are urothelial carcinomas). They are one of the most aggressive neoplasms encountered in these species, with approximately 20% of patients having detectable metastasis at the time of diagnosis (often pulmonary); see page 212 (prostate) for a more detailed description of the cytological appearance, but

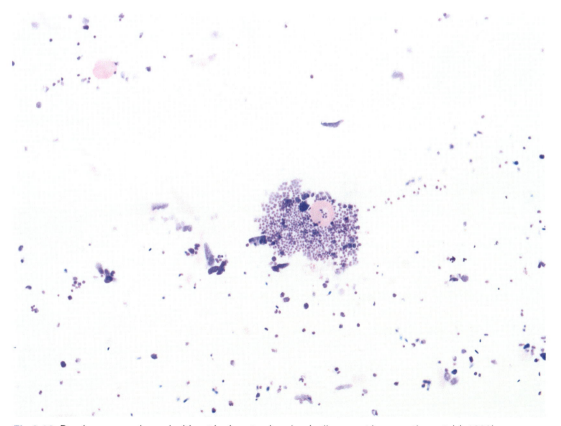

Fig 8.10 Poorly preserved cocci without leukocytes in urine (cell present is an erythrocyte) (×1000)

the cells in urine can be challenging to assess due to the effect of urine on preservation; epithelial cells often swell and rupture in urine samples, making them appear pleomorphic and disorganised.

More reliable features of malignancy in urine are the presence of multinucleate cells or Melamed-Wolinska bodies (round usually eosinophilic inclusions within the cytoplasm of epithelial cells – see Fig 8.11). Neither of these features are likely to be caused by poor preservation in urine, although neither are absolutely specific for neoplasia and can occur with marked dysplasia secondary to inflammation/infection. The presence of high numbers of multinucleate cells or Melamed-Wolinska bodies, in the absence of any inflammation, raises significant concern for neoplasia, however.

Other neoplastic cells are only rarely found within the urine. The author has occasionally encountered identifiable lymphoma on urine samples.

Bladder

Neoplasia

Urothelial carcinoma (FIG 8.11)
Neoplasm type: epithelial
Age: middle-aged to older
Gross appearance: usually mass in the trigone region (caudal ventral bladder)
Species/breed predispositions: common in dogs, uncommon in cats; more common in neutered dogs; Scottish terriers have 20-fold higher risk
Cytological appearance/further comments: As mentioned above (page XX), urothelial carcinoma is the most common bladder neoplasm by far; Diagnosis can occasionally be made in the urine, but direct aspiration or traumatic bladder catheterisation (see page 24 for technique) are usually more diagnostically useful. Direct aspiration runs some risk of seeding neoplastic cells along the line of aspiration, but this risk is usually outweighed by the seriousness of the diagnosis and the limited treatment

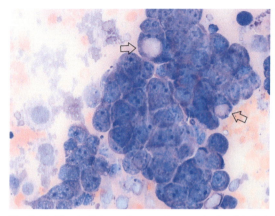

Fig 8.11 Urothelial carcinoma; the atypical epithelial cells sometimes contain pale pink *Melamed-Wolinska* bodies (open arrows) (×1000)

options for even a single mass within the bladder wall.

Cytologically, urothelial cell carcinomas can appear similar to other carcinomas (see page 92 for general features), but they often display markedly atypical features, with pleomorphism, multinucleation and disorganisation all common.

Melamed-Wolinska bodies are sometimes found, and occasionally in high numbers; these are round eosinophilic (pink to red) inclusions found within the cytoplasm of some neoplastic cells, occasionally displacing the nucleus. They are not pathognomonic for urothelial carcinomas (they can occasionally be seen in markedly inflamed transitional epithelium, and rare similar inclusions can be found in other epithelial neoplasms (for instance, mammary carcinomas, in the author's experience) but their presence should raise strong suspicion for urothelial carcinoma.

Other neoplasms
Other bladder neoplasms are relatively rare, but occasional adenomas are found within the bladder wall. Adenomas resemble well-differentiated transitional epithelial cells cytologically, and they can be challenging to distinguish from hyperplasia (which can sometimes be polypoid)

secondary to inflammation. Other rare tumours include squamous cell carcinoma and mesenchymal tumours (such as leiomyoma/leiomyosarcoma, fibroma, haemangiosarcoma).

> **Key points**
>
> **Urine and bladder**
> - Urine cytology is most useful to assess the morphology of epithelial cells when they are identified on sediment analysis; crystal analysis is more useful on urine sediment exam
> - Degenerate neutrophils are often markedly degenerate within urine, losing their characteristic nuclear shape and developing round nuclei
> - Urothelial (transitional cell) carcinoma is the most common bladder neoplasm in dogs and cats by a large margin
> - *Melamed-Wolinska* bodies are sometimes found in urothelial carcinoma, occasionally in high numbers

Prostate

The prostate is an accessible location for direct aspiration. In the author's experience, the cytological quality of direct aspirates is far superior to samples retrieved via prostatic wash (Fig 8.12). Additionally, prostatic wash samples often only harvest the transitional epithelial cells which line the prostatic urethra, and are sometimes not representative of the prostate gland. Concerns remain, however, on the risk of neoplastic cells tracking along the line of aspiration, particularly with urothelial carcinoma. In the author's opinion, the risk of this is relatively low, and given the poor clinical outcome of urothelial carcinoma regardless of location, the superior diagnostic quality of samples must be weighed against the relatively low risk of direct aspiration. This remains a clinical decision for the veterinarian.

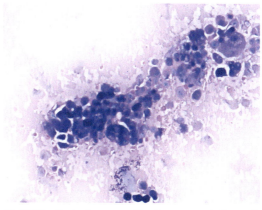

Fig 8.12a Typical preservation from a prostatic wash sample (×500)

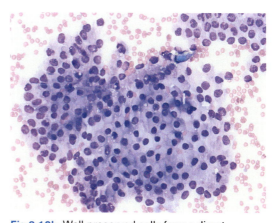

Fig 8.12b Well-preserved cells from a direct prostatic aspirate (×500)

'Normal' appearance

The 'normal' prostate is small, and so true samples of completely normal prostatic epithelium are relatively rare. Well-differentiated prostatic epithelium has a characteristic appearance, however – the cells are cuboidal to columnar, with small uniform nuclei roughly 1.5 erythrocytes in diameter, coarse chromatin and occasionally a single dark round nucleolus. The cells have moderate amounts of pale pink cytoplasm and may contain high numbers of vacuoles. In clusters, the cells form a tessellating hexagonal pattern, easily recognisable as prostatic epithelium (Fig 8.13).

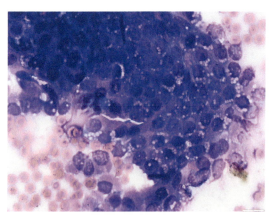

Fig 8.13 Well-differentiated prostatic epithelium (×1000)

Moderate amounts of blood are also often present, and spermatozoa may be found in intact male dogs, where they appear similar to spermatozoa found in the urine (see page 210).

Prostatic wash samples harvest similar material, although cellularity and preservation are often poorer. Sometimes prostatic wash samples harvest only transitional epithelial cells. These cells are so called as they appear as something of a cytological middle ground between cuboidal and squamous epithelial cells. Cytologically, they appear as clusters of cells, smaller and more cuboidal in the centre, maturing and enlarging to more squamous-appearing cells peripherally, and are often accompanied by individual larger squamous-like cells.

Prostatic inflammation

Prostatitis is a relatively common finding on prostatic samples; samples generally contain a mixture of well-differentiated prostatic epithelial cells and intense neutrophilic inflammation. Bacteria are often present, often phagocytosed within neutrophils, which confirms bacterial infection. With very intense inflammation, the epithelial cells can undergo dysplastic features which can mimic malignancy, and care must be taken to interpret the presence of neoplasia when there is marked concurrent inflammation.

Resampling following appropriate treatment of inflammation is often useful to aid assessment of the epithelial cells.

Prostatic neoplasia

Urothelial (transitional cell) carcinoma
(FIG 8.14)
Neoplasm type: epithelial
Age: middle-aged to older
Gross appearance: usually large irregular mass within prostate
Species/breed predispositions: common in dogs; more common in neutered dogs; Scottish terriers have 20-fold higher risk; very rare in cats
Cytological appearance/further comments: true primary prostatic carcinomas are very rare in dogs, and almost never seen in cats. Instead, most prostatic tumours are urothelial in origin, with similar predispositions to bladder wall tumours. The cytological appearance is similar to urothelial carcinoma elsewhere (see page 212).

Squamous metaplasia

This is an uncommon but highly recognisable cytological finding. With this condition, the normally cuboidal to columnar epithelial cells have undergone transition to squamous epithelial cells. Aspirates from prostates with squamous metaplasia resemble aspirates from the epidermis or oral cavity (without the bacteria). Preparations contain often high numbers of otherwise unremarkable squamous epithelial cells (Fig 8.15).

The typical hexagonal pattern of the prostatic epithelial cell is not present, and there are usually no 'normal' prostatic epithelial cells present. Misdiagnosis can sometimes occur when there is significant contamination from the dermis during sampling (the presence of both squamous and more normal prostatic epithelial cells may raise the cytologist's suspicion of this possibility).

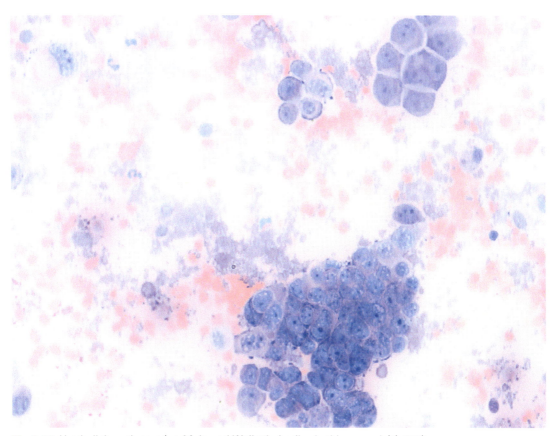

Fig 8.14 Urothelial carcinoma (no *Melamed-Wolinska* bodies in this example) (×500)

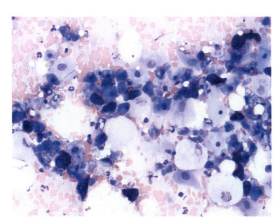

Fig 8.15 Squamous metaplasia of the prostate (×500)

It is a useful finding because it greatly narrows the differential list; the most common reason by far for this transformation of epithelial cells is the presence of a testicular tumour, usually a Sertoli cell tumour (rarely, interstitial cell tumours (Leydig cell tumours) due to the production of oestrogen. If squamous metaplasia is found in an apparently castrated male, it may be useful to investigate the possibility of cryptorchidism.

Much less commonly, squamous metaplasia can occur as a consequence of prolonged inflammation within the prostate gland.

Chapter 8 – take home messages

- 'Normal' kidneys often exfoliate poorly and contain scattered renal epithelial cells with occasional tubules and glomeruli.
- A common feature of renal carcinoma is the presence of prominent pink smooth secretory material, sometimes in large amounts.
- Urine cytology is most useful to assess the morphology of epithelial cells when they are identified on sediment analysis.
- Degenerate neutrophils are often markedly degenerate within urine, sometimes losing their characteristic nuclear shape altogether, developing round nuclei somewhat reminiscent of lymphocytes.
- Squamous metaplasia of the prostate is most commonly caused by testicular tumours.

Chapter 9

Respiratory system

Cytological preparations from the respiratory system are acquired in two ways: flushing/lavage and direct aspiration (usually for lung masses or consolidation, occasionally nasal or laryngeal masses). Techniques for respiratory washes are described on page 22. As elsewhere in this book, the focus is primarily on the most commonly and easily sampled areas – in this location, nasal flushes, broncho-alveolar lavage (BAL) and direct lung aspirates.

Nose

'Normal' appearance

The external nares are covered in keratinised squamous epithelium, which rapidly transitions

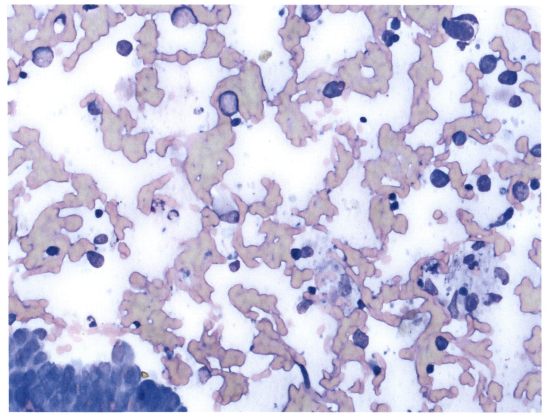

Fig 9.1 Lymphoma in a nasal wash; low numbers of epithelial cells are evident in the bottom left (×500)

through non-keratinised squamous epithelium to columnar epithelium, with characteristic cilia, persisting down to the terminal alveoli.

Nasal flushes often produce a mix of a small number of both types of epithelium, as well as commensal bacteria, including *Conchiformibius*, the large distinctive colonies of which are helpful to distinguish commensals from pathogens (see page 107, Fig 5.1b). Neutrophils are often present. As with other locations, bacteria present within neutrophils confirm the presence of infection, although this finding is often less helpful in nasal flushes, as primary bacterial rhinitis is uncommon in both dogs and cats, and the finding is usually secondary to another pathological process.

Neoplasia and fungal organisms exfoliate only rarely with nasal flushes, even when large masses or fungal plaques are evident. The most commonly exfoliative neoplasm is lymphoma in cats, which appears similar to elsewhere in the body (see page 86) although preservation is often suboptimal in nasal washes. Direct aspirates of suspect lesions are usually preferable where possible, although unforgiving nasal anatomy often makes this challenging.

Nasal masses

Direct aspiration of nasal lesions often yields higher numbers of better preserved and more relevant cells than nasal flushing. Common neoplasms include lymphoma (Fig 9.1), usually in cats (see page 86), carcinomas in dogs (see

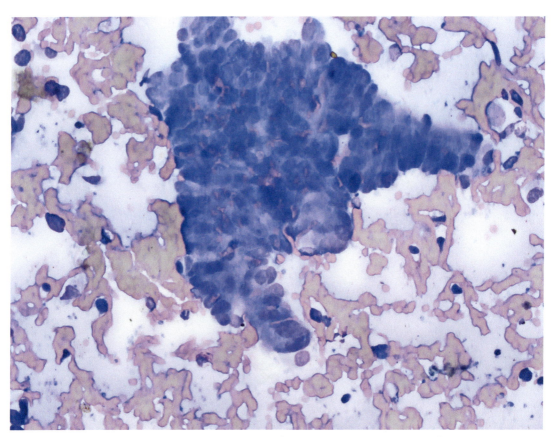

Fig 9.2 Dysplastic but non-neoplastic nasal epithelium (moderate nuclear size variation (anisokaryosis), occasional prominent nucleoli) (×500)

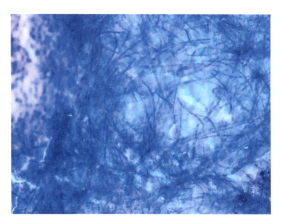

Fig 9.3 Mat of fungal hyphae in a nasal flush (*Aspergillus sp.*) (×500)

> **Key points**
>
> **Nose**
> - Primary bacterial rhinitis is uncommon in both dogs and cats
> - Most nasal tumours are malignant (usually by local invasion); metastasis is less common at the time of diagnosis
> - Inflammation in the nasal cavity can lead to marked dysplasia in nasal epithelium which can resemble malignancy

page 92) and sarcomas in both (see page 78). Most nasal tumours are malignant, although occasional adenomas or papillomas occur. Regardless of this, metastasis is not usually present at the time of diagnosis (local invasion is more common). Neuroendocrine and blastic tumours are rare but have been reported.

A challenging feature of nasal cytology is that epithelial cells often display much more marked dysplastic features when significant inflammation is present, and these cells can strongly mimic malignancy – features such as disorganisation, marked variations in size and shape, and atypical nuclear features can all be seen more prominently in inflamed nasal epithelium than elsewhere in the body (Fig 9.2). The reason is unclear, although it could reflect the enclosed limited space of the nasal cavities. Regardless, cytologists should have a higher bar for malignant features in nasal epithelium than elsewhere in the body, particularly when inflammation is present.

Fungal plaques appear similar to elsewhere in the body (see page 116) – significant inflammation, either macrophagic (granulomatous) or neutrophilic/macrophagic (pyogranulomatous) is generally present. Aspergillus is the most commonly implicated organism, usually appearing in hyphal form (see page 117) (Fig 9.3).

Broncho-alveolar lavage (BAL) and trans-tracheal wash (TTW)

See page 22 for one technique for performing these procedures – BAL is much more commonly performed in practice. The cytological results are similar for both techniques, although TTW usually yields cells/inflammation from higher in the respiratory tract, which should be borne in mind when interpreting the findings.

Cytological examination of airway samples is useful to identify patterns of inflammation and, less commonly, aetiological agents (such as bacteria, fungi and parasites). Cytology is less useful, however, for non-inflammatory conditions. Exfoliation of neoplasia is variable and unpredictable, but neoplastic cells occasionally can be found in respiratory washes (most commonly lymphoma or bronchial carcinoma). Cytobrush techniques (not described here) are often slightly less sensitive for detecting inflammation, although it is possible, they are more sensitive at detecting neoplasia within the airways.

'Normal' findings

Wash samples from the lower respiratory tract usually contain respiratory epithelium (ciliated columnar epithelial cells) in variable numbers (Figs 9.4 and 9.5). Blood may be present

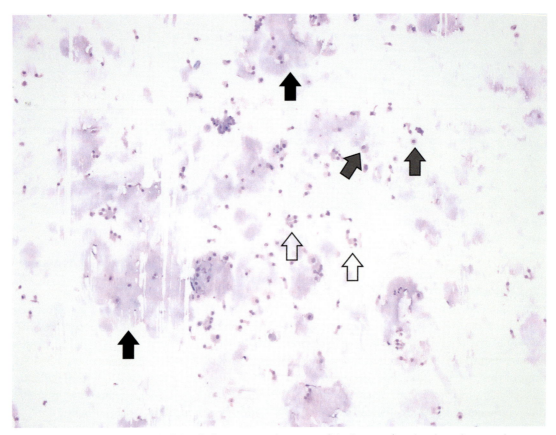

Fig 9.4 Ciliated columnar epithelial cells (open arrows); mucous (black arrows) and activated macrophages (grey arrows) are also present (×100)

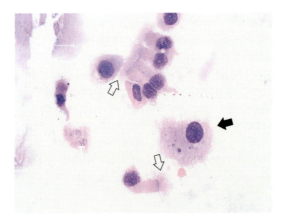

Fig 9.5 Ciliated columnar epithelial cells; at this magnification the cilia are clearly visible (open arrow); an activated macrophage is also present (×1000)

if haemorrhage occurred during sampling. Macrophages are normal residents of the lower respiratory tract – this makes assessment of macrophagic inflammation on wash samples challenging.

Other normal cytological findings include goblet cells (columnar to slightly cuboidal epithelial cells containing large blue-purple rounded droplets of mucous), although increased numbers of goblet cells could reflect chronic inflammation (goblet cell hyperplasia) (Fig 9.6). In some samples, the cilia detach from the surface of the cell and can be mistaken for rod-shaped bacteria – they are paler and more irregular than true bacterial organisms, however.

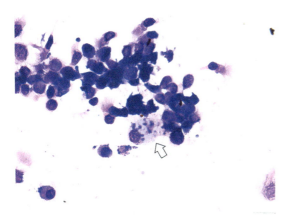

Fig 9.6 Goblet cell with droplets of mucous within the cytoplasm (open arrow) (×1000)

Oropharyngeal contamination (FIG 9.7)

Even in normal situations, the oropharynx contains high numbers of mixed bacteria, as well as high numbers of neutrophils. Contamination of airway samples with material from the oropharynx therefore makes assessment very challenging and can lead to misinterpretation of inflammation or bacterial infection.

The presence of keratinised squamous epithelial cells or mixed morphology bacterial organisms should raise the cytologist's suspicion of oropharyngeal contamination. *Conchiformibius* organisms are commensals in the oropharynx with almost no pathogenic potential; they have a distinctive large tablet-like shape (which actually comprises high numbers of closely associated rod-shaped bacteria), and their presence confirms oropharyngeal origin (see page 107, Fig 5.1b).

> Note samples from cases of aspiration pneumonia can resemble oropharyngeal contamination, although there is usually an intense inflammatory response in these cases.

Haemorrhage prior to sampling (FIG 9.8)

Evidence of prior haemorrhage includes red blood cells, especially when phagocytosed within macrophages, as well as haematoidin crystals and haemosiderin granules. Macrophages containing haemosiderin granules are consistent with haemorrhage prior to sampling. They have occasionally been described as 'heart failure' cells due to their perceived association with cardiac disease. However, recent studies have shown that the finding is not very specific, especially in cats – nearly 65% of feline BAL samples were reported to contain haemosiderophages.

Possibilities for haemorrhage into the airway include lungworm, heart disease (presumably due to lung congestion), bleeding disorders and other causes of inflammation.

'Normal' BAL figures

Cell counts of 250–500/mL have been reported in clinically normal patients (although see above regarding exfoliation of samples) See Table 9.1 for reported leukocyte proportions (although see note on page x regarding caution when using differential counts and percentages in cytological specimens).

Mucous may also be seen as patches of amorphous bluish-purple material, often containing embedded leukocytes (Fig 9.9).

Neoplasia

Neoplasia exfoliates only rarely into respiratory washes, although occasional bronchial carcinomas or lymphomas can be found. The appearance of bronchial carcinoma is similar to that found on direct lung aspirates (see page 228), although preservation is often poor. Regardless, the presence of dense basophilic clusters of cells raises concern for a carcinoma. Lymphoma exfoliates as high numbers of monomorphic lymphocytes, similar to its appearance elsewhere.

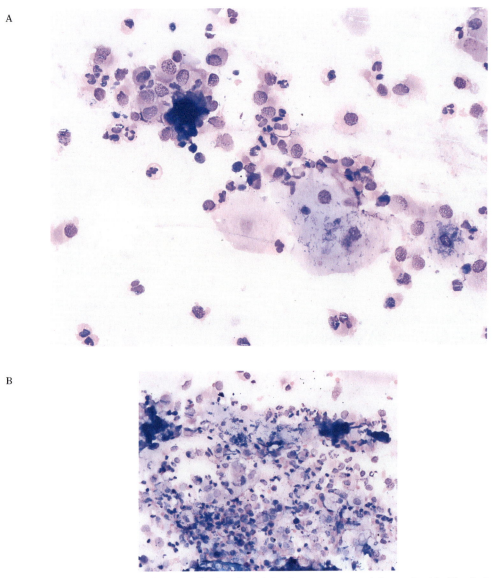

Figs 9.7a and b Oropharyngealy contamination; keratinised squames containing embedded bacteria (including *Conchiformibius*) are present (×1000)

Inflammation

Inflammatory patterns are similar to other areas of the body, with similar causes. Other findings consistent with chronic inflammation irritation include increased amounts of mucous and/or goblet cell hyperplasia (represented by increased numbers of goblet cells) and Curschmann's spirals (inspissated mucous which appears as dense basophilic spirals on cytology).

Neutrophilic inflammation

Even low numbers of neutrophils interspersed with respiratory epithelium are consistent with respiratory epithelium (Fig 9.10), although assessment of inflammation can be complicated by oropharyngeal contamination and

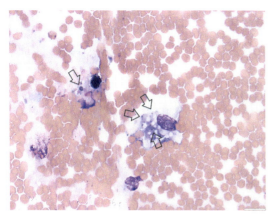

Fig 9.8 Haemosiderophages: Macrophages containing dark pigment granules (haemosiderin, open arrows) indicate haemorrhage prior to sampling (×1000)

Table 9.1 'Normal' BAL leukocyte proportions

Leukocyte	Dog	Cat
Macrophages	70–80%	70–80%
Lymphocytes	6–14%	<5%
Neutrophils	<5%	<5%
Eosinophils*	<5%	<25%

*studies have reported eosinophil proportions of up to 25% in feline BAL preparations as 'normal', although in the author's experience this is unusual and in practice, proportions greater than 15–20% are likely to be significant

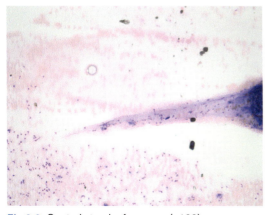

Fig 9.9 Central streak of mucous (×100)

haemorrhage during sampling, both of which introduce neutrophils to the specimen that were not present in the respiratory tract.

As with other cytological specimens, the presence of degenerate neutrophils raises suspicion for infection, although this can be harder to assess due to the often poor preservation of airway samples. Phagocytosed bacteria confirm the suspicion (Fig 9.11) (although a delay in sample preparation can lead to this occurring *in vitro*).

The normally pale granulation of neutrophils can become darker and more prominent in airway samples; added to the fact that eosinophil granules occasionally become paler brown and slightly harder to visualise, it can sometimes be surprisingly difficult to distinguish between neutrophils and eosinophils on airway preparations (Fig 9.12). Spending time finding both types of leukocytes in the same visual field greatly helps in identification.

Eosinophilic Inflammation (FIG 9.13)

Eosinophils are found in higher proportions in feline airway samples – proportions up to 25% are reported to be normal (see table 9.1 – although in the author's experience proportions of 15–20% or above are likely to be significant). In dogs, proportions >5% are considered abnormal.

As elsewhere in the body, eosinophils are associated with parasitism and hypersensitivity. The presence of lungworm larvae confirms infestation; even in the absence of larvae, high numbers of eosinophils as well as evidence of prior haemorrhage in canine BAL samples should raise suspicion for lungworm (Fig 9.14).

Eosinophilic inflammation is also commonly associated with feline asthma and canine eosinophilic bronchopneumopathy, although it is worth remembering that the use of corticosteroids prior to sampling will drastically reduce eosinophil numbers. Mixed inflammatory patterns comprising neutrophils and eosinophils are sometimes associated with bacterial infection secondary to hypersensitivity (particularly

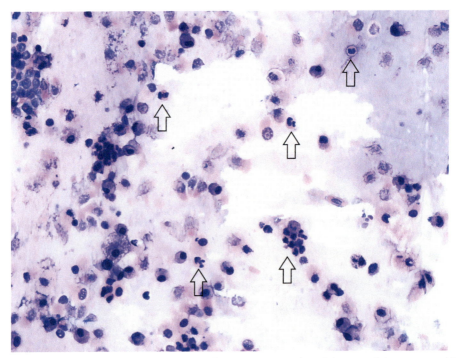

Fig 9.10 Neutrophilic inflammation on BAL, note the poor preservation of the material, not unusual for respiratory washes, but neutrophils are still identifiable (open arrows and other examples) (×500)

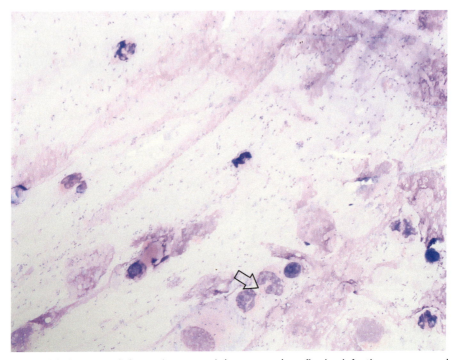

Fig 9.11 Bacterial phagocytosis in respiratory wash (open arrow) confirming infection; many more bacteria are visible in the background (×1000)

Mycoplasma sp., which are extremely challenging to identify on cytology samples due to their small size).

Macrophagic (granulomatous) and neutrophilic/macrophagic (pyogranulomatous) inflammation

Macrophages are normal residents of the lower airway, and this makes identification of 'true' macrophagic inflammation difficult. Increased numbers of leukocytes can be an indicator, but perhaps more reliable is the presence of increased numbers of activated macrophages (see page 62). These cells have expanded and often vacuolated cytoplasm, and occasional multinucleate cells may be present (Fig 9.15).

Macrophages are associated with chronic inflammation (Fig 9.16) and this pattern of

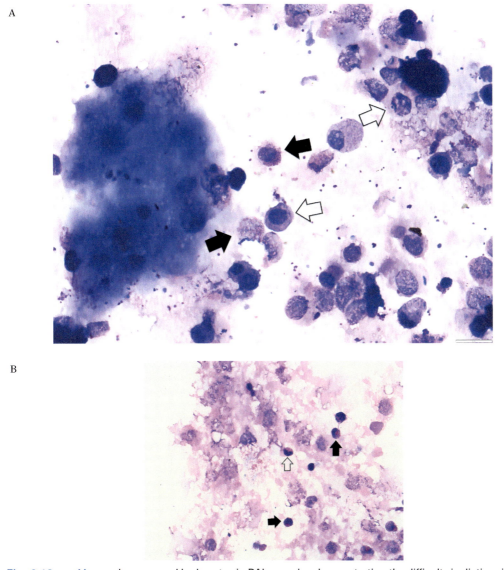

Figs 9.12a and b poorly preserved leukocytes in BAL samples demonstrating the difficulty in distinguishing between neutrophils (open arrows) and eosinophils (black arrows) (×1000)

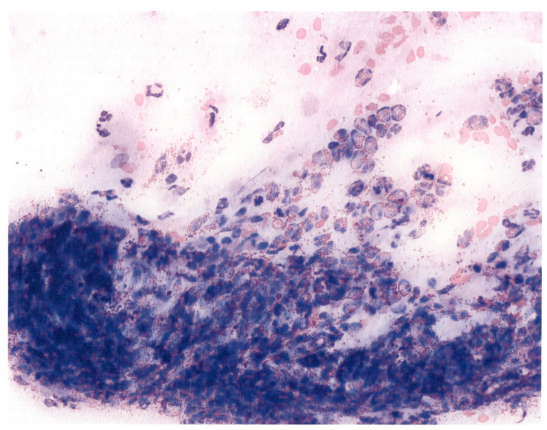

Fig 9.13 Eosinophilic inflammation in respiratory wash (×500)

inflammation raises concern for more challenging infectious organisms. Mycobacterial infection is a significant concern in feline patients, especially due to the zoonotic potential, and suspected cases should have air-dried samples submitted for closer examination and Ziehl Neelsen (ZN) staining (Fig 9.17). Fungal organisms can also cause this inflammatory pattern in both dogs and cats, as well as other causes of prolonged inflammation.

Infectious agents

Bacteria (and oropharyngeal contamination) have been discussed elsewhere. Fungal infections are very rare in the UK, but the presence of organisms phagocytosed within macrophages is diagnostic. Helminth parasites (most commonly

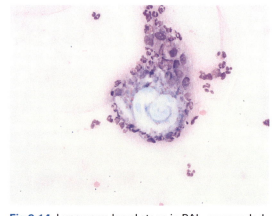

Fig 9.14 Lungworm larval stage in BAL, surrounded by eosinophils and macrophages; as is common, the larva is curled, making identification via tail morphology challenging (×500)

angiostrongylus and *crenosoma* in dogs, *aelurostrongylus* in cats) have large larvae that are easier to identify on lower power, and often elicit significant eosinophilic inflammation.

Protozoal infections are occasionally seen, although they can be hard to identify cytologically. *Toxoplasma gondii* tachyzoites are small banana-shaped organisms found free in the background and phagocytosed within macrophages. *Pneumocystis jirovecii* (previously *carinii*) have small, elongated tachyzoites, and bradyzoites are round structures with central and radial dots – they can be relatively easily mistaken for large platelets. This organism is usually found in CKCSs and dachshunds, and usually associated with an inherited immune disorder.

> **Key points**
>
> **Respiratory washes**
> - Macrophages are normally present in the lower respiratory tract, but the presence of increased numbers or, particularly, increased activation, aids a diagnosis of macrophagic inflammation
> - Keratinised squamous epithelial cells and mixed morphology bacterial organisms are suggestive of oropharyngeal contamination
> - It is sometimes difficult to distinguish between neutrophils and eosinophils on airway preparations
> - Use of corticosteroids prior to sampling will drastically reduce eosinophil numbers on washes

Lung

Direct lung aspirates are relatively low-risk and often rewarding, although generally more so for neoplastic lesions than inflammatory (the opposite of respiratory washes). As with other locations (particularly the prostate/bladder), some studies have found a risk of tumour implantation along the line of sampling, and this slight

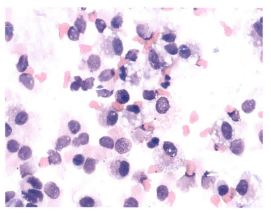

Fig 9.15 Increased activated macrophages; most of the macrophages have abundant vacuolated cytoplasm (×1000)

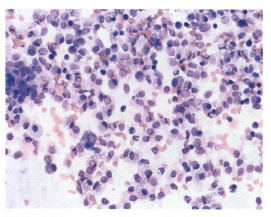

Fig 9.16 Macrophagic inflammation in respiratory wash; increased numbers of highly vacuolated macrophages (×100)

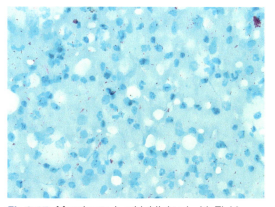

Fig 9.17 *Mycobacterium* highlighted with Ziehl Neelsen stain (purple rod-shaped structures) on feline respiratory wash (×500)

risk must be weighed against the diagnostic utility. Pneumothorax is extremely unlikely using needles of cytologically-appropriate gauge.

'Normal' findings

Typical lung aspirates have low cellularity, mostly comprising scattered small clusters of epithelial cells. These cells usually appear cuboidal to columnar, rather than the ciliated columnar epithelial cells present on washes, as they represent the terminal alveolar epithelial cells. Aspirates often also contain low numbers of macrophages, sometimes activated, as well as small amounts of blood (and associated leukocytes, usually neutrophils) and occasional small sheets of mesothelium.

Given the typically poor cellular harvest of lung aspirates, increased cellularity alone can raise the cytologist's suspicion of a pathological process. It is sometimes challenging to distinguish between sheets of epithelioid macrophages and epithelial cells within lung aspirates; in general, very highly cellular aspirates of cells which appear predominantly epithelial are more likely to represent neoplasia such as a carcinoma rather than normal anatomy or inflammation.

Neoplasia

The most common neoplastic lesions aspirated from the lung are discussed below.

Metastatic neoplasia

Neoplasm type: variable
Age: variable
Gross appearance: variable
Species/breed predispositions: common in dogs and cats
Cytological appearance/further comments: metastatic disease is more common than primary neoplasia in lung aspirates – the lungs are a frequent site of metastasis for many neoplasms, including many carcinomas, haemangiosarcoma, osteosarcoma, and other high-grade tumours.

Despite this, in the author's experience, metastatic neoplasia is less commonly sampled as it is more typical to sample the primary lesion, or the primary lesion alongside the lungs. If only lung masses are present, then primary lung neoplasia is more likely (see below).

The cytological appearance of metastatic lesions is similar to their appearance in the primary lesion. It is often challenging to discern the cell of origin of metastatic neoplasia but close examination and the basic morphology of different cell types (see page 72, Table 4.2) will often at least narrow down the possibilities.

Primary pulmonary carcinoma (FIG 9.18, 9.19)

Neoplasm type: epithelial
Age: middle-aged to older (slightly younger in cats)
Gross appearance: single or diffuse masses throughout lungs
Species/breed predispositions: slightly more common in cats
Cytological appearance/further comments: primary neoplasia is less common than metastatic disease within the lungs, but of these, primary pulmonary carcinomas are the most common, and these lesions are perhaps more commonly sampled than metastatic disease.

Cytologically, these lesions usually exfoliate well; indeed, the increased cellularity of these aspirates compared to normal lung samples raises some concern for neoplasia by itself. The cells are cuboidal to columnar and often arranged in papillary (finger-like) clusters of cells, sometimes appearing surprisingly bland cytologically; atypical features can vary from mild anisokaryosis to much more obviously atypical features. They are generally interspersed with low to moderate numbers of activated macrophages.

Other neoplasms

Any part of lung tissue can potentially become neoplastic, and primary lung sarcomas, adenomas or

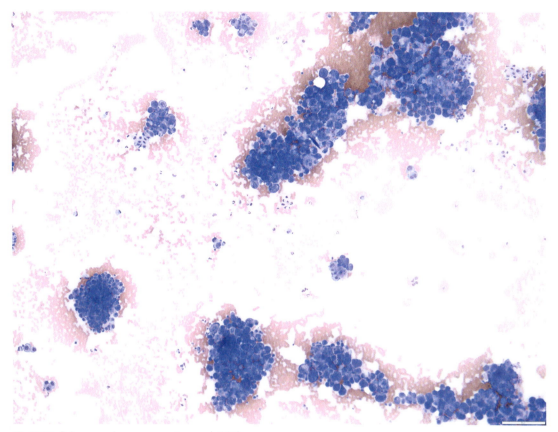

Fig 9.18 Primary pulmonary carcinoma (×100)

other tumours sometimes occur. They are, however, much rarer than primary carcinomas.

Inflammation

Inflammatory types and causes are similar to those from washes (see page 222); infectious organisms are slightly less likely to be present but can sometimes be found, especially in granulomas caused by *Mycobacterium*. As with washes, the presence of high numbers of activated macrophages from a granuloma-like lesion in a cat should raise some concerns for mycobacterial infection, and close examination for negative-staining organisms (see page 114) and/or ZN stain should be considered, as well as the possibility of zoonosis from the patient and samples.

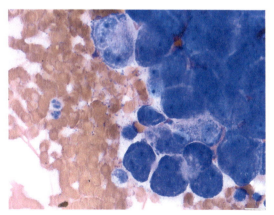

Fig 9.19 Primary pulmonary carcinoma (×1000)

Accidentally Sampling Through the Diaphragm

When an unusual population of epithelial cells is found on lung aspirates with a bland appearance (i.e. uniform size and shape) but with more cytoplasm than expected for pulmonary epithelium, one potential explanation to consider is accidental sampling of the liver through the diaphragm. The liver extends much more cranially than the last rib, and this sampling error is surprisingly easy.

Hepatocytes appear similar to those directly aspirated from the liver (see page 186), and great care must be taken when interpreting the presence of a neoplasm when there are cells resembling well-differentiated hepatocytes. If blue-green cytoplasmic pigment is present, aspiration of the liver is confirmed. An alternative explanation for hepatocytes unexpectedly appearing in aspirates from the thoracic cavity is diaphragmatic herniation of the liver.

Chapter 9 – take home messages

- Primary bacterial rhinitis is uncommon in both dogs and cats.
- Squamous epithelial cells, mixed bacteria and (particularly) *Conchiformibius* on respiratory samples is suggestive of contamination from the oral cavity during sampling.
- Macrophagic inflammation can be difficult to diagnose on respiratory washes, but if found in cat samples it raises concern for *Mycobacterium*.
- Direct lung aspirates are usually poorly cellular; high numbers of epithelial cells raises suspicion for neoplasia.

Chapter 10

Lymph nodes, spleen and thymus

This chapter discusses the cytological evaluation of the easily accessible lymphoid organs for sampling – essentially, the lymph nodes and spleen. The spleen is also an organ of secondary haematopoiesis; evaluation of bone marrow, the primary site of haematopoiesis, is not discussed here. Bone marrow sampling is technically challenging, and cytological assessment of bone marrow involves detailed knowledge of haemopoietic cells. It is largely beyond the scope of in-house evaluation and, therefore, this textbook.

Lymph nodes

Lymph nodes are aspirated for a number of different reasons:

- assessing whether enlarged lymph nodes are neoplastic or hyperplastic/reactive
- assessing the type and (ideally) cause of inflammation, where present
- staging nearby neoplasms by checking for metastatic disease
- monitoring ongoing lymphoma.

Sampling

When peripheral lymph nodes are enlarged, sampling is relatively simple, although lymphocytes, particularly neoplastic lymphocytes, are fragile and often rupture during sampling or spreading. The preservation of samples from enlarged lymph nodes may be improved by sampling without suction (fenestration – see page 17) and by careful spreading of sampled material.

It is also worth considering that the mandibular lymph nodes are often exposed to a large variety of antigens originating in the oral cavity, and consequently they are often more reactive and slightly harder to assess than other nodes. When given a choice, aspirates from prescapular or popliteal nodes are generally preferable. When nodes are markedly enlarged, samples taken from the periphery, rather than the centre, often have improved preservation.

Internal lymph nodes usually require ultrasound or other imaging for accurate sampling. As always with the use of ultrasound-guided biopsy, care must be taken not to introduce too much contact gel into the sample, as it obscures cytological specimens and can ruin otherwise diagnostic preparations. Due to the more challenging sampling, internal lymph node samples often have lower cellularity and worse preservation, but their cytological appearance is otherwise the same as peripheral nodes.

Sampling of non-enlarged nodes (i.e. for staging of tumours) is much more difficult, as the nodes are not usually palpable and it is very common even for experienced clinicians to sample fat (perinodal adipose tissue) or salivary glands (instead of mandibular nodes) instead of procuring a decent lymphoid harvest.

When multiple lymph nodes are enlarged, then sampling of multiple nodes spanning the diaphragm is recommended, to assess whether all nodes are enlarged for the same reason, and to help stage neoplasia such as lymphoma, where present.

Facial lymph nodes

Samples from the facial (or 'buccal') lymph nodes are relatively common, mostly because only a small percentage of dogs (9%) and no cats have them. When present, they are found over the nose, slightly more than midway between the medial commissure of the eye and the nasal planum (Fig 10.1). When aspirates from unexpected growths in this region yield a harvest of mixed and mostly small lymphocytes, it is very likely that a reactive facial lymph node has been sampled.

'Normal' lymph nodes

Normal cytological findings

It is worth spending some time discussing the appearance of a 'normal' (that is, non-neoplastic, non-inflamed) lymph node, as the assessment of lymph node samples depends as much on the balance of cells as their cytological appearance. Familiarity with the normal proportion of cells is very important to rapidly identify where changes are present.

As with other areas of cytology, a stepwise and logical approach greatly aids evaluation of lymph node aspirates – first assess the lymphoid population, and then concentrate on non-lymphoid cells.

Lymphoid component

Although lymphocytes can be classified into multiple different categories and subdivisions (i.e. *centrocytes*, *immunoblasts* etc.), from a practical perspective the most useful task is to assess the proportions of small, intermediate and large lymphocytes.

It is also important to assess whether the lymphocytes are atypical or morphologically unremarkable (see page 86 on lymphoma for examples). In some cases, differential count of these cells may be helpful to completely assess the population, although uneven spread of cells and difficulty in absolutely accurately assessing cell size in densely packed preparations limits the usefulness.

As discussed above, sampling a 'normal' lymph node is challenging; almost all aspirates examined by cytologists are actually from enlarged nodes. Regardless, aspirates from a non-inflamed, non-reactive and non-neoplastic node should contain mostly lymphocytes, and these lymphocytes should be mostly small (Fig 10.2).

Small lymphocytes have a minimalist aesthetic. They basically contain as small a nucleus as it is possible to have which contains all the genetic material of the patient tightly compacted into a small dense dot, as well as a thin rim of pale blue cytoplasm, and that's it. When people complain that cytology involves 'Just looking at little blue dots', they're complaining about small lymphocytes. They have nuclei that are only just bigger than a red blood cell (about 1.5 red blood cells in diameter, in fact, or smaller than a neutrophil), but their strength is in their potential. Within their ranks they have the capacity to react to practically any possible protein sequence that can ever find its way into a living organism.

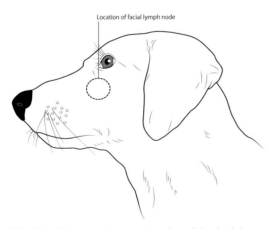

Fig 10.1 Diagram showing location of the facial lymph node

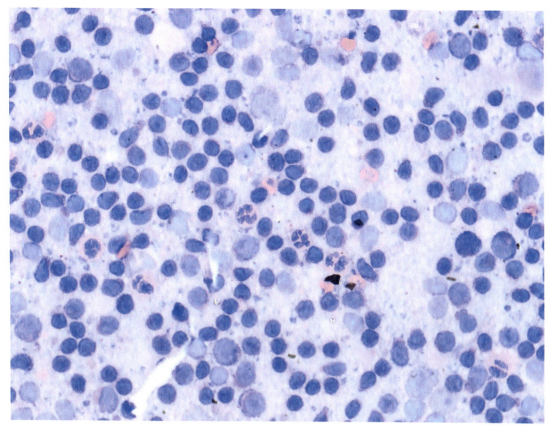

Fig 10.2 Small lymphocytes, slightly smaller than neutrophils (×1000)

The majority of lymphocytes within a node are immature and naive, waiting for the protein sequence that is specific for their near-unique reception – the key that unlocks them. This is why most cells in a 'normal' lymph node are 'unremarkable' small lymphocytes. Stated percentages vary but for a normal node, 70% or more of lymphocytes should be small (although if *all* the lymphocytes are small, this is a concern – see small cell lymphoma on page 240, below).

Intermediate and large lymphocytes should also be present – these are cells which have been exposed to their longed-for antigen and that are in the process of maturing. Intermediate cells have nuclei that are roughly the size of a neutrophil and have slightly more 'open' chromatin (slightly paler; as nuclei become more active and proteins are transcribed from loops of DNA, the chromatin unwinds and becomes less dense – the paler the nucleus of a cell is, the more active it is).

Large lymphocytes, which should be even less common than intermediate cells, have nuclei that are larger than a neutrophil. They have more open chromatin and occasional nucleoli (see page 31) may also be present. They often have more deeply-blue cytoplasm (often indicating protein synthesis and again an indication of a more active cell) (Fig 10.3).

Plasma cells should also be present (see page 68, Fig 4.18); these are the final mature stage of B-lymphocytes, and the cells which produce antibodies. They have a distinctive appearance and are a sign that normal follicular activity (B cells maturing from small lymphocytes into

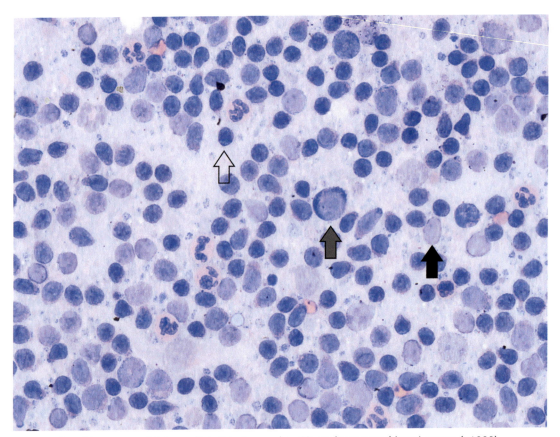

Fig 10.3 Small (open arrow), intermediate (black arrow) and large (grey arrow) lymphocytes (×1000)

plasma cells) is occurring within the sampled node (Fig 10.4). Occasional Mott cells can also be seen (see page 71, Fig 4.21) – these are 'constipated' plasma cells, containing large clumps of immunoglobulins (known as 'Russell bodies'). When found in low numbers, they are pretty but cytologically not significant (Fig 10.5).

> **Key point**
>
> - A 'normal' lymph node contains a mixed and predominantly small population of lymphocytes.

Non-lymphoid component

Other 'normal' resident nucleated cells of lymph nodes include 'tingible body' macrophages (activated macrophages containing phagocytosed cellular debris) (Fig 10.6); these are more commonly found accompanying lymphoma (as neoplastic lymphocytes tend to be more fragile),

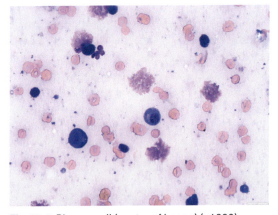

Fig 10.4 Plasma cell (centre of image) (×1000)

Lymph nodes, spleen and thymus | Chapter 10

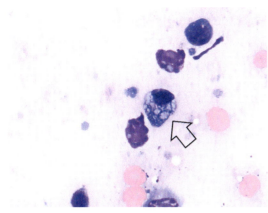

Fig 10.5 Mott cell (open arrow) (×1000)

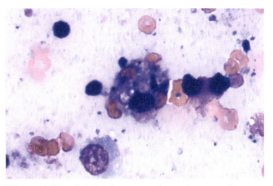

Fig 10.6 Tingible body macrophage (centre of image) containing phagocytosed erythrocyte and debris (×1000)

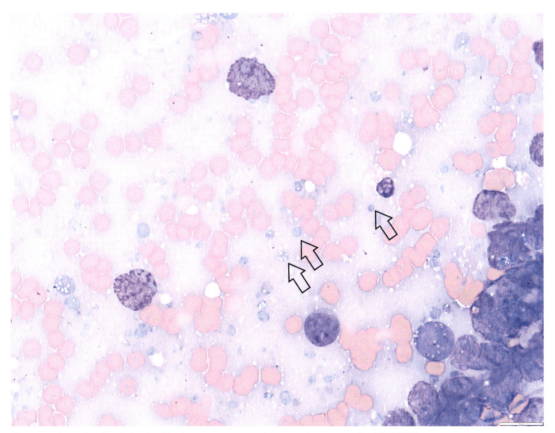

Fig 10.7 Lymphoglandular bodies (open arrows and many other examples) (×1000)

but low numbers are often seen in otherwise unremarkable lymph nodes.

Lymph node aspirates also frequently contain high numbers of 'lymphoglandular bodies' – these are small irregular pale grey fragments of cytoplasm stripped from the fragile lymphocytes (Fig 10.7). When observed in the presence of high numbers of unidentifiable cells, lymphoglandular bodies strongly suggest (but don't absolutely confirm) that the ruptured cells were once lymphocytes. Given that they are not completely specific to lymphocytes, however, some pathologists prefer the term 'cytoplasmic fragments' instead.

Other cells, such as other leukocytes, epithelial or mesenchymal cells, are not expected to be found in significant numbers within 'normal' lymph nodes.

Reactive lymph node

'Reactive' lymph nodes are those which have been exposed to antigens in excess of 'normal', and which have enlarged in response to increased blood flow, antigen traffic, and enlargement and expansion of the resident lymphocyte population. Reactive lymph nodes occur due to nearby inflammation, infection, necrosis or other forms of damage; the crucial cytological distinction is that these nodes are not enlarged due to the presence of neoplastic lymphocytes.

Reactive lymph nodes are like normal lymph nodes, only more so. That is, they should contain a mixed population of lymphocytes, similar to above, but the cell population will be *more* mixed than previously. Small lymphocytes are still the most prominent cell, but as more lymphocytes mature, the proportion of small lymphocytes decreases, with a concurrent expansion of intermediate and large cells, and increased numbers of plasma cells (Fig 10.8). Even in a very reactive lymph node (Fig 10.9), however, small lymphocytes are unlikely to drop significantly below 60% of the lymphocytes present. Inflammation and melanin incontinence (see below) may also be present).

There are many causes for reactivity or hyperplasia of nodes; the most common include draining sites of inflammation or neoplasia. Generalised lymphadenopathy is not exclusive to lymphoma – it is also seen with generalised or systemic inflammation (such as FIV, leishmania) and immune-mediated disease. In fact, in feline patients (unlike dogs), generalised lym-

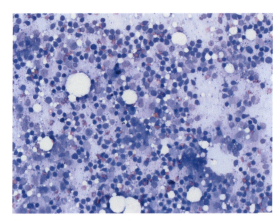

Fig 10.8 Reactive lymph node with expanded intermediate and large lymphocytes; note the mixed nature of the lymphoid harvest. Melanin pigment is also present scattered throughout the background (×500)

phadenopathy is more commonly associated with inflammation than with lymphoma.

Melanin incontinence

This term, despite the peculiar mental images it may produce, actually refers to the presence of melanin within lymph nodes. It is a consequence of inflammation in pigmented areas such as the skin or the mouth. The melanin is visible as small dark pigment granules scattered (sometimes liberally) throughout the specimens, and occasionally phagocytosed within macrophages (Fig 10.10). It is a relatively common finding in nodes draining areas of dermatitis. It can be a concerning discovery when examining lymph nodes for the staging of malignant melanomas but it is not, in itself, evidence of metastatic disease.

Neoplasia

Lymphoma is the most commonly encountered neoplasm in lymph nodes and, indeed, one of the most commonly encountered in many locations. For this reason, the following section on lymphoma is more detailed than many other neoplasms discussed previously.

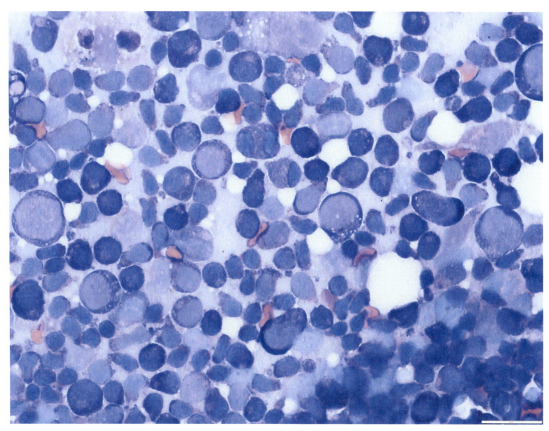

Fig 10.9 Markedly reactive lymph node (×1000); very mixed population of lymphocytes as well as plasma cells, a Mott cell and a dividing binucleate cell (×1000)

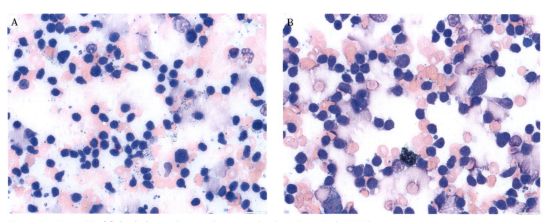

Figs 10.10a and b Melanin incontinence in a reactive lymph node (×1000)

Lymphoma (FIG 10.11)

Lymphoma (interchangeably termed *lymphosarcoma*) is caused by uncontrolled clonal expansion of lymphocytes; because the neoplastic cells are clones, they are morphologically similar. For many neoplasms, a population of cells displaying marked differences to each other raises significant concerns for malignancy, whereas with

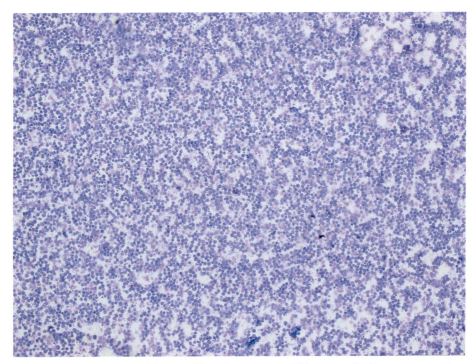

Fig 10.11 Low power appearance of large cell lymphoma; even at this power, the homogenous nature of the lymphocytes can be appreciated (×100)

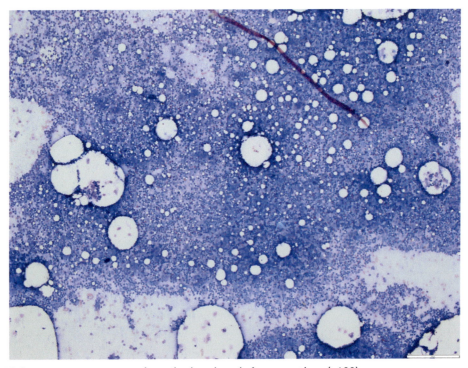

Fig 10.12 Low power appearance of reactive lymph node for comparison (×100)

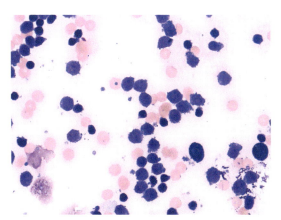

Fig 10.13 Lymphoma (large monomorphic cells) interspersed with small lymphocytes (×1000)

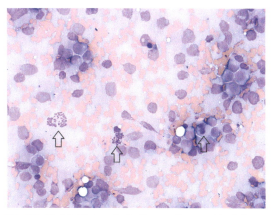

Fig 10.14 Multiple mitotic figures (two on the left ruptured but recognisable) in lymphoma (×500)

lymphoma, a population of lymphocytes that appear nearly identical, rather than the mixed pattern found in reactive nodes (Fig 10.12), raises the cytologist's suspicion of cancer.

The many sub classifications of lymphoma which have been described are beyond the scope of this chapter. The majority of them do not have specific treatment protocols currently developed for them, and are mainly useful for prognostic purposes (those interested are directed to the *Veterinary Pathology* article on classification of canine malignant lymphomas according to the World Health Organization criteria (*Valli* et al., 2011)).

For practical in-house purposes, the important thing is to recognise that a homogenous population of lymphocytes, particularly when plasma cells and other indications of reactivity are absent or greatly reduced, is consistent with lymphoma. This is relatively straightforward when the neoplastic cells are large and in high numbers but can be more challenging in early disease when mixed with non-neoplastic cells (Fig 10.13), or when the cells are small (see following section).

Small cell versus large cell lymphoma and mitotic index

Although it can be challenging to distinguish between lymphoma subtypes, the size of the neoplastic cells is often (but not always) an indication of the grade of the tumour – in general, the larger the cell, the higher the grade of the tumour. Lymphocytes are classified as small, intermediate and large, but 'intermediate cell lymphoma' is not a useful cytological interpretation.

The cytologist's task is to assess whether the cells are mostly small to intermediate (roughly smaller than or the same size as a neutrophil), in which case a lower-grade tumour may be a consideration, or intermediate to large (the same size as a neutrophil or larger), in which case a higher-grade tumour is more likely.

Mitotic figures are also a strong indication of the grade – increased mitotic figures almost always correlate with a higher-grade tumour (Fig 10.14). The author is, as ever, wary of a specific definition for 'increased mitotic figures' as cellularity is variable on cytological samples, but Raskin (see references) has suggested the following scheme:

Count the mitotic figures in 10 highly cellular fields using 40× or 50× objective.
<three Low mitotic index
Three to five Moderate mitotic index
>five High mitotic index

Large cell lymphoma (FIG 10.15)

Diffuse large cell lymphoma is the most common lymphoma observed in dogs – clinically,

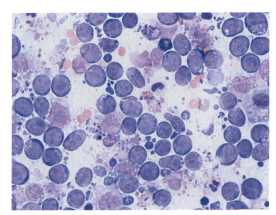

Fig 10.15 Large cell lymphoma; the lymphocytes are dominated by a population of large cells (>2.5 erythrocytes) with dispersed chromatin and multiple prominent nucleoli, as well as multiple small clear cytoplasmic vacuoles. There are also bare nuclei and a single macrophage (centre right) (×1000)

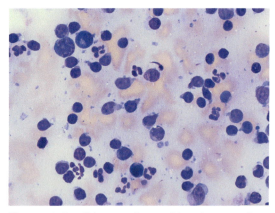

Fig 10.16 Small-intermediate cell lymphoma; cells have slightly atypically clumped chromatin, and frequent hand mirror forms; note there are also occasional plasma cells (upper left) – although plasma cells suggest reactivity, they do not exclude lymphoma (×1000)

the disease generally presents as generalised lymphadenopathy, and cytologically the specimens contain >30% (and often >50%) monomorphic large lymphocytes, usually with open or 'dispersed' chromatin, and frequently with prominent nucleoli. Mitotic figures may be increased.

Small cell lymphoma (FIG 10.16)

Clonal expansions of small lymphocytes are much more challenging to identify cytologically – the cells often appear as unremarkable small lymphocytes, although they are often slightly larger than typical small cells, and occasionally have slightly more open or clumped chromatin patterns. High numbers of uropods ('hand mirror' lymphocytes, with a tapering cytoplasmic projection) are concerning but not absolutely exclusive for lymphoma (as certain types of hyperplasia also produce this pattern). As above, high numbers of small lymphocytes with limited evidence of reactivity (i.e. very few intermediate to large cells, reduced or no plasma cells) raise suspicion for lymphoma.

A subset of small cell lymphoma – T-zone lymphoma – is 'indolent' – these cells multiply and spread very slowly, which has a number of consequences. Firstly, survival times are often longer, and secondly, these tumours are much less responsive to chemotherapy, although there appear to be variants of this disease that behave more aggressively, not as indolent as first thought.

T-zone lymphoma appears cytologically as a monomorphic population of small to intermediate cells with high numbers of uropods (Fig 10.17), and often occurs initially in a single markedly enlarged lymph node, usually the mandibular node.

B-cells versus T-cells

B lymphocytes and T lymphocytes are named for the location in which they were first discovered (the Bursa (in avians) and the Thymus, respectively). They have different functions within the body (B-cells produce antibodies, whereas T-cells are involved in cell-mediated immunity, as well as modifying and suppressing immune responses, although this is an oversimplification).

From the perspective of general practice, the question of whether lymphoma is of B-cell or T-cell lineage is relevant, as B-cell lymphoma is often slightly less aggressive than T-cell (not always – see T-zone lymphoma, above), and

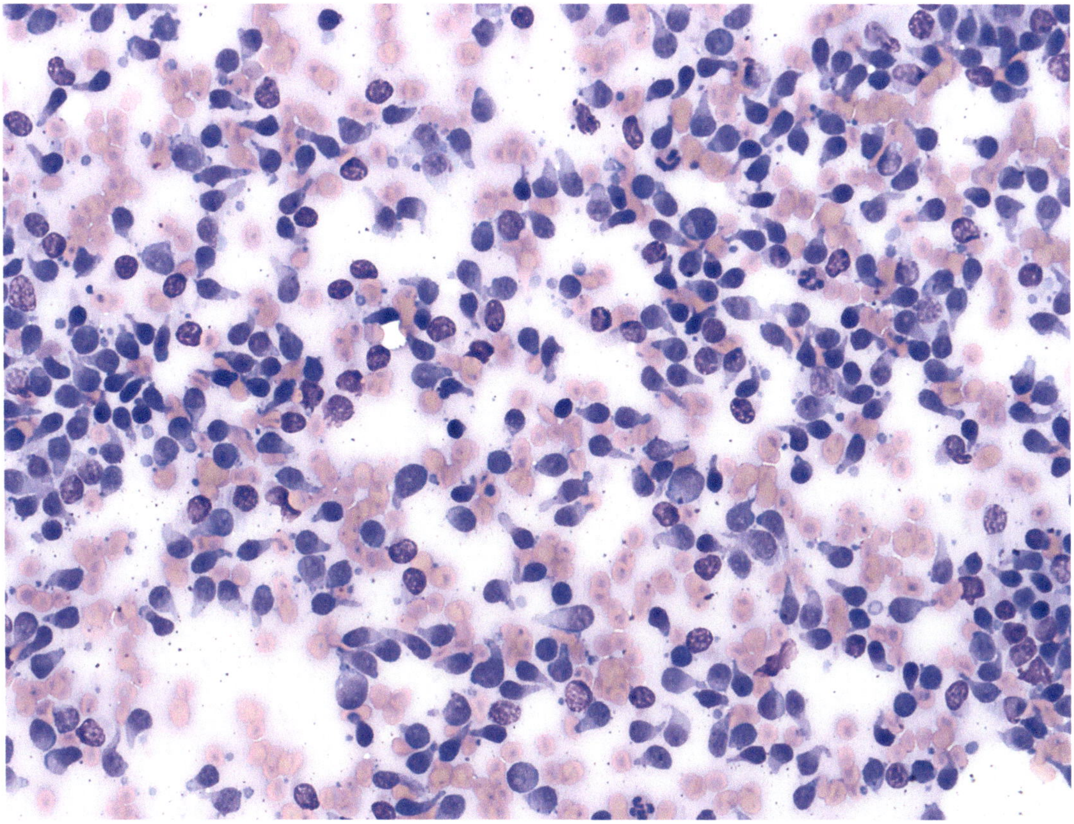

Fig 10.17 T-zone lymphoma; cells are smaller or the same size as a neutrophil and have frequent uropods (a triangular cytoplasmic projection – their shape is slightly reminiscent of hand mirrors) (×500)

different chemotherapy protocols have been developed for the different types of lymphoma. Unfortunately, however, it is difficult to be confident about the lineage of lymphocytes cytologically. There are some features which are more associated with B-cells: specifically, the presence of rounded nuclei, deeply basophilic (blue) cytoplasm and a prominent clear area next to the nucleus (representing the Golgi apparatus) (Fig 10.18). In contrast, T-cells are more associated with eccentric and more polygonal/amorphous nuclei, paler cytoplasm and uropods (hand mirror forms) (Fig 10.19). The features are not entirely reliable, however.

Cytoplasmic granulation is usually a clear indication of T-cell (or NK-cell) origin, and if most cells have granules then this is likely, but the absence of granules does not exclude T-cell origin, and the author has even experienced low numbers of small granules in confirmed B-cell lymphoma. Further testing is required for confident assessment of lymphoma lineage.

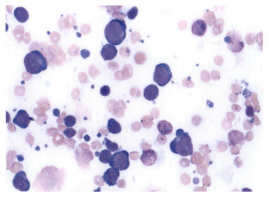

Fig 10.18 B-cell lymphoma (confirmed with immunocytochemistry)

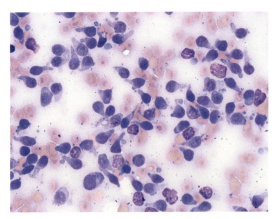

Fig 10.19 T-cell lymphoma (confirmed with immunocytochemistry)

Other neoplastic features (FIG 10.20)

Atypical lymphocyte features are less common in lymphoma than in other neoplasms, but when present and particularly when replicated many times across the observed cell population raise concerns for neoplasia. Such features include:

- Atypical mitotic figures
- Irregular, convoluted or 'cleaved' nuclei
- Binucleate or multinucleate cells
- Prominent cytoplasmic vacuolation (in the author's experience, this seems especially common in large cell intestinal lymphoma in cats)

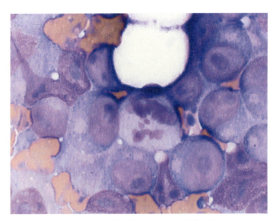

Fig 10.20 Atypical mitotic figure with 'lag' chromosomes (found individually rather than part of the bipolar cell spindle (×1000)

- Prominent cytoplasmic granulation (particularly when granules are large and irregular – in cats, this raises concern from *large granular lymphoma*, a highly aggressive variant which again originates in the gastrointestinal tract) (Fig 10.21).

Further testing for lymphoma

Several further tests are available for lymphoma, either to confirm the diagnosis in more challenging cases, or to further characterise the neoplasm.

PARR (**P**CR for **A**ntigen **R**eceptor **R**earrangement) can be performed on pre-stained slides and can confirm the presence of a clonal (as opposed to mixed) population of cells. The presence of clonal lymphocytes raises strong suspicion for lymphoma, although a negative result does not entirely rule it out. Although reports include which receptor (B or T cell) has undergone clonal expansion, it is most useful in identifying the presence of a neoplasm rather than identifying the lineage of a tumour (as cells can be genetically identified as B-cells but phenotypically express T-cell behaviour).

Immunophenotyping (such as immunocytochemistry, which again can be performed in some labs on pre-stained preparations) identifies the surface markers on cells, and so is more useful to confirm the neoplasm's lineage (i.e. B or T cell). Non-lymphoid markers can also be assessed, for tumours which are hard to distinguish from each other (such as myeloid leukaemia versus lymphoma, histiocytic sarcoma versus pleomorphic lymphoma, etc.).

Metastatic disease

Assessment for metastatic disease of an already identified neoplasm is a common reason for aspiration of lymph nodes. Metastasis is suspected when cells are present which are not normally observed within lymph nodes (such as epithelial cells) or when cells normally only present occasionally are found in high numbers (such as mast cells).

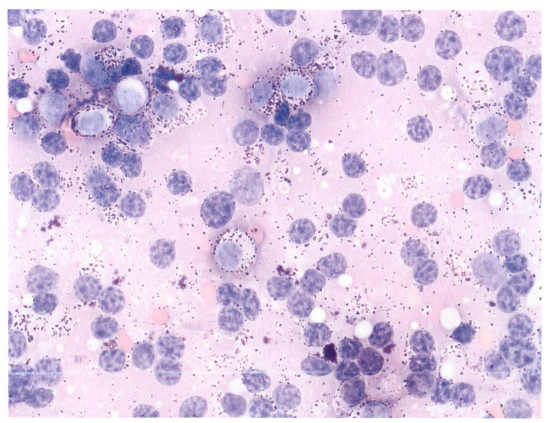

Fig 10.21 Large granular lymphoma, feline; the intact lymphocytes are packed with large and slightly irregular purple granules. The background is also filled with these granules from ruptured cells (×1000)

The cytological appearance of metastatic disease can vary from finding occasional small clusters of atypical cells to complete effacement of the node with atypical cells and no obvious lymphoid component. In the latter cases, it is important to know exactly where (anatomically) the aspirate was taken from, as it is no longer possible to confirm lymph node aspiration on the cytological appearance.

Common metastatic tumours within lymph nodes include carcinomas, mast cell tumours and melanomas – sarcomas are rarely found within lymph nodes (except via local invasion) as they usually metastasise via blood vessels rather than lymphoid channels. If high numbers of mesenchymal cells are found within a node, fibrosis may be more likely than a sarcoma, but, as ever in cytology, context is important. If there is no other inflammation and no obvious reason for fibrosis, then sarcoma remains a concern.

The presence of the invading neoplasm often produces a reactive population of lymphocytes and, occasionally, inflammation. Necrosis can also be found, although this is not specific for neoplasia as it can also be found in very inflamed nodes.

Mast cell tumour metastasis can be difficult to identify in the early stages, as low numbers of mast cells can be found in reactive nodes, particularly those draining areas of skin disease or non-metastatic mast cell tumours. Atypical features (such as reduced granulation, binucleation and pleomorphism) and/or the presence of mast cells in aggregates, rather than individually, should raise the cytologist's suspicion of metastatic disease (Figs 10.22, 10.23).

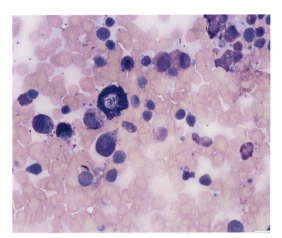

Fig 10.22 Mast cell tumour metastasis (×1000); note the irregular and often poorly granular mast cells, often found in small aggregates

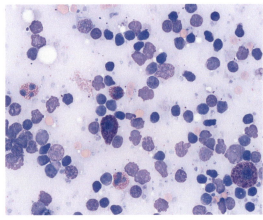

Fig 10.23 Normal mast cell trafficking for comparison (×1000); the mast cells are found individually, with central nuclei and regular granulation

Metastasis of melanoma (Fig 10.24) can also be challenging in the early stages, particularly if melanin incontinence (see page 68, Fig 4.18) is present; the presence of melanin alone is not in itself an indication of metastasis.

Carcinomas commonly metastasise to lymph nodes. Epithelial cells are not found in normal nodes, and so the presence of clusters of epithelial cells raises significant concern for carcinoma metastasis (Figs 10.25, 10.26). Note, however, that metastatic carcinomas usually display significant atypical features (see page XX).

The presence of relatively bland epithelium could reflect concurrent inadvertent aspiration of an adjacent site (such as the salivary glands in the submandibular lymph nodes (Fig 10.27), or liver, for abdominal lymph nodes). Abdominal lymph nodes can also contain sheets of mesothelium, which can appear very similar to epithelium. Finally, lymphocytes in nodes can occasionally clump together in a manner very similar to epithelial clusters (Figs 10.28 and 10.29); care should be taken in diagnosing metastatic disease based on poorly-preserved or unremarkable-appearing clusters.

Many other tumours can invade lymph nodes; other common tumours include histiocytic sarcoma (which appears similar to elsewhere in the body) and plasma cell tumours (Fig 10.30). Single cutaneous plasma cell tumours are unlikely to metastasise, but multiple myeloma can sometimes enter nodes.

Multiple myeloma is the malignant version of plasma cell neoplasia and, unusually, has a much blander cytological appearance than the more benign version; therefore, the presence of high numbers of unremarkable plasma cells within a lymph node raises some concern for this, although some areas of the node (the medullary chords) contain higher numbers of plasma cells, so further context (i.e. the presence of lytic bone lesions, hypercalcaemia, hyperglobulinaemia, peripheral cytopenias) is important, as is further investigation.

Inflammation

Actual inflammation within a lymph node is cytologically challenging to distinguish from the presence of increased leukocytes passing through the node on the way to or from an area of significant inflammation, but it is not usually necessary or clinically useful to do so. Practically, when leukocytes within a node (other than lymphocytes) appear in numbers much higher than expected for the amount of blood present, then inflammation either within or near the node is

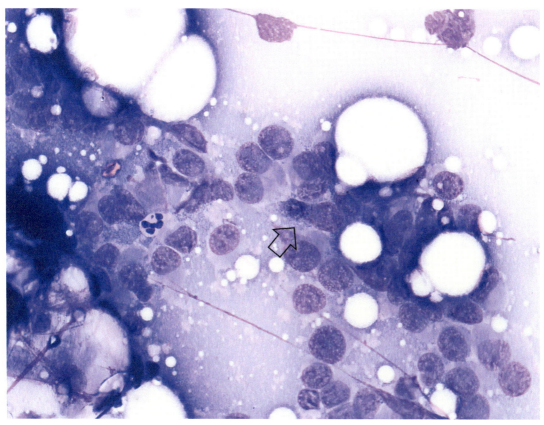

Fig 10.24 Melanoma metastasis to lymph node; rare intact cells contain scattered melanin pigment (open arrow) (×1000)

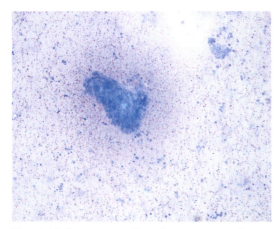

Fig 10.25 Squamous cell carcinoma metastasis to lymph node (×100)

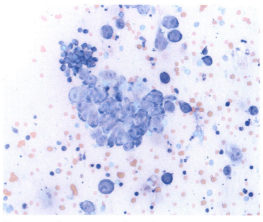

Fig 10.26 Squamous cell carcinoma metastasis to lymph node (×500)

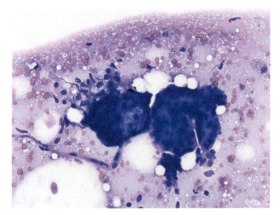

Fig 10.27 Salivary material from submandibular salivary gland aspirated whilst attempting to sample mandibular lymph node (×500)

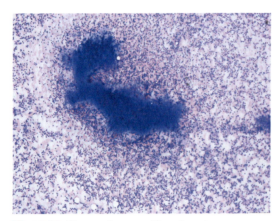

Fig 10.28 Clump of ruptured lymphocytes mimicking epithelium in a lymph node (×100)

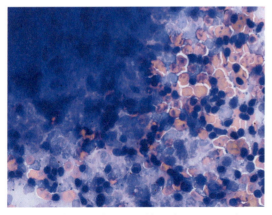

Fig 10.29 Clump of ruptured lymphocytes as above at high power; at the edge of the clump, bare nuclei and occasional intact lymphocytes are visible (×500)

likely, and the term 'lymphadenitis' is warranted (although this can only be absolutely confirmed on histopathology).

Neutrophilic lymphadenitis (FIG 10.31)

Neutrophils are usually the most numerous leukocyte in dogs and cats, which makes this pattern of inflammation especially difficult to interpret when there is a large amount of peripheral blood present.

As with other tissues, neutrophilic inflammation within a node is often caused by bacterial infection, either within the node itself or in an area drained by the node. Neutrophils may be degenerate or non-degenerate (see earlier section on neutrophilic inflammation), and bacteria may or may not be present. Other causes include generalised inflammation, immune-mediated disease or underlying neoplasia (again, either in a region drained by the node or metastatic within the node itself).

Eosinophilic lymphadenitis (FIG 10.32)

The most common reasons for eosinophilic inflammation within a node are hypersensitivity or external parasites. In peripheral nodes, it is often seen in nodes draining areas of skin disease (such as atopy or flea allergic dermatitis), and often accompanied with melanin incontinence.

In abdominal lymph nodes, the pattern is more commonly seen as a reflection of eosinophilic inflammation within the intestines (i.e. IBD).

Other causes include eosinophilic granuloma, hypereosinophilic syndrome (accompanied with a significant circulating eosinophilia) or as a paraneoplastic syndrome (most commonly due to mast cell tumours or lymphoma).

Macrophagic (granulomatous) lymphadenitis (FIG 10.33)

Low numbers of tingible body macrophages are normal residents within lymph nodes, but increased numbers, or the presence of multinucleate or epithelioid macrophages indicate

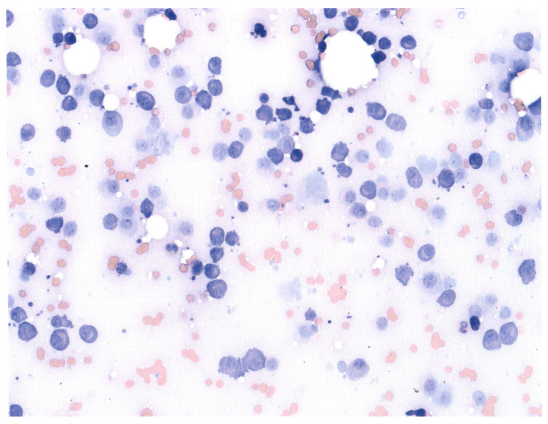

Fig 10.30 High numbers of plasma cells in the lymph node of a cat with myeloma-related disorder (×500)

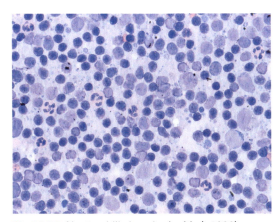

Fig 10.31 Neutrophilic lymphadenitis (×1000)

Fig 10.32 Eosinophilic lymphadenitis (×1000)

granulomatous or *'histiocytic'* inflammation. Causes in dogs include fungal infections, Leishmaniosis (see page 120), or immune-mediated disease – springer spaniels, in particular, are prone to a sterile (and probably immune mediated) granulomatous or pyogranulomatous inflammation, often affecting multiple nodes (Fig 10.34). The inflammation can be very

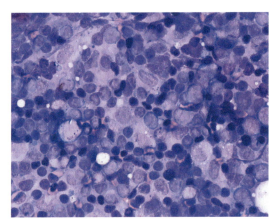

Fig 10.33 Macrophagic lymphadenitis (×1000)

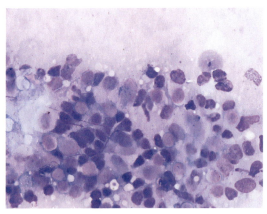

Fig 10.34 Sterile granulomatous lymphadenitis, springer spaniel (×1000)

> **Key points**
>
> **Lymph node**
> - A 'normal' lymph node contains a mixed and predominantly small population of lymphocytes (usually >70%)
> - Reactive lymph nodes have expanded intermediate and large lymphocytes and increased plasma cells; small cells are still usually >60% of total
> - In cats, generalised lymphadenopathy is more commonly associated with inflammation than with lymphoma
> - Lymphoma appears as a monomorphic homogenous population of lymphocytes, sometimes within a mixed population, sometimes replacing the mixed population
> - Increased cell size and increased mitotic figures are usually correlated with increased grade of lymphoma
> - Sarcomas very rarely metastasise to lymph nodes
> - Springer spaniels are prone to sterile (and probably immune mediated) granulomatous or pyogranulomatous inflammation, often affecting multiple nodes

marked and these nodes can often contain mesenchymal cells, sometimes in high numbers, which can initially appear similar to a sarcoma.

In cats, mycobacterial infection, viral infections (such as FIP, particularly abdominal nodes) or fungal infection are more commonly causes of granulomatous or pyogranulomatous inflammation.

Well-differentiated histiocytic sarcoma can sometimes be challenging to distinguish from granulomatous inflammation. Histopathological examination of nodes containing an otherwise unexplained large population of macrophages is worthwhile in susceptible dog breeds (e.g. flat-coat retrievers, Bernese mountain dogs, also Rottweilers and schnauzers).

Spleen

The spleen is a commonly sampled internal organ, partially because of the relative ease of sampling and ultrasound examination. Unfortunately, it is also a complex organ containing large amounts of lymphoid tissue and haemopoietic cells, as well as a large amount of blood – cytological samples from the spleen are generally very bloody and contain very mixed cells.

Nodular hyperplasia is common within it but challenging to distinguish from more sinister lesions via imaging, and thus many aspirates of nodular hyperplasia will find their way to the cytologist's desk. Because of all this, it is a rare splenic aspirate which clarifies a more generalised problem.

'Normal' appearance

As mentioned above, the most prominent feature of a splenic aspirate is blood, densely packed and sometimes containing large platelet clumps. Embedded within the blood, there should also be islands of stroma – splenic connective tissue. Cytologically, this appears as aggregates of mesenchymal cells as well as lymphocytes, low numbers of mast cells, and occasional macrophages. The overall appearance of stroma is indistinct but vaguely mesenchymal, studded with lymphocytes and ruptured purple blobs (mast cells) (Figs 10.35, 10.36).

Interspersed with the stroma are lymphocytes, mixed and mostly small, as with lymph nodes, as well as low numbers of intermediate lymphocytes and rare large lymphocytes, and plasma cells. Overall lymphocyte numbers may be quite low in 'normal' spleen due to the diluting effect of the blood. Neutrophils and occasional macrophages may also be present (Figs 10.37, 10.38).

Aspirates of completely normal appearing spleen are relatively uncommon, however – many samples contain evidence of extra-medullary haematopoiesis or lymphoid hyperplasia (see below).

Extra-medullary haematopoiesis (EMH)

A complicating factor of many splenic aspirates is the presence of extra-medullary haematopoiesis (EMH) – the formation of blood cells and platelets outside of the bone marrow. EMH can actually be observed in practically any tissue sampled, but it is most commonly seen in the spleen (and, occasionally, the liver).

Cytologically, extra-medullary haematopoiesis comprises early and late myeloid (white blood cell) and erythroid (red blood cell) precursors, as well as the giant-sized megakaryocytes, from whose creeping pseudopods platelets are born. Megakaryocytes are useful as they are easily visible on a low-power scan and alert the cytologist to the presence of EMH.

The myeloid line consists of everything from the large myeloblasts to mature neutrophils, and the erythroid line everything from large

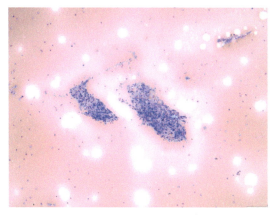

Fig 10.35 Splenic stroma, low power (×100)

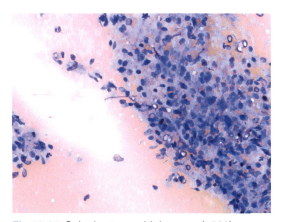

Fig 10.36 Splenic stroma, high power (×500)

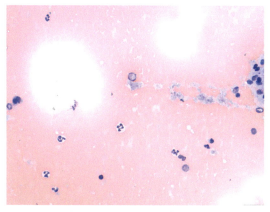

Fig 10.37 Mixed nucleated cells (neutrophils, small lymphocytes) in a typical splenic aspirate (×500)

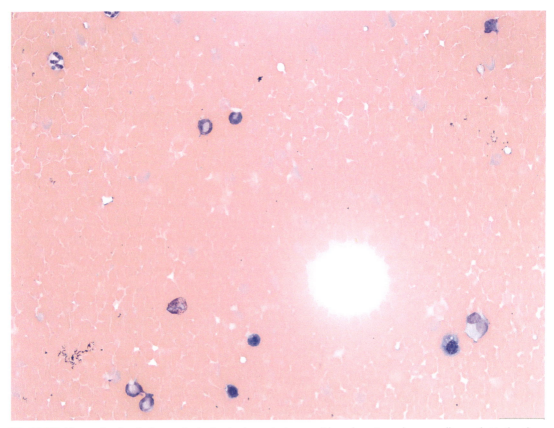

Fig 10.38 More mixed cells from a typical splenic aspirate: small lymphocytes, plasma cells, nucleated red blood cell (bottom of image) (×500)

erythroblasts to nucleated red blood cells and erythrocytes (Figs 10.39, 10.40, 10.41). The difficulty, cytologically, is that when EMH is present, it means that the cells are very mixed and it is challenging to definitively identify every cell present, let alone pick out a potentially atypical population.

Identifying all of the stages of the myeloid and erythroid lines is a specialist task, but here are some general principles.

- The proportions of the cell lines should be an inverse pyramid; that is, the later stages (neutrophils and nucleated red blood cells) should be most numerous, with progressively fewer cells down the line. Myeloblasts and erythroblasts should be the rarest cells and therefore the hardest to find.

- Myeloblasts and erythroblasts strongly resemble large lymphocytes, although there are a few differences: blastic cells usually have more prominent nucleoli than large lymphocytes; erythroblasts have deeply blue cytoplasm with very rounded central nuclei; myeloblasts have paler and more amorphic/polygonal nuclei, sometimes eccentric.
- Neither blastic population should have cytoplasmic granules (these occur later in development in the myeloid line, and not at all in the erythroid line).

EMH is a non-specific finding within the spleen and is rarely useful diagnostically.

Its presence can explain nodular lesions within the spleen, as they are likely to represent nodular hyperplasia. Markedly reactive spleens

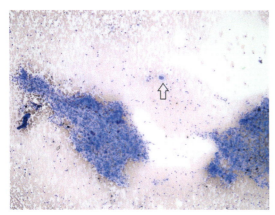

Fig 10.39 EMH in the spleen, low power, showing splenic stroma and a megakaryocyte (open arrow) (×100)

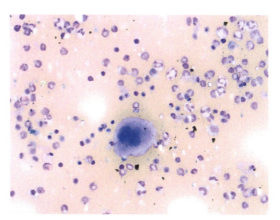

Fig 10.40 EMH in the spleen, high power, showing very mixed cells including a megakaryocyte (×500)

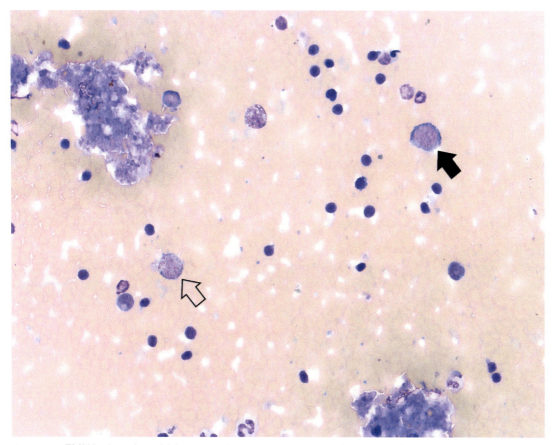

Fig 10.41 EMH in the spleen, high power, showing a promyelocyte (open arrow) and an erythroid precursor (black arrow) (×500)

can have very prominent EMH, with high numbers of blast cells which can raise significant concern for neoplasia. A diagnosis of round cell neoplasia or lymphoma must be made with care when significant EMH is present.

Lymphoid hyperplasia

Some splenic aspirates contain very high numbers of lymphocytes, often streaked towards the middle of the preparation and surrounded by blood (in contrast to the more even distribution of cells seen on lymph node aspirates). This generally indicates aspiration of an area of lymphoid hyperplasia, another explanation for nodular lesions observed via imaging.

In reactive spleens, the proportion of intermediate lymphocytes can be markedly increased – in some areas they can form the majority of nucleated cells (Figs 10.42, 10.43). These intermediate lymphocytes are often *marginal zone* lymphocytes, with a characteristic prominent large single nucleolus (10.44). It can be extremely difficult to distinguish between marked lymphoid hyperplasia with an expanded intermediate lymphoid population and marginal zone lymphoma (a relatively low-grade and often indolent lymphoma subtype – see below (page 254).

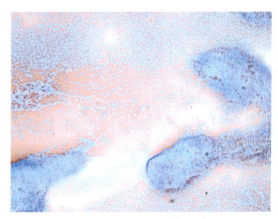

Fig 10.42 Lymphoid hyperplasia (×100)

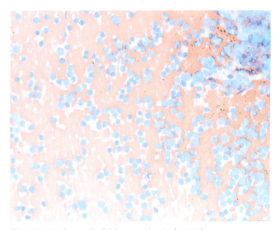

Fig 10.43 Lymphoid hyperplasia (×500)

Erythrophagia in the spleen

One of the functions of the spleen is the removal of old, damaged or other blood cells from the circulation. Consequently it is not uncommon to see red blood cells phagocytosed within macrophages, as well as occasional haemosiderin-laden macrophages (see page 98). The clinical significance of this is therefore uncertain as it is a normal function of the spleen, but when many macrophages are found containing phagocytosed erythrocytes and/or haemosiderin, it is likely to be an indication of increased red-cell turnover (this potentially supports a diagnosis of immune-mediated haemolytic anaemia, but it is not a specific finding.

Neoplasia

The most common splenic neoplasms are listed below. As elsewhere in this book, they are listed in rough order of commonality, with the most common tumours at the top of the list. The list is not exclusive but covers the neoplasms most likely to be encountered in practice.

Haemangiosarcoma (FIG 10.45)

Neoplasm type: mesenchymal
Age: middle-aged to older
Gross appearance: one or more variably-sized cavitated masses within splenic parenchyma
Species/breed predispositions: the most common splenic neoplasm in dogs; uncommon in cats.

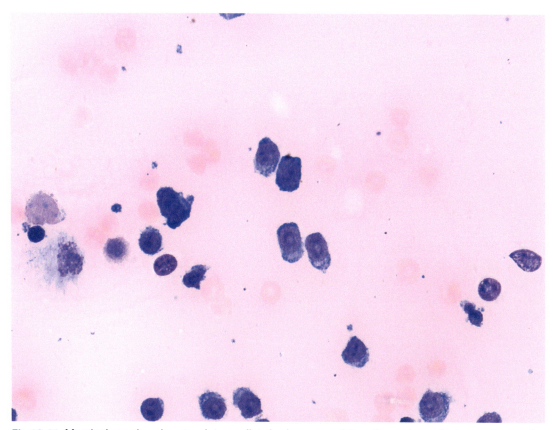

Fig 10.44 Marginal zone lymphocytes: intermediate in size, many of them have a large single prominent pale central nucleolus (×1000)

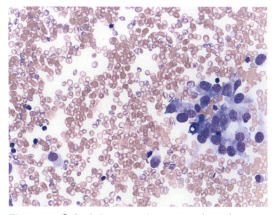

Fig 10.45 Splenic haemangiosarcoma (×500)

Labrador and German shepherd reportedly predisposed.
Cytological appearance/further comments: haemangiosarcoma can be challenging to diagnose cytologically as samples often contain large amounts of blood and relatively few neoplastic cells. The appearance is similar to elsewhere in the body (see page 147): low numbers of large blue angular mesenchymal cells, found individually or in aggregates.

It is also difficult to determine cytologically whether these lesions are primary or represent metastasis, but a diagnosis of haemangiosarcoma in the spleen should prompt a search for other lesions, particularly in the heart and liver.

Haematoma

Neoplasm type: see below
Age: any
Gross appearance: usually single variably-sized lesions within parenchyma

Species/breed predispositions: common in dogs, rare in cats

Cytological appearance/further comments: these lesions appear cytologically as blood as well as macrophages containing phagocytosed red blood cells and red-cell breakdown products such as haemosiderin (see page 98). They are not a true neoplasm but occur as a result of physical disruption to splenic vessels. Trauma, underlying neoplasia (such as haemangiosarcoma) and underlying hyperplasia (such as lymphoid hyperplasia) are all aetiological considerations. The main diagnostic challenge of these lesions is the difficulty distinguishing them from haemangiosarcoma via imaging, and often with cytology. Histopathology is often required when neoplastic cells (indicating haemangiosarcoma) are not evident cytologically.

Lymphoma (FIG 10.46)

Neoplasm type: round cell

Age: variable; can be quite young

Gross appearance: often diffuse enlargement

Species/breed predispositions: uncommon in cats, rare in dogs

Cytological appearance/further comments: lymphoma in the spleen is difficult to diagnose, due to the very mixed nature of normal splenic aspirates, and the fact that aspirates from reactive lymphoid hyperplasia often contain increased numbers of intermediate lymphocytes. As elsewhere in the body, the presence of a monomorphic, rather than mixed, population of cells, raises concern for lymphoma.

Marginal zone lymphoma: is an indolent (slow-growing) subtype found within the spleen, comprising increased numbers of intermediate cells with prominent round central

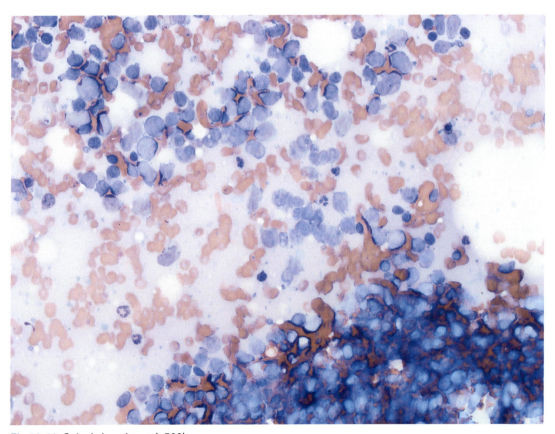

Fig 10.46 Splenic lymphoma (×500)

nucleoli. Unlike diffuse lymphoma, it is often present in small nodules, and is extremely difficult to distinguish cytologically from lymphoid hyperplasia. Further ultrasound monitoring of such lesions may be the most useful method of management, with further testing if the nodule grows or spreads.

Metastatic neoplasia (FIG 10.47, 10.48)
Neoplasm type: varies
Age: varies
Gross appearance: varies, often diffuse
Species/breed predispositions: varies
Cytological appearance/further comments: although the spleen has a large blood supply, metastasis is perhaps less common than may be expected compared with other organs. Lymphoid and myeloid lesions such as lymphoma (see above) and myeloid leukaemia often disseminate throughout the spleen, and primary lymphoma can also occur – these lesions are sometimes difficult to diagnose due to the mixed leukocytes present in normal splenic aspirates. As with lymph nodes, the presence of a monomorphic population of cells, rather than mixed, raises concern for neoplasia. Other metastatic tumours include mast cell tumours, multiple myeloma, carcinomas and mesenchymal tumours. Appearance is similar to elsewhere within the body.

Stromal sarcoma (FIG 10.49)
Neoplasm type: mesenchymal
Age: 3+
Gross appearance: usually large discrete masses
Species/breed predispositions: uncommon in dogs, rare in cats
Cytological appearance/further comments: this is a group of neoplasms including fibrosarcoma, myxosarcoma, liposarcoma and leiomyosarcoma; each individual subtype is rare but together they form a reasonable proportion of splenic primary tumours in dogs.

The cytological appearance is similar to other sarcomas elsewhere in the body (see page 78), although it can be challenging to distinguish normal stromal aggregates from neoplastic

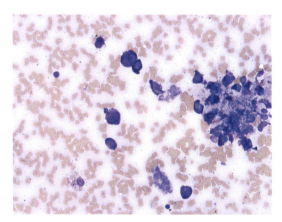

Fig 10.47 Mast cell tumour metastasis to the spleen (×500)

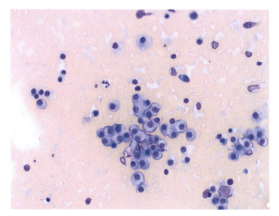

Fig 10.48 Plasma cell neoplasia, spleen (×500)

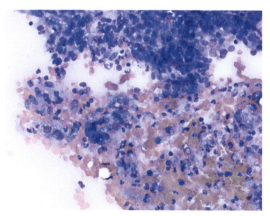

Fig 10.49 Stromal sarcoma (×500)

mesenchymal cells. In general, neoplastic mesenchymal cells are better-defined and more obviously comprise mesenchymal cells than the more indistinct splenic stroma.

Myelolipoma (FIG 10.50)

Neoplasm type: mesenchymal
Age: usually older
Gross appearance: vary from large single mass to smaller multiple masses
Species/breed predispositions: rare in both dogs and cats
Cytological appearance/further comments: these are rare benign lesions, usually splenic but occasionally found in other locations. Cytologically, they contain a mixture of both adipocytes and haemopoietic cells; they appear as a lipoma containing extra-medullary haematopoiesis. Excision, if required, is curative.

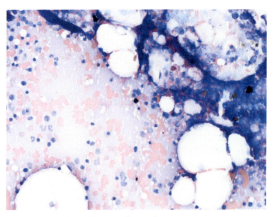

Fig 10.50 Myelolipoma (×500)

Splenitis (FIG 10.51)

Inflammation within the spleen is challenging to discern cytologically, as aspirates from non-inflamed spleens generally contain mixed

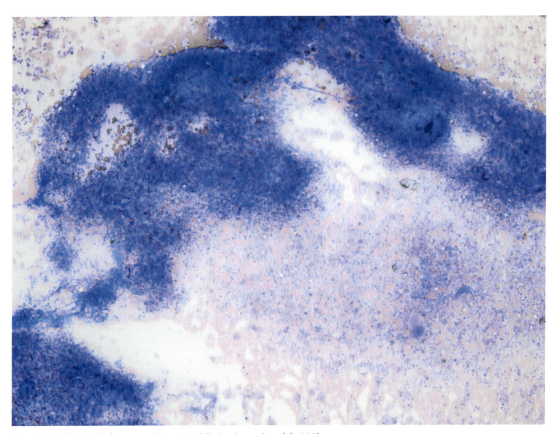

Fig 10.51 Splenitis (increased neutrophils in the spleen) (×500)

leukocytes, sometimes in high numbers, and the large amount of blood that is usually present makes it difficult to determine whether leukocytes originated in the blood or the spleen.

As with elsewhere in the body, one reliable indicator is the presence of neutrophils phagocytosed within macrophages, which confirms neutrophilic or neutrophilic/macrophagic inflammation.

Increased numbers of macrophages, particularly when they are activated (with abundant foamy cytoplasm) raises suspicion of granulomatous (macrophagic) inflammation, and a careful search of macrophages for infectious organisms (see chapter 5) is usually recommended in these cases, particularly in patients with history of travelling outside of the UK.

> **Key points**
>
> **Spleen**
> - Splenic aspirates are usually very bloody and contain very mixed nucleated cells
> - Extramedullary haematopoiesis is often present, complicating assessment
> - Splenic lymphoid hyperplasia often contains very increased intermediate marginal zone lymphocytes; it is very difficult to distinguish between lymphoid hyperplasia and marginal zone lymphoma
> - Splenitis is also hard to assess, but neutrophils phagocytosed by macrophages will confirm this

Thymus

The thymus, present in the cranial mediastinum, regresses with age, and so is very rarely sampled except when it is neoplastic. The main diagnostic challenge of masses in the cranial mediastinum is distinguishing between thymoma (a mostly surgical condition) and lymphoma (a mostly medical condition); both contain increased lymphocytes. Lymphoma appears similar as it does in other locations of the body. Thymoma is discussed below.

Thymoma and thymic carcinoma

Neoplasm type: epithelial
Age: middle-aged to older (usually 10+ years)
Gross appearance: appears on imaging as a mass in the cranial mediastinum, can be large and displace the heart caudally
Species/breed predispositions: uncommon in dogs and cats
Cytological appearance/further comments: thymomas are usually aspirated in an attempt to distinguish between masses in the cranial mediastinum; for such masses, the chief differentials are thymoma and lymphoma (in the cranial mediastinal lymph node).

This is why it is frustrating that, although thymoma is an epithelial tumour, it often contains high numbers of lymphocytes. In fact, lymphocytes are not uncommonly the most numerous cell present, with only small amounts of thymic epithelium (occasionally, no epithelium at all is found).

The epithelial cells in thymoma have moderate amounts of pale cytoplasm with small dense nuclei, usually with a single prominent nucleolus; the small clusters often resemble *epithelioid macrophages* (Fig 10.52, 10.53) (see page 68, Fig 4.15).

The associated material is often more distinctive than the epithelial cells. As discussed, thymoma aspirates often contain high numbers of lymphocytes, but the population is not quite like a reactive population, nor is it especially consistent with lymphoma. In thymoma, the lymphocytes are mixed but often *dimorphic* – that is, there are two populations of cells, mostly small lymphocytes but with a significant population of intermediate to large lymphocytes, usually with not much in between and not many more typical large lymphocytes. Plasma cells are only very rarely found, unlike reactive lymph nodes.

Thymoma aspirates also often contain significant numbers of mast cells. They are morphologically normal and found individually (rather

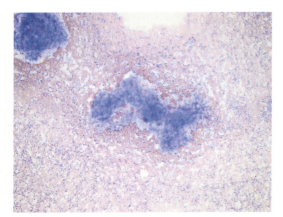

Fig 10.52 Cluster of epithelium in thymoma (×100)

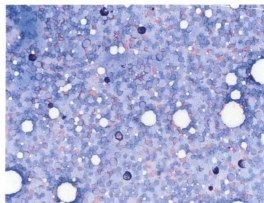

Fig 10.54 Thymoma without significant epithelium; note the increased mast cells; small and large lymphocytes are present with very few intermediate cells ('dimorphic population') (×500)

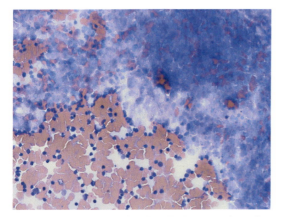

Fig 10.53 Cluster of epithelium in thymoma (×500)

than in groups); as many as 20 per ×50 HPF may be present.

On their own, none of these elements are completely specific – differentials for the various elements above include epithelioid macrophages, reactive lymph nodes, lymphoma, mast cell trafficking and mast cell tumour metastasis. Because of this, it is hard to confidently diagnose thymoma, especially when the epithelium is absent or rare, but the neoplasm can be strongly suspected when aspirates from a cranial thoracic mass yield dimorphic lymphocytes with few plasma cells and increased mast cells (Fig 10.54).

Thymic carcinoma is the malignant counterpart of thymoma. It is much rarer. Cytologically, it appears similar to thymoma, although the epithelium present displays often prominently atypical features (see page 92 for a general discussion of atypia).

Chapter 10 – take home messages

- Normal and reactive lymph nodes contain very mixed lymphocytes, most of which should be small.
- Lymphoma appears as a proliferation of monomorphic lymphocytes replacing the normal mixed appearance of nodes.
- Generalised lymphadenopathy in cats is more commonly associated with inflammation than neoplasia.
- As a general rule, larger neoplastic lymphocytes have a higher grade than smaller ones.
- Splenic aspirates can be hard to interpret due to the large amounts of blood, mixed harvest and frequent present of extra-medullary haematopoiesis.
- Thymoma aspirates often contain little (or no) epithelium, and often contain mostly lymphocytes and mast cells.

Chapter 11

Muscle, bone and synovial fluid

Bone and muscle are almost never sampled as a normal tissue; usually they are either inadvertently aspirated during sampling of another lesion, or directly sampled due to the presence of a lesion suspected to be neoplastic. Synovial fluid is usually sampled to assess the pattern of inflammation within it (most commonly to investigate the possibility of infection or immune mediated disease).

Muscle

'Normal' appearance

Muscle is a mesenchymal tissue. Skeletal muscle is much more commonly sampled than smooth muscle, although neither generally exfoliate well, in common with most other mesenchymal tissues. Skeletal muscle (see page 134) is deeply basophilic (blue) and is usually found in small aggregates, often with faint striations which are just visible on high-power examination (often more visible when slowly shifting in and out of focus) (Figs 11.1, 11.2). The nuclei in skeletal muscle should be nearly parallel with each other. Smooth muscle, in contrast, is paler blue than skeletal muscle and contains nuclei perpendicular to each other or present in a haphazard arrangement (Figs 11.3, 11.4).

Neoplasia

Primary muscle neoplasia is uncommon or rare in both dogs and cats, but muscle tumours can be aggressive when present. The muscle is also an uncommon site of metastatic disease, but local invasion of tumours occurs relatively frequently.

Skeletal muscle – rhabdomyoma and rhabdomyosarcoma

Neoplasm type: mesenchymal
Age: rhabdomyosarcoma – often very young patients (less than 1 year old)
Gross appearance: usually solitary mass lesion
Location: commonly around the head, especially laryngeal region
Species/breed predispositions: rare but seen more often in dogs; rhabdomyosarcoma usually seen, rhabdomyoma very rare in both species
Cytological appearance/further comments: rhabdomyosarcoma is the most common primary skeletal muscle tumour in dogs and cats, but it is still encountered only rarely. Although they

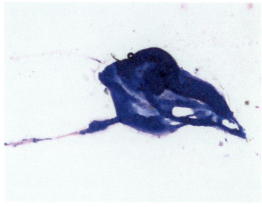

Fig 11.1 Skeletal muscle aggregate (low power) (×100)

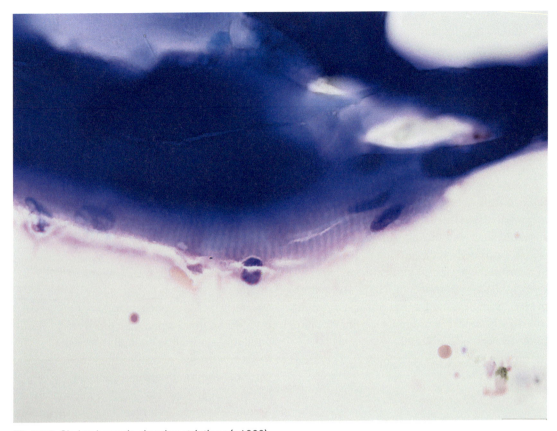

Fig 11.2 Skeletal muscle showing striations (×1000)

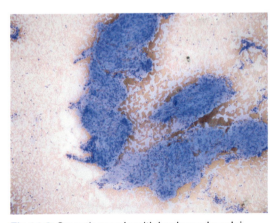

Fig 11.3 Smooth muscle with haphazard nuclei (×100)

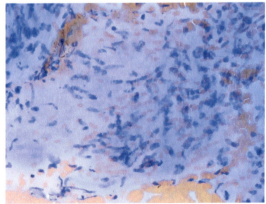

Fig 11.4 Smooth muscle (×500)

can occur in older patients, they are often seen in animals less than a year old.

Cytologically, they resemble other mesenchymal tumours, although they are often markedly pleomorphic and show multiple malignant features. Some cells may contain faint striations, and some multinucleate cells may contain nuclei lined up in a row, like peas in a pod ('strap cells'); these features can indicate to the cytologist that skeletal muscle was the origin of the neoplasm.

Rhabdomyomas are very rare, and more typically occur in adults, usually around the head and neck.

Cardiac muscle – haemangiosarcoma

Haemangiosarcoma is covered elsewhere (see page 147) but, although it is not a primary muscle tumour, it is worth considering that it is the most common neoplasm of cardiac muscle. Lymphoma and metastatic carcinomas can also be found on aspirates, although both are relatively uncommon.

Smooth muscle – leiomyoma and leiomyosarcoma (FIG 11.5)

Neoplasm type: mesenchymal
Age: usually older (10 years +)
Gross appearance: usually large single mass, can be multiple masses when metastasised
Species/breed predispositions: uncommon in dogs, rare in cats
Cytological appearance/further comments: leiomyosarcomas are more common than their benign counterparts, occurring most common in the gastrointestinal tract, in the female genital tract (usually the external genitalia), or, rarely, in the bladder. As with many mesenchymal tumours, these lesions often exfoliate poorly. Cytologically they strongly resemble other mesenchymal tumours and, in particular, are very challenging to distinguish from Gastro Intestinal Stromal Tumours (GISTs). Both GISTs and leiomyosarcomas can metastasise, often to the liver; histopathology is often required to distinguish between the possibilities.

Inflammation

Inflamed muscle sometimes exfoliates more readily than normal muscle. The cytological appearance is as may be expected: aggregates of muscle interspersed with inflammatory cells. The cytological challenge is often to associate the inflammation with muscle, as even though exfoliation may be better in inflamed muscle, the muscle aggregates are likely to be far less numerous than inflammatory cells.

Morphology of the muscle cells can be helpful; inflamed/degenerate muscle may appear more disorganised, and skeletal muscle can lose its characteristic striations and have overall smoother appearance. Neutrophilic inflammation is the most common, but inflammation within the muscle has similar causes to inflammation elsewhere (neutrophils for acute inflammation, macrophages for more chronic inflammation, lymphocytes in younger patients or with antigenic stimulation, eosinophils with hypersensitivity or parasitism – see page XX for a more general discussion of inflammation).

Bone

'Normal' appearance

As may be expected, normal bone is very poorly cellular; samples from the region of normal bone usually only harvest blood and scraps of debris. If a good cytological yield can be harvested from bone, then it is unlikely to be normal bone.

Bone remodelling

This is a relatively common finding in aspirates from lesions near or within bone. Cytologically,

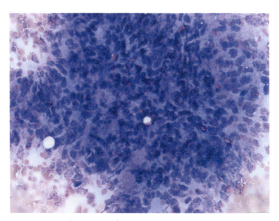

Fig 11.5 Leiomyoma/leiomyosarcoma – appearance is very similar to smooth muscle (z500)

aspirates comprise osteoblasts (mesenchymal cells which produce the mineralised bony matrix) and osteoclasts (large specialised multinucleate macrophages which break down bone and regulate the behaviour of the osteoblasts). The cytological appearance of both cells belies their origins.

Osteoblasts are caudate mesenchymal cells – that is, they have an oval shape with eccentric oval nuclei at one pole of the cell. The nuclei are also oval and are generally orientated perpendicular to the line of the cell (see picture). They have mid to deeply blue cytoplasm, similar to plasma cells and sometimes have a small clear area next to the nucleus (Fig 11.6), again similar to plasma cells (it can sometimes be challenging to distinguish between plasma cells and osteoblasts – the main differences is that osteoblasts are larger and much more oval, rather than the more rounded plasma cells).

Osteoblasts produce osteoid, which appears as small amounts of pink or faintly purple extra-cellular matrix (Fig 11.7), and it can sometimes also be visualised as small reddish granules within the cytoplasm of osteoblasts.

Osteoclasts are large multinucleate cells, often with a characteristic pink cytoplasm and many nuclei (Fig 11.8). Osteoclasts can be alarming at first glance as they can resemble neo-

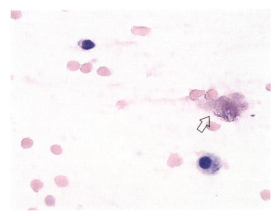

Fig 11.7 Osteoid (pink material, open arrow) with osteoblast and probable small lymphocyte (×1000)

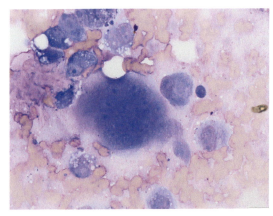

Fig 11.8 Osteoclast (×1000)

plastic cells (Fig 11.9); the biggest clue to their non-neoplastic nature is the nuclei within them; many neoplastic multinucleate cells have variably-sized nuclei (anisokaryosis), often markedly so, whereas osteoclasts have uniform-sized nuclei (typically 1.5–2 erythrocytes in diameter) no matter how many they have.

Bone remodelling is seen in cases where bone has been damaged and is repairing – it is therefore not a specific finding but can be seen secondary to trauma, other inflammation or neoplasia. It is a valuable but potentially misleading finding (as the large osteoclasts can initially be mistaken for neoplastic cells).

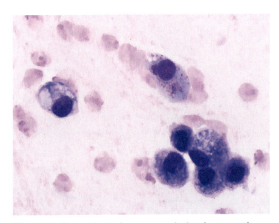

Fig 11.6 Osteoblasts (note granulation in central cell) (×1000)

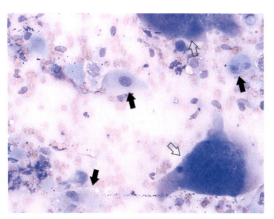

Fig 11.9 Bone remodelling in a squamous cell carcinoma; the large multinucleate cells are non-neoplastic osteoclasts (open arrows), whereas the nucleated squamous cells are neoplastic (black arrows) (×1000)

Bone marrow

Rarely, samples from lesions on or near bone can harvest bone marrow; in the author's experience this most commonly occurs with rib lesions. The cytological appearance is typical of bone marrow, and similar to extra-medullary haematopoiesis (see page 249). Whenever a cytologist is examining samples from a bony lesion which contains highly varied round cells, nucleated red blood cells and megakaryocytes, then inadvertent aspiration of bone marrow is likely (and probably indicates some erosion of the surrounding bone).

Neoplasia

Bone is a relatively uncommon site of metastasis; the most common bone neoplasia is osteosarcoma (see below). Other bone neoplasia includes invasive sarcoma such as soft tissue sarcoma, chondrosarcoma, histiocytic sarcoma (often around joints) or occasional carcinomas, although any neoplasm can potentially invade bone – the appearance of other lesions is as described elsewhere.

Osteosarcoma (FIGS 11.10, 11.11)
Neoplasm type: mesenchymal
Age: middle-aged to older, low numbers in young dogs (one to two years old), average age lower in giant breed dogs
Gross appearance: usually large single mass, can be multiple masses when metastasised
Location: appendicular skeleton most common, forelimbs more common in dogs 'away from the elbow and towards the knee' (distal radius, proximal humerus, distal femur). Sites in cats are less well-defined but possible hindlimbs more likely; very rare extra-skeletally except with metastasis
Species/breed predispositions: most common primary bone tumour in dogs and cats
Cytological appearance/further comments: osteosarcoma is a neoplasm of osteoblasts and can present some cytological challenges. The osteoblasts can vary from well-differentiated (see page 262, Fig 11.6) and relatively easy to identify to markedly atypical cells with multiple features of malignancy (see page 92).

When the neoplastic cells are well-differentiated, it can be difficult to distinguish them from osteomyelitis (see below), and when they are markedly atypical, it can be difficult to identify their origin as osteoblasts. Osteoclasts are also generally present, but this is true of any neoplasia within bone.

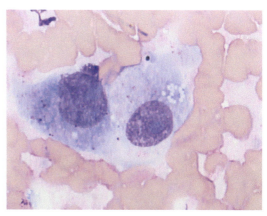

Fig 11.10 Osteosarcoma; atypical osteoblasts (×500)

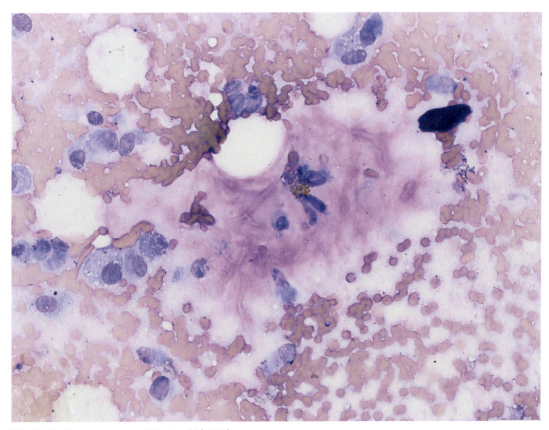

Fig 11.11 Osteosarcoma with osteoid (×500)

Osteosarcoma and other bony lesions can also be complicated by the presence of varying amounts of fibrous tissue and cartilage. Histopathology is usually required to distinguish between different types of osteosarcoma and rarer bone lesions (such as mutlilobular osteochondrosarcoma, typically seen in flat bones on the head and with slightly lower metastatic potential than osteosarcoma).

Osteomyelitis

One of the key reasons for sampling bone lesions is to attempt to differentiate between osteomyelitis and neoplasia (usually suspected osteosarcoma) and it is frustrating, therefore, that this can be a challenging cytological task. Osteomyelitic lesions contain high numbers of leukocytes, usually neutrophils and macrophages. Infectious agents may be present (when macrophages predominate, a careful search for fungal organisms is prudent). Osteoblasts and osteoclasts will also be present in variable numbers.

The osteoclasts are typically cytologically unremarkable but the osteoblasts can display some atypical features such as binucleate and mild pleomorphism (variation in shape and size). It can be extremely challenging, therefore, to distinguish between inflamed bone and well-differentiated osteosarcoma.

To further complicate matters, bone neoplasia often stimulates osteomyelitis around it. For this reason, it is helpful to aspirate the centre of bone lesions, rather than the periphery, to try to avoid osteomyelitis (this is in contrast to the advice for other large lesions, where sampling at the periphery can avoid central necrosis). The key message here is that, as with many other mesenchymal lesions, bone neoplasia should be interpreted with great care in the presence of significant inflammation.

> **Key points**
>
> **Muscle and bone**
> - Primary muscle tumours are rare, but rhabdomyosarcoma can occur in very young dogs (often <1 year old), usually around the head or neck
> - Bone remodelling (well-differentiated osteoblasts and osteoclasts) can be seen following bone damage; it can be confused with neoplasia or inflammation
> - It can be challenging to distinguish between osteomyelitis and neoplasia; sampling bony lesions at the centre is recommended to avoid peripheral inflammation

Synovial fluid

Synovial fluid is typically sampled to assess the presence of inflammation – usually, to assess whether neutrophils are present or not.

'Normal' appearance (FIG 11.12)

Synovial fluid is distinctive because of its bright pink background, often stippled and generally containing protein clefts (see page 99, Fig 4.81). This is because of the dense background of glycosaminoglycans present in the fluid. It is viscous and poorly cellular – the few cells present are often 'windrowing' (lined up in rows – see page 52).

The cells are generally 'mononuclear' cells – synovial cells which are cytologically identical to macrophages, and most of them are inactive. Occasional aggregates of synovial lining cells (a combination of mesenchymal cells and mononuclear cells) are sometimes found (Fig 11.13).

'Normal' synovial fluid should contain no blood and very few neutrophils (reportedly <10%, but in a completely normal joint no neutrophils should be present).

It can be challenging to distinguish between synovial fluid and material aspirated from myxomas/myxosarcomas – see chapter 155 for more discussion on this.

Haemodilution (FIGS 11.14, 11.15)

Blood is the bane of synovial fluid samples. True *haemarthrosis* (blood present in the synovial space prior to sampling) is rare – it can be recognised, as elsewhere in the body, by the presence of macrophages/mononuclear cells containing phagocytosed erythrocytes or, most convincingly, red-cell breakdown products such as haemosiderin or haematoidin. It can occur following trauma, underlying neoplasia or bleeding disorders.

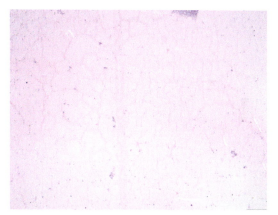

Fig 11.12a Synovial fluid (×100)

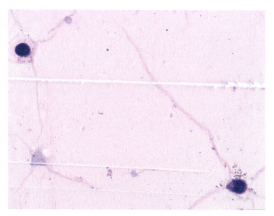

Fig 11.12b Synovial fluid (×1000)

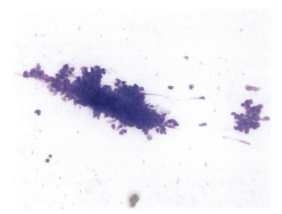

Fig 11.13 Aggregate of synovial lining cells (×100)

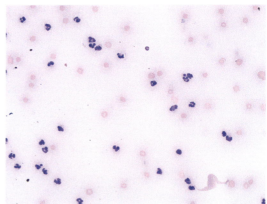

Fig 11.15 Haemodiluted joint; neutrophil numbers are increased for the amount of blood (×500)

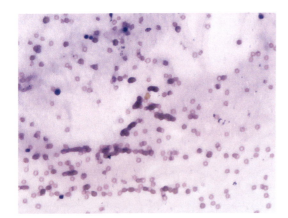

Fig 11.14 Haemodiluted joint; note windrowing of erythrocytes (×500)

Much more common, however, is the presence of blood contamination that occurs during sampling; it is understandable given the difficult of sampling joints, but it greatly complicates the examination. Even a sample that appears to be a clean 'stick' grossly can contain blood microscopically. Blood makes assessment of synovial fluid very difficult; the principal purpose of synovial fluid examination is to decide whether neutrophils are present (see below). If significant red cells are present, it can be very difficult to discern whether the neutrophils are blood-derived or were present in the joint before sampling. Blood also dilutes the synovial fluid, reduces the viscosity and obscures the view.

Neoplasia

Neoplasia is rarely found on synovial fluid samples; even when tumours are present (such as histiocytic sarcoma or synovial cell sarcoma) they rarely exfoliate into joint fluid. Direct aspiration of the mass lesion is much more likely to produce a diagnostic sample. Histiocytic sarcoma is discussed elsewhere; synovial cell sarcoma is rare but appears broadly similar to high-grade sarcoma in other locations, although small clusters of cells resembling epithelial cells may also be found.

Even when high numbers of mesenchymal-appearing cells are harvested in synovial fluid, they are more likely to represent proliferating synovial lining cells due to inflammation rather than neoplasia.

Inflammation

Inflammation in joints is almost always either mononuclear or neutrophilic; exceptions are rare and can sometimes be difficult to interpret, but the context of the case is likely to help explain unexpected eosinophils or lymphocytes within synovial fluid.

Mononuclear inflammation (FIG 11.16)

This is the most common type of inflammation found within joints, and it is almost always

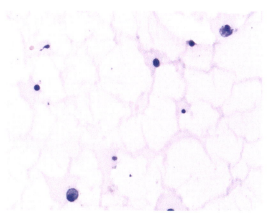

Fig 11.16 Mononuclear inflammation; increased cellularity with increased activation (×500)

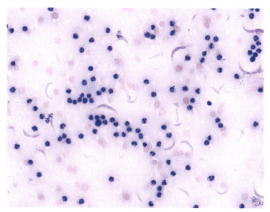

Fig 11.17 Marked neutrophilic inflammation (×500)

associated with degenerative joint disease. It can be recognised by either increased numbers of mononuclear cells (>3 cells/×500 HPF in well-spread fluid) or by increased activation (expanded vacuolated cytoplasm) of the cells (>20% of cells). Interestingly, the degree of degenerative joint disease appears to have relatively little effect on the number of cells – very severely arthritic joints can contain only slightly increased cell numbers. The degree of activation and, particularly, the presence of multinucleate cells may be more associated with disease severity.

Neutrophilic inflammation (FIG 11.17)

Less common but often more clinically relevant, neutrophilic inflammation is defined as >10% neutrophils within synovial fluid (although this is complicated by the presence of blood; when haemodilution is present, the cytologist should not rely on percentages but instead on subjective judgement as to whether neutrophils are increased compared to the amount of blood).

Very marked neutrophilic inflammation within a single joint is usually associated with septic arthritis. A search should be made for infectious organisms, although they are rarely found even with confirmed infection – not finding them does not exclude the possibility. Even with septic arthritis, neutrophils are usually non-degenerate.

Marked neutrophilic inflammation in multiple joints, in contrast, is much more commonly associated with immune-mediated disease (usually IMPA); infection is not impossible but very unlikely. Underlying neoplasia can also produce this pattern. As ever, the clinical context is important.

Lower-grade neutrophilic inflammation is more challenging. If it is present in multiple joints, then immune mediated disease is still likely. In a single joint, trauma or underlying neoplasia may be considerations.

Ragocytes and LE cells

These are associated with neutrophilic inflammation due to immune-mediated disease. *Ragocytes* are neutrophils containing phagocytosed immunoglobulins – bluish-purple inclusions that can resemble bacteria, but much more irregularly sized. *LE cells* are neutrophils that contain the phagocytosed nucleus of another neutrophil – these appear as large pale purple or pink inclusions within the neutrophil cytoplasm, often displacing the nucleus to the periphery of the cell.

Both findings are very rare, but when present can aid diagnosis of immune-mediated disease.

Chapter 11 – take home messages

- Aspirate bony lesions at the centre, rather than the periphery, to try to avoid osteomyelitis.
- Mononuclear inflammation in synovial fluid is usually associated with degenerative joint disease.
- Marked neutrophilic inflammation in a single joint is most often due to septic arthritis.
- Neutrophilic inflammation in multiple joints is more often due to immune-mediated disease.

Chapter 12

Cavity effusions

Fluid accumulates in body cavities (principally the peritoneum, pleural and pericardial cavities) for a number of reasons – the main purpose of fluid analysis is to distinguish between transudates (formed due to alterations in hydrostatic forces) and exudates (formed by changes in vascular permeability due to inflammation). In certain cases, more specific causes (e.g. chylothorax) or definitive diagnoses (e.g. neoplastic effusions) can be made.

Fluid analysis

Assessment of fluid involves assessing the following features, all of which offer clues to the type of fluid sampled:

Macroscopic appearance

Colour
Very pale, watery effusions may be transudates; pinkish to red fluid often indicates the presence of blood. Yellowish effusions can indicate either transudates or exudates.

Turbidity
Turbidity is a description of opacity, ranging from hazy or with suspended particles, to completely opaque. As a general rule, the more turbid a fluid is, the more cellular it is likely to be, although completely opaque effusions most often contain triglycerides (chylous effusions – see below).

Viscosity
A measure of the resistance to deformation of a fluid, roughly corresponding to the 'thickness'; in general, increasing viscosity approximates increasing protein within fluids, although cellularity also has a slight effect.

Cell count (FIGS 12.1, 12.2)

This is a very important part of fluid assessment. It can be broadly assessed from the cytological preparations but some haematology machines can give cell counts; the manufacturer's advice should be sought but attempting cell counts on very viscous fluid often gives inaccurate results.

When assessing cellularity of fluid cytologically, it is important to use direct smears (i.e. smears of unaltered fluid); concentrated smears (made by centrifugation or leaving cells to settle and pouring off excess fluid) by definition give a false impression of cellularity – when examining preparations made by other clinicians it is important to know whether they are concentrated or not.

Cytological estimates of fluid cellularity on direct smears are subjective, and this improves with experience. Whilst learning, it is useful to get into the habit of assessing direct smears of fluids with known cell counts. Examples of poorly and highly cellular direct fluid preparations are below.

Protein

The amount of protein within a fluid is also very important for classification. Refractometers can

Fig 12.1 Poorly cellular fluid, direct preparation (×500)

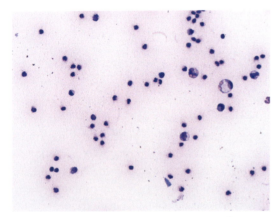

Fig 12.2 Highly cellular fluid, direct preparation; mostly neutrophils with activated macrophages (sometimes containing phagocytosed erythrocytes) (×500)

give a broad indication of protein content (total protein), although they can underestimate at lower values. More accurate values can be achieved using well-spun supernatant in in-practice automated chemistry analysers, which can also distinguish between albumin and globulin (the majority of globulins encountered are immunoglobulins, mostly associated with inflammation).

In general, transudates have lower protein, exudates have higher protein (see below).

Other biochemistry

Other biochemical values can be calculated by many in-practice analysers; evaluation of triglycerides, bilirubin, glucose and others can all aid interpretation, especially when compared with serum values. These are best assessed when specific types of fluid are suspected and are most useful when compared to serum values.

Triglycerides/cholesterol: used to assess whether an effusion is chylous; chylous effusions are rich in triglycerides from the intestine – details are below but in general, chylous effusions have higher triglycerides than serum values, and lower cholesterol.

Bilirubin: bilirubin concentration above serum levels is most suggestive of leakage of bile into the cavity (usually the peritoneum).

Glucose: glucose concentrations *below* serum levels suggest utilisation of glucose within the fluid. This is suggestive of the presence of bacteria, but not absolutely specific for it – in some cases, neoplastic cells can also utilise glucose with effusions.

Urea/creatinine: used to assess the possibility of urine within the cavity; with uroperitoneum, urea and creatinine are much higher than serum levels, and comparable with urine.

Cytological assessment

As elsewhere, a stepwise approach to fluid cytology assessment is useful. Initially, examine a direct preparation of the fluid – this gives a true idea of the background of the fluid, and is useful to assess cellularity.

Fluid backgrounds (FIGS 12.3–5)

Pure transudates (with very low protein) have largely clear backgrounds. As protein increases, the background to the fluid becomes denser and pinker, and increasingly stippled (small greyish dots become visible, increasing in number as protein increases). Protein clefts (see page 99, Fig 4.81) are apparent in highly proteinaceous samples.

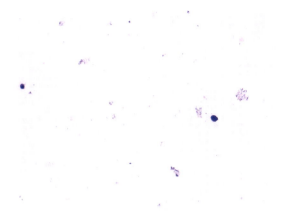
Fig 12.3 Low protein background (mostly clear with small amounts of debris) (×500)

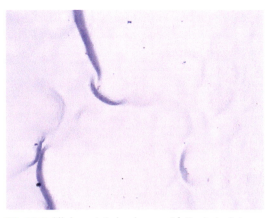
Fig 12.4 High protein background (stippled, pink, with protein crescents/clefts) (×500)

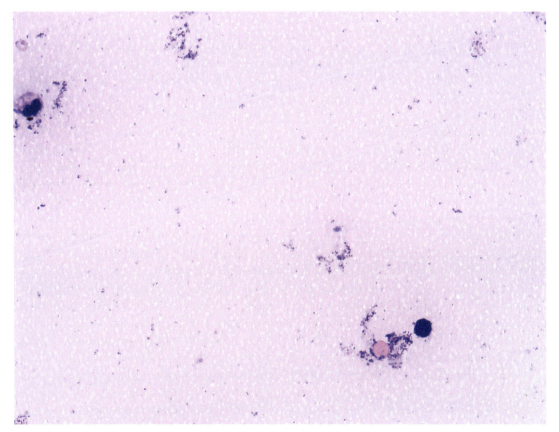
Fig 12.5 Chylous effusion background (pink with high numbers of small clear vacuoles – fat spaces due to triglycerides) (×1000)

Fluids rich in triglycerides often have high numbers of very small vacuoles just visible at high magnification. Bile is sometimes visible as patches of dark granulation (see full description below). With septic effusions, free bacteria can sometimes be seen.

Cells

In highly cellular fluids, the cellular component can be assessed on direct preparations, but for most effusions, concentrated preparations (see page 21) are useful to examine many nucleated cells at once.

For the majority of fluids, the cells are usually neutrophils and macrophages in varying numbers. The macrophages are usually active, as they organise and remove the fluid. Other fluids contain different cells (see below for more specific details), but one common finding deserves a section all to itself – mesothelium.

Mesothelium

The body cavities are lined with mesothelium – these cells are derived from embryonic mesoderm and are arranged as a thin sheet attached to a basement membrane. They express both epithelial and mesenchymal biochemical markers (cytokeratin, for epithelium, and vimentin for mesothelium).

Despite this seemingly innocent description, mesothelial cells cause great confusion and frustration amongst cytologists. They present a diagnostic challenge because they become markedly reactive in the presence of inflammation or in long-standing fluids, and the reactive changes strongly mimic features of malignancy. They are large mononuclear cells, usually found individually or in small sheets. Their nuclei are usually central and they have a clear to reddish-magenta fringe with 'wrinkled' borders (Fig 12.6). When reactive, their mitotic rate increases dramati-

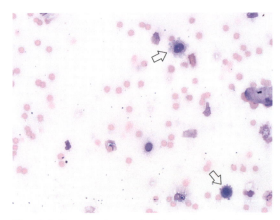

Fig 12.6 Scattered mesothelial cells in pleural effusion (open arrows); note the central nuclei, irregular/wrinkled or slightly blebbed membrane with a faint pink-red (eosinophilic) halo (×1000)

cally, the cells enlarge, and binucleate and multinucleate cells become common (Fig 12.7).

In most cavity effusions, mesothelial cells are relatively scarce, and increased numbers of cohesive clusters of cells raise concern for neoplasia rather than reactivity. However, reactive mesothelial cells are frequent and markedly reactive in pericardial effusions and, in the author's experience, in pleural effusions from patients which have had pericardial disease or pericardectomy. In practice, it is almost impossible to distinguish between markedly reactive mesothelial cells and neoplastic cells cytologically (Figs 12.8–12.10).

For this reason, neoplasia should be diagnosed with some caution in body cavity fluids, especially in pericardial fluid. It is sometimes more helpful to consider the number of cells rather than their appearance – is there an obvious explanation why a particular fluid should contain many large cells resembling reactive mesothelium (such as a history of pericardial disease when examining pleural fluid)? If not, then neoplasia should be a consideration.

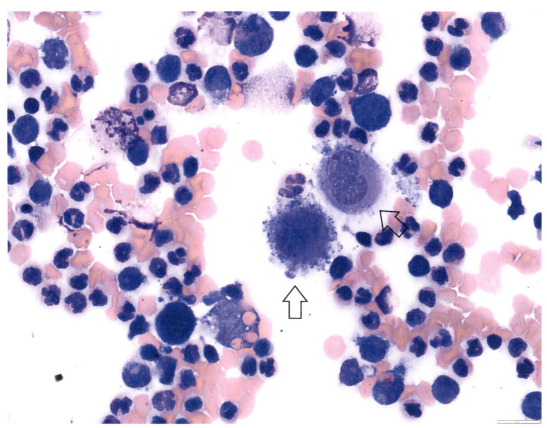

Fig 12.7 Reactive mesothelial cells in pericardial effusion (open arrows); binucleation and multiple nucleoli are present (×1000)

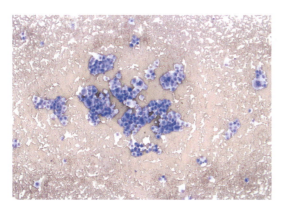

Fig 12.8 Sheets of reactive mesothelium resembling epithelium in pericardial effusion (×100)

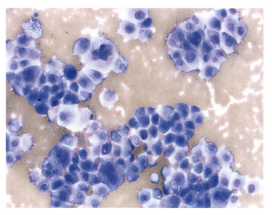

Fig 12.9 Sheets of reactive mesothelium resembling epithelium in pericardial effusion (×500)

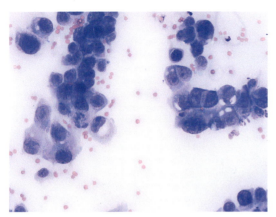

Fig 12.10 Sheets of epithelium from a carcinoma in pleural effusion (×1000)

Fluid assessment – take home messages

- Fluid analysis is largely used to distinguish between transudates and exudates, and to assess for the presence of neoplastic cells
- Always look at direct fluid preparations (not concentrated) when assessing cellularity
- Take great care when diagnosing neoplasia in pericardial effusions – they often contain high numbers of mesothelial cells which can appear markedly atypical

Fluid classification

'Normal' fluid is not assessed clinically, as there is too little to collect in the absence of pathology. When assessed experimentally, it has a clear/pale straw colour, with low cellularity and low to moderate protein.

There are several proposed methods of fluid classification, none of which are ideal. Pathological fluids are classified according to their protein and cellularity, and as with many biological processes, there is considerable overlap between the classifications. Correct interpretation does not involve classifying using protein and cellularity alone; clinicians should take the history, clinical picture and other relevant factors into consideration.

This textbook follows the most common classification method of dividing fluids into transudates, modified transudates and effusions, whilst recognising its imperfections, especially where fluid values are at the borderline between fluid types.

Transudates (FIG 12.11)

Macroscopic appearance: clear
S.G. <1.015
Total Protein <25g/L
Nucleated Cell Count very low (<1×10^9/l) – mesothelial cells, macrophages, neutrophils

'Pure' transudates have very low protein and cellularity. They are usually caused by reduced oncotic pressure due to low serum albumin (<14g/L, more often <10g/L), often in combination with increased hydrostatic pressure. Severe liver disease such as cirrhosis combines reduced albumin production with increased portal venous pressure, and so it is a common cause of peritoneal transudates. Other causes include renal disease (nephrotic syndrome due to renal protein loss), protein-losing enteropathy, or underlying neoplasia (although this is a relatively uncommon cause).

Fig 12.11 Clear background in a pure transudate (×500)

Finding a transudate within a body cavity should prompt assessment of a patient's serum protein levels.

'Modified' or 'high-protein' transudates

Macroscopic appearance: yellow to clear, occasionally slightly turbid
SG 1.015–1.022
Total Protein >25g/L
Nucleated Cell Count moderate($1-5\times10^9$/L) – mesothelial cells, macrophages, neutrophils, occasionally lymphocytes & other leukocytes

Although still formed by transudation (alterations in hydrostatic forces), these effusions are 'modified' by increased protein and, usually, increased cellularity. Many of these effusions represent transudates which have been present long enough to elicit mild irritation/inflammation (hence the increased cellularity). They are the least specific of the effusions; common causes include heart disease, increased venous pressure (often due to liver disease), or underlying neoplasia or inflammation (such as pancreatitis, hepatitis, or lung lobe torsion).

Exudates (FIGS 12.12, 12.13)

Macroscopic appearance: turbid and usually opaque; red-pink-yellow
SG >1.022
Total Protein >25g/L (often much higher)
Nucleated Cell Count – usually high (>5×10^9/L, often significantly higher)

Exudates are formed from increased vascular and mesothelial permeability due to inflammation, allowing large proteins and cells to enter the cavity. Sepsis (septic peritonitis, pyothorax) is the most common cause, and in these cases the majority of cells present will be degenerate neutrophils, alongside activated macrophages and reactive mesothelial cells. Free bacteria may be present, and the presence of phagocytosed bacterial organisms confirms bacterial infection.

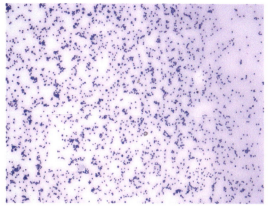

Fig 12.12 Direct preparation from an inflammatory exudate (×100)

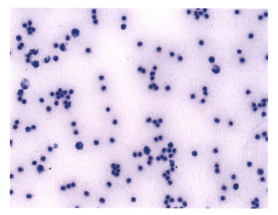

Fig 12.13 Direct preparation from an inflammatory exudate; note the stippling in the background due to increased protein (×500)

For suspected exudates, always take a sample in a sterile plain tube for culture. The bacterial morphology may guide empirical therapy – mixed morphology bacteria, including cocci and long rods, suggest anaerobic infection and GI rupture.

Sterile exudates contain non-degenerate neutrophils or, occasionally, other leukocytes – causes include underlying neoplasia, inflammation or foreign body. The presence of an otherwise unexplained sterile exudate raises significant concern for underlying neoplasia, and a careful search of the fluid for neoplastic cells is recommended (although note the above section on mesothelial cells).

Note: as the protein in exudates reflects the patient's serum protein, significantly hypoproteinaemic patients can have low-protein exudates.

Poorly-Cellular Exudates and FIP
(FIGS 12.14, 12.15)

In some situations, an effusion can have significantly high protein but a relatively low cell count ($<1\times10^9$/l). Although this could equally be classified as a 'high-protein poorly-cellular transudate', the underlying cause is often an increase in vascular permeability. The cytological appearance is of a fluid with a highly stippled background containing scattered and usually poorly preserved cells.

FIP is the most common cause of this effusion and is described in some sources as unique for this disease, although the author has also occasionally encountered it in cases of poorly exfoliative underlying inflammatory disease, particularly pancreatitis, or in other causes of vasculitis (such as toxoplasmosis).

These effusions will often have a low albumin:globulin ratio, consistent with inflammation. Albumin:globulin ratios <0.4 are strongly suggestive of (but not pathognomonic for) FIP. Identifying coronavirus within the fluid (either via PCR or immunohistochemistry) lends further strong support for FIP.

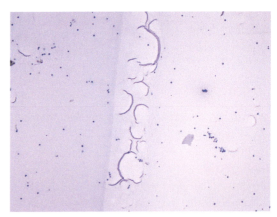

Fig 12.14 Pink background and high numbers of protein clefts consistent with a highly proteinaceous background in FIP (×100)

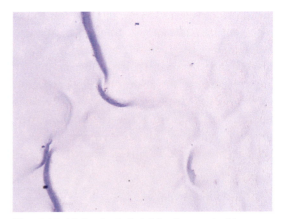

Fig 12.15 High stippled pink background with protein clefts in FIP (×500)

Note: however, that FIP effusions can also, occasionally be highly cellular and more typical of normal inflammatory exudates (albeit with markedly reduced albumin: globulin ration, as above).

Specific effusions

Haemorrhagic effusions (FIGS 12.16, 12.17)
Macroscopic Appearance: Turbid-red
Protein and cell count varied but usually high (compare with peripheral blood)
PCV usually >5% (often much higher – again, varies and depends upon peripheral blood value)

Fig 12.16 Haemorrhagic effusion; no platelet clumps are visible (×100)

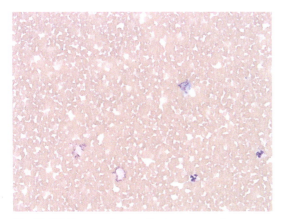

Fig 12.17 Haemorrhagic effusion; macrophages contain phagocytosed erythrocytes (×500)

Cellularity: mostly RBCs with neutrophils, macrophages and mesothelial cells

It is crucial to distinguish between true haemorrhagic effusions (with erythrophagia and possibly haemosiderin/hematoidin) and blood contamination during sampling (containing platelets – see earlier boxed text). Note that, due to the fibrinolytic activity of mesothelium, haemorrhagic effusions will not form clots within them after sampling (unlike accidental sampling of peripheral blood).

Causes of haemorrhagic effusions include bleeding disorders (including infectious causes such as *Angiostrongylus vasorum* or *Dirofilaria immitis*, trauma, torsion (e.g. liver or spleen, followed by rupture) or underlying haemorrhagic neoplasia (most commonly haemangiosarcomas). Aspirates of pericardial effusions are most commonly haemorrhagic, and these effusions frequently contain high numbers of reactive mesothelial cells, often displaying multiple features resembling malignant neoplasia.

Chylous effusions (FIG 12.18)

Macroscopic appearance: milky/opaque
Total Protein: variable but usually high (>25g/L)
Triglyceride >serum level (and usually >1.1mmol/L (100mg/dL))
Cholesterol <serum level
Nucleated cell count – moderate to high (>1.5×10^9/L) – mostly small lymphocytes (early) with neutrophils and macrophages (later), variable mesothelial cells

Chylous effusions form due to reduced lymphoid drainage or rupture of lymphatic ducts, and in small animals are most commonly found within the thoracic cavity. The elevated triglyceride level comes from chylomicrons, formed from intestinal lipids and absorbed into the lymphatics, and which also gives chyle its characteristic milky opacity.

Cytologically, chyle often has a background containing high numbers of small indistinct vacuoles (only usually appreciated on higher power magnification) and contains high numbers of lymphocytes, most of which should be unremarkable small lymphocytes (Fig 12.19). In more established chylous effusions, the irritant effects of the chyle causes a mixed inflammatory influx (mostly macrophages and neutrophils) along with reactive mesothelial cells.

Heart disease, underlying neoplasia and trauma are the most common causes of chylous effusions, although they are also frequently idiopathic.

Lymphorrhagic effusions (lymphocyte-rich effusions) (FIGS 12.20, 12.21)

These are uncommon effusions formed via reduced drainage from rupture of lymphatics which do not contain chylomicrons (i.e. which do not drain the intestines), or in patients with markedly reduced food intake. They have similar characteristics to modified transudates but contain high numbers of small lymphocytes; causes are similar to those of chylous effusions.

Both lymphocyte-rich types of effusion can sometimes be challenging to distinguish from lymphoma, especially small cell lymphoma. Further testing (especially PARR or flow cytometry) is sometimes required for definitive information.

Pseudochylous effusions

These effusions are rare in veterinary practice. Although they appear grossly similar to chyle,

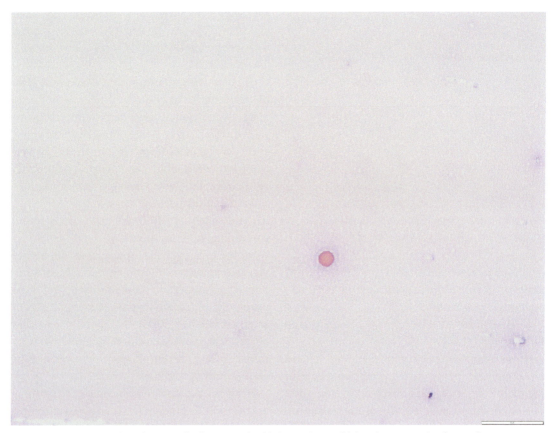

Fig 12.18 Background of chylous effusion; note the high numbers of faint clear vacuoles (×1000)

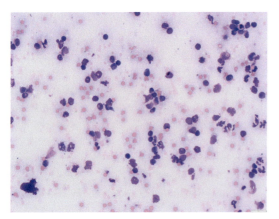

Fig 12.19 Mixed lymphocytes and bare nuclei in chylous effusion (concentrated preparation) (×500)

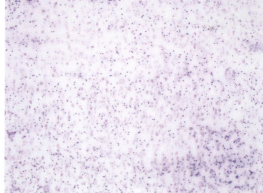

Fig 12.20 Lymphocyte-rich effusion (low power) (×100)

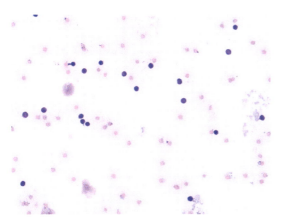

Fig 12.21 Lymphocyte-rich effusion; lymphocytes are mixed and mostly small (high power) (×500)

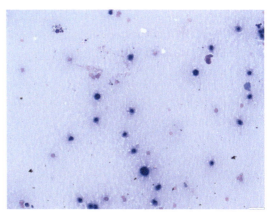

Fig 12.22 Greyish-blue background in bile peritonitis, reminiscent of chylous background but darker – the actual amount of bile can be considerably less than this as it is diluted by influxes of fluid from the exudate it stimulates; note the poorly preserved and largely unidentifiable leukocytes (direct preparation, ×100)

they are rich in cholesterol, rather than triglycerides (the cholesterol is formed from the breakdown of cell membranes), often due to chronic inflammation of the serosa.

Bile peritonitis (Fig 12.22)

Macroscopic appearance: yellow-orange, occ. greenish, variably turbid
Protein and cellularity high (as with exudate)
Bilirubin high (>serum level, often much higher)

Bile is irritant and quickly elicits an inflammatory response – the influx of fluid often masks the initial greenish colour of the fluid. Bile peritonitis can be suspected from the history, or if bile is observed on cytological examination. It may be seen as a greyish-blue to black material, free in the background or phagocytosed within macrophages, although in fluids of longer duration, much of the bile will have been converted to rhomboidal golden crystals of pigment (Fig 12.23). In some cases, the bile effusion also contains amorphous bluish-grey cloudy mucinous material (sometimes termed 'white bile') – if this is the only material present, bilirubin in the fluid may not be increased.

The inflammatory response typically comprises high numbers of neutrophils and macrophages as well as reactive mesothelial cells.

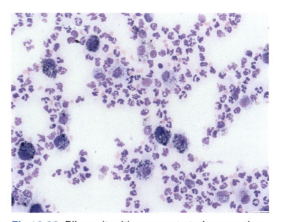

Fig 12.23 Bile peritonitis, concentrated preparation; bile pigment is phagocytosed within macrophages, which appear similar to haemosiderophages as bile pigments and haemosiderin are analogous substances (×500)

Uroabdomen

Macroscopic Appearance: clear to pale yellow
Protein and cellularity low (as transudate or modified transudate)
Urea and creatinine high (>serum level, usually much higher)

Urine is also irritating to the abdomen, but there is a continued influx of urine, diluting cellularity and protein; an exudate will eventually form in long-standing uroabdomen. Occasionally, urine crystals may be present.

Creatinine equilibrates more slowly than urea, and so is more likely to be elevated, although usually both urea and creatinine are significantly increased from serum values.

Neoplastic effusions

Most neoplasms exfoliate poorly into fluid, so the majority of effusions secondary to neoplasia do not contain neoplastic cells. The most common exceptions are lymphoma (in cats) and carcinomas (in dogs) (Fig 12.24, 12.25), although care must always be taken to avoid misdiagnosing reactive mesothelial cells as neoplastic (see earlier).

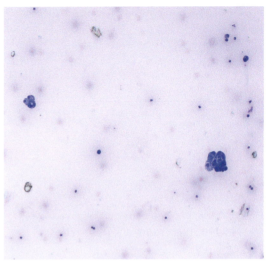

Fig 12.24 Cluster of atypical epithelium in pleural effusion (direct preparation) (×100)

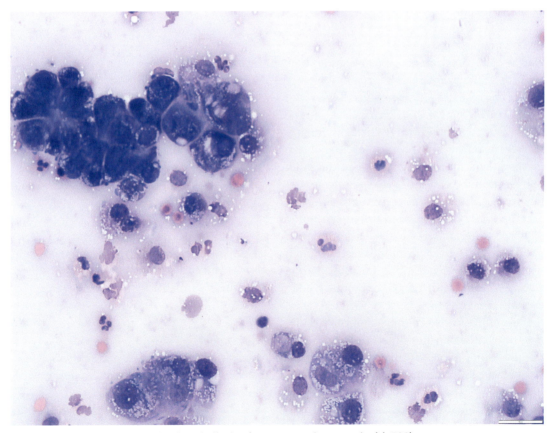

Fig 12.25 Atypical epithelium in pleural effusion (concentrated preparation) (×500)

Chapter 12 – take home messages

- Effusions are broadly classified as transudates or exudates (inflammatory)
- Transudates are caused by low oncotic pressure (usually low serum protein), increased hydrostatic pressure or, usually, both
- Modified transudates have higher protein and cellularity; they have the least specific causes
- Exudates are caused by increased vascular permeability due to inflammation
- The presence of an otherwise unexplained sterile exudate raises significant concern for underlying neoplasia
- Aspirates of pericardial effusions are most commonly haemorrhagic, and these effusions frequently contain high numbers of reactive mesothelial cells, often displaying multiple features resembling malignant neoplasia.

Chapter 13

Blood films

Microscopic examination of blood films is a large topic – large enough for a textbook by itself. This chapter is necessarily limited in scope and concentrates on the most common and useful reasons for examining blood films, to give information beyond that provided by automated haematology machines.

Blood film preparation

Why examine blood films?

Automated haematology machines provide a huge amount of information to clinicians; they count hundreds of thousands of cells and, when cell size and morphology is close to normal, produce extremely accurate differential counts and measurements. At the current stage of technology, however, there remain a number of situations where errors occur. Sometimes the errors are flagged by the analyser for checking, sometimes not. Blood film examination can often identify and correct these errors. Such situations include:

- platelet clumps leading to falsely low platelet counts
- misclassification of platelets as small red blood cells in cats
- misclassification of band neutrophils and lymphocytes or other leukocytes
- misclassification of atypical circulating cells as other 'normal' leukocytes.

Additionally, although some modern analysers provide details and images of circulating cells, this remains a rarity currently; without these analysers, examination of blood films is the only way to examine the morphology of cells, which can reveal details such as the presence of spherocytes, Heinz bodies, toxic change in neutrophils and circulating neoplasia.

Blood film examination can also reveal whether anaemia is regenerative or not – probably the most important question to answer when faced with an anaemic patient – in analysers which do not provide reticulocyte counts.

Blood film preparation (FIG 13.1)

Here, as with most skills, practice makes perfect. The author has their own legacy of sadly discarded and useless blood films and is certainly not in a position to judge anyone else's efforts. It can help, when making films, to keep in mind the most important areas required for a comprehensive blood film examination. These are:

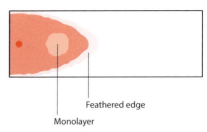

Fig 13.1 Anatomy of a blood film – the feathered edge and the monolayer (diagram)

The Feathered Edge (FIG 13.3)

The 'feathered edge' is the 'tail' of the blood film. This part of the film is important to examine as many heavier cells will finish their journey here, including mast cells, atypical cells, and platelet clumps.

The blood film does not need to be particularly long – in fact, long blood films often have their feathered edge right at the end of the slide, which can lead to some cells falling off the edge (Fig 13.2). And when automated stainers are used (as they will be when submitting to external labs), the feathered edge can be beyond the stainable portion of the slide.

The Monolayer (FIG 13.4)

The 'monolayer' is the section of blood film usually just behind the tail where the red blood cells are present in a single thin layer, spaced out

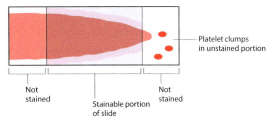

Fig 13.2 Blood film extending beyond the typically stained portion of a slide on an automatic stainer (platelet clumps are missed) (diagram)

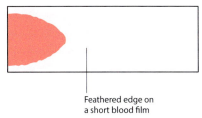

Fig 13.3 Feathered edge on a short blood film (diagram)

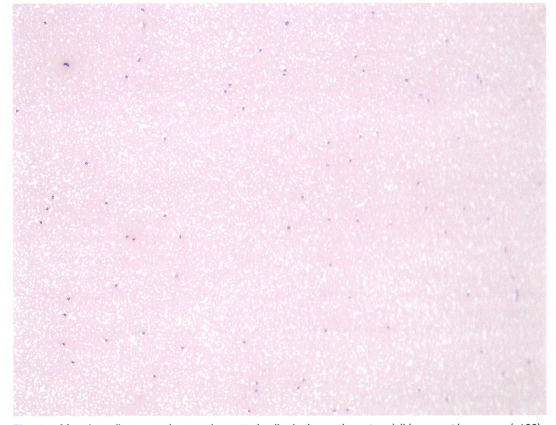

Fig 13.4 Monolayer (low power) – note the central pallor in the erythrocytes visible even at low power (×100)

evenly. The monolayer is very important as it is where examination of red blood cell morphology is most useful, and where platelet numbers can be most easily estimated.

In dogs, the monolayer is the area behind the feathered edge where most of the red blood cells have a clear obvious area of central pallor. It can be harder to locate in cats as their blood cells have limited central pallor visible but can often be found by scrolling the slide back towards the point of origin from the feathered edge until the red blood cells are spaced out evenly.

Fresh films vs. older films (FIG 13.5)

Morphological changes within white and red blood cells start to occur relatively quickly after sampling. In particular, neutrophil nuclei begin to swell, making them appear similar to band neutrophils, and changes resembling toxic change (see page 301, below) (in particular, basophilic structures resembling Döhle bodies) begin to appear.

It can be challenging to distinguish between a neutrophilic left shift with toxic change and sample ageing when blood films are not made quickly. Prolonged delay in making blood films (two+ days, depending on temperature and other conditions) can lead to complete degeneration of white cells, making them impossible to identify.

Red cell morphology is also affected by sample ageing – red cells will shrink and become crenated (wrinkled), leading to increased numbers of echinocytes (small red blood cells with spikes) throughout the film. Further degeneration leads to formation of haemoglobin crystals and makes assessment of morphology almost impossible.

Platelets are more likely to be present in clumps in older samples; platelet clumps make platelet numbers challenging for analysers to assess, although clumps are easily identifiable on blood films and this helps to rule out immune mediated thrombocytopenia (which is very unlikely to be present when platelet clumps are seen).

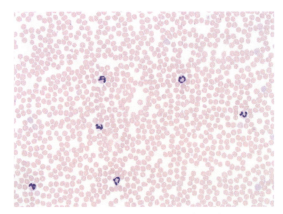

Fig 13.5a Fresh blood film (canine) (×500)

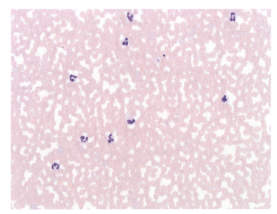

Fig 13.5b Aged blood film (same case as 13.5a) – note the decreased segmentation of neutrophils, causing them to resemble band neutrophils in some cases (×500)

For these reasons, blood films should be made as soon as possible after sampling, and ideally within two hours.

Making the blood film – procedure (FIG 13.6)

- Using a microhaematocrit tube, place a small drop of blood (well-mixed) at one end of a clean glass slide (several centimetres from the end of the slide, or just past the frosted portion when frosted glass slides are used).
- Hold the slide in one hand or place on a flat clean surface.
- Take a second clean glass slide (the 'spreader' slide) and hold at a 30–45 degree angle to the first.

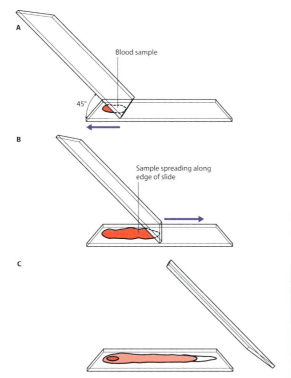

Fig 13.6 Making a blood film (diagram)

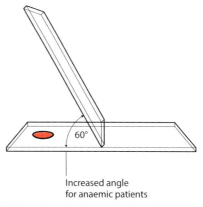

Fig 13.7 Altered angle for anaemic patients (diagram)

- Reverse the slide onto the drop of blood.
- As soon as the blood spreads along the back side of the spreader slide, rapidly move it forwards.
- Dry the film immediately, either in the air or using a hairdryer on a cool or very slightly warm setting (not hot).

This should produce a smear thick around the drop of blood with a monolayer of cells just behind the feathered edge. If smears are too thick, monolayers are hard to find. If smears are too thin it can affect the white cell preservation, as well as make the film too long for the slide. Anaemic patients have thinner blood, and so smears are longer. For these patients (the blood is often visibly more watery than normal), hold the slide in a more upright position to shorten the film (and therefore make it thicker) (Fig 13.7).

> **Key points**
>
> **Blood film preparation**
> - The most important parts of the blood film are the feathered edge (where many heavier cells are present) and the monolayer (to assess platelet numbers) and red cell morphology
> - Blood films should be made as soon as possible after sampling, and ideally within 2 hours, to prevent morphological changes in red and white cells; blood films made later are still useful so long as these changes are borne in mind

Blood film evaluation

Initial evaluation

Suggested approach:

- Low power assessment (quality and preservation)
- Platelets (low and high power)
- Erythrocytes (low and high power)
- Leukocytes (low and high power).

An initial low power examination (4× or 10× objective) of the film is used to assess how successful the blood film has been (is preservation good enough for morphological assessment? Is there a monolayer? Is the feathered edge entirely on the slide?) and to assess more general features ('Are large platelet clumps present? 'Are red cells or white cells increased or decreased?' – see sections below for more detail on this). Microfilariae are also more easily spotted at low power.

After the initial assessment, perform a more detailed assessment (at low and high power) of platelets, red cells and white cells in turn. An alternative approach would be to assess all low power details at first (platelets, erythrocytes and leukocytes) and then repeat the process at high power. Whilst potentially more efficient (as it avoids constantly changing from low to high power), the author finds it difficult to concentrate on more than one thing at once, and therefore prefers the stepwise approach.

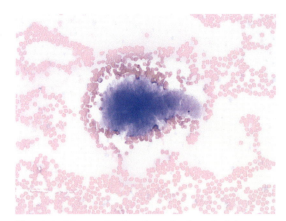

Fig 13.8 A large platelet clump in the tail of the blood film (×500)

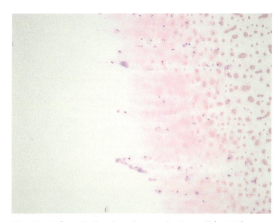

Fig 13.9 Small platelet clumps in the tail (×100)

Platelets

One of the most common and useful reasons for blood film examination is to check whether an analyser-reported thrombocytopenia is genuine, or to check platelet numbers in patients displaying signs of a bleeding disorder.

Low power assessment – platelet clumps
(FIGS 13.8, 13.9)

Platelet clumps are very useful to find on blood films; although they make accurate platelet estimate very difficult, the presence of any platelet clumps at all on a film means that clinically significant thrombocytopenia (i.e. platelet numbers low enough to allow spontaneous haemorrhage – typically $<20 \times 10^9/l$) is extremely unlikely.

Platelet clumps can be found anywhere in the film, but as they are usually larger and heavier than most individual cells, they are usually pushed along to the feathered edge or the sides of the film. This is why it is important to have a film short enough to enable examination of the whole of the feathered edge – platelet clumps may otherwise fall off the edge of the slide and a misdiagnosis of thrombocytopenia may result.

Record the size and frequency of platelet clumps for reference later (such as 'numerous small platelet clumps' or 'occasional large clumps') rather than simply recording the presence or absence of clumps.

High power assessment – platelet number estimation

To estimate platelet numbers, count platelets in 10–20 fields in the monolayer using ×100 objective (×1000 magnification) (Fig 13.10). Take the mean number of platelets from these fields and multiply by 15 (to give a low end) and 20 (high end) to give an estimate range of platelets (in $\times 10^9/l$).

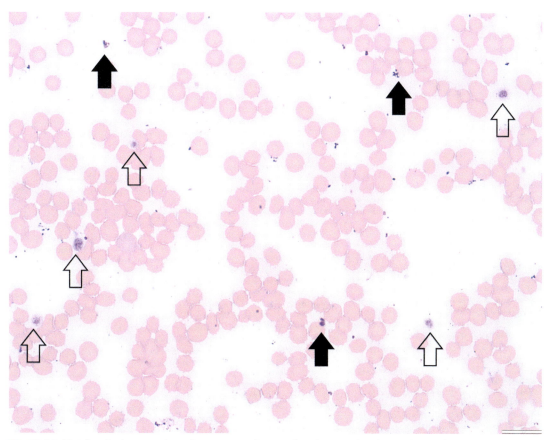

Fig 13.10 Platelets in the monolayer (open arrows); note also clumps of stain precipitate (black arrows) (×500)

Platelet estimate (×10^9/l) = mean number of platelets (from 10–20 ×100 HPF) × 15–20

High power assessment – morphology: giant platelets and protoplatelets

These are larger platelets than normal – the actual definition of the two is slightly variable among pathologists. The author uses the following: *giant platelets* are large platelets, larger than red blood cells, but which otherwise appear unremarkable. They are relevant because they can be miscounted by analysers as red blood cells, particularly in cats. *Macroplatelets* are similar except they do not exceed the size of a red cell, they're just larger than most platelets. Many pathologists do not make this distinction and use giant platelets and macroplatelets as synonyms (Fig 13.11).

Giant platelets and macroplatelets can make platelet number estimates misleading, because these larger platelets increase the overall platelet mass (the plateletcrit, or PCV) more than a normal platelet, and thus a patient with many large platelets can have a low platelet count but still have perfectly effective platelet function. Therefore, the presence of large platelets should be recorded, as with platelet clumps, along with platelet estimates.

Cavalier King Charles spaniels, in particular, often have high numbers of giant platelets with a mild-moderate asymptomatic thrombocytopenia. Other breeds such as the Japanese breeds have been reported as having thrombocytope-

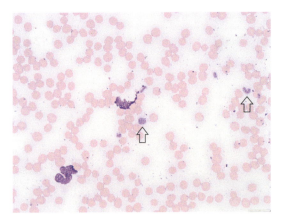

Fig 13.11a Macroplatelets (open arrows) (×1000)

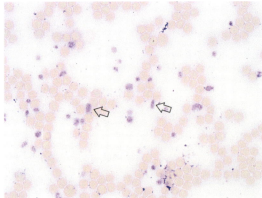

Fig 13.12 Linear platelets (open arrows) (×1000)

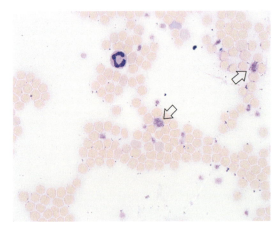

Fig 13.11b Giant platelets (open arrows) (×1000)

nia accompanied with large elongated platelets (resembling protoplatelets – see below), again with no clinical signs.

Protoplatelets are platelets released early from megakaryocytes. Rather than the more typical round shape, protoplatelets have 'elongated' linear structures (Fig 13.12). They have a similar effect on platelet numbers and counts to other larger platelets, but their presence is also a possible indication of early release from the bone marrow in response to increased demand (similar to band neutrophils – see below).

Final note on thrombocytopenia

Before thrombocytopenia is diagnosed on the basis of a blood film examination, it is important to check the syringe and/or blood tube for the presence of any large clots which will have consumed platelets post-sampling and record that clots have been checked for grossly.

> **Key points**
>
> **Platelets**
>
> - Platelet clumps make assessment of numbers difficult, but also make clinically significant thrombocytopenia very unlikely
> - Platelet numbers should be assessed at high power (×1000) in the monolayer
> - Always check for clots within the sample before diagnosing significant thrombocytopenia

Erythrocytes

Low power assessment – anaemia (FIG 13.13)
Scanning at low power gives the cytologist a rough idea of if anaemia is present based upon how densely packed the red cells are; the further apart the red cells are, the more likely it is that anaemia is present. This is a skill which requires experience to acquire, as well as some familiarity with how a particular smear has been made; it can be useful to practise assessing films of known haematocrit to become familiar with the appearance of anaemia of differing severity.

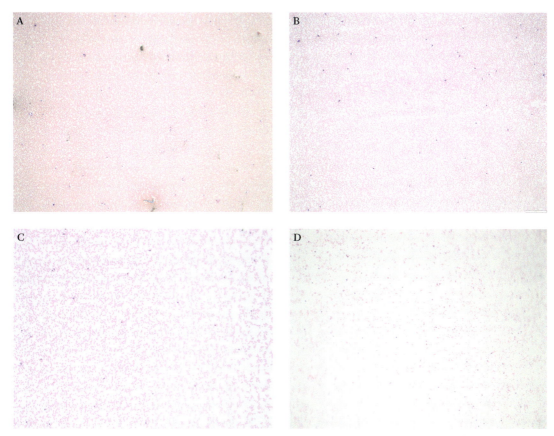

Figs 13.13a, b, c and d No anaemia, mild anaemia, moderate anaemia and severe anaemia (all ×100)

High power assessment – polychromasia and nucleated red blood cells

Polychromasia and regeneration

Once anaemia is established, the next most important question is: is it regenerative or non-regenerative? This can be determined by examination of blood films at high power and enumerating *polychromatophils* (and so assessing the degree of polychromasia). These are early-released red blood cells which are yet to be fully haemoglobinised.

They are roughly equivalent to *reticulocytes*, which are early red blood cells containing fragments of RNA; reticulocytes are evaluated by automated analysers or manually via a special cytological stains (New Methylene Blue (NMB)), whereas polychromatophils can be seen using Romanowsky stains. The picture is slightly more complicated in cats, as they have both punctuate and aggregate reticulocytes, but polychromatophils remain roughly equivalent to aggregate reticulocytes in cats and are still a valuable guide to the presence of regeneration.

Polychromatophils are larger than typical red blood cells (as they have been released earlier in the cell division cycle) and bluer (because they contain less haemoglobin). As a general rule, the presence of one or more polychromatophils per ×1000 high power field in cats (Fig 13.14), or two or more in dogs (Fig 13.15), is consistent with regeneration (dogs release red blood cells from the marrow earlier than cats – it is normal to have low numbers of polychromatophils present, hence the slightly higher bar for regeneration in dogs).

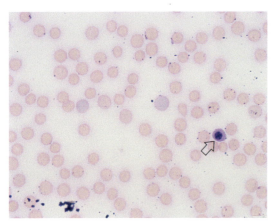

Fig 13.14 Regenerative anaemia (cat); note also nucleated red blood cell (metarubricyte, open arrow) (×1000)

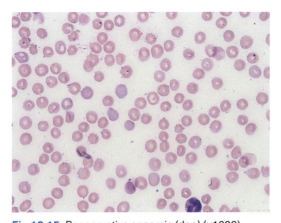

Fig 13.15 Regenerative anaemia (dog) (×1000)

The degree of polychromasia should mirror the degree of regeneration – mild anaemia should produce mild polychromasia, and so on. Polychromasia takes three to five days following blood loss to be apparent on blood smears.

Nucleated red blood cells (nRBCs) (FIGS 13.16)

Nucleated red blood cells (nRBCs) are an even earlier step in the cell division cycle and start to appear on blood films with marked regeneration. The numbers of nucleated red cells should be much lower than polychromatophils, and of those red blood cells (Fig 13.16), most should be *metarubricytes*, with small dense nuclei and similar cytoplasm colour to polychromatophils.

As cells are released even earlier, occasional *rubricytes* will start to appear; these have larger nuclei with slightly more open chromatin and bluer cytoplasm (Fig 13.17).

Nucleated red blood cells can sometimes be challenging to distinguish from small lymphocytes. The most useful differences are that nRBCs usually have more cytoplasm, and the pattern of chromatin is 'cracked', similar to plasma cells, whereas lymphocytes generally have dense black chromatin.

The presence of nRBCS without significant polychromasia, or in the wrong proportion (i.e. with rubricytes outnumbering metarubricytes or polychromatophils) should alert the cytologist to the possibility of bone marrow damage leading to leakage of the cells into the blood. The most common causes of this 'inappropriate rubricytosis' are heatstroke, lead poisoning or, in cats, erythroid leukaemia (typically accompanied by bizarre-appearing nucleated red blood cells. It is usually caused by feline leukaemia virus).

Splenectomised dogs also have higher numbers of circulating nRBCs due to reduced clearance.

Low-high power assessment – agglutination and rouleaux

A combination of low and high power examination can help identify the presence of two similar-appearing but very different phenomena involving adhered red blood cells: agglutination and rouleaux. Both should be checked for in the monolayer, as some degree of rouleaux is typically seen in most blood films at the denser end of the film (that is, towards where the blood drop was initially placed) and is unlikely to be clinically relevant here.

Rouleaux (from the French word meaning 'rolls') is seen as red blood cells stacked up in short rows, similar in appearance to *windrowing* (see page 52) but with the cells overlapping. (Fig 13.18)

Red blood cells normally resist this stacking because they are negatively charged, and

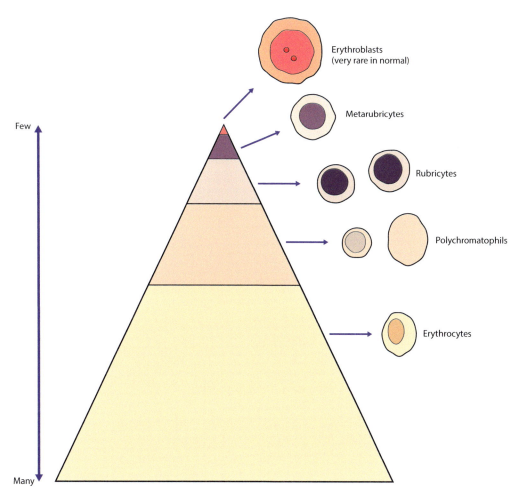

Fig 13.16 Pyramid displaying expected proportions of erythrocytes and erythrocyte precursors (diagram); in a normal situation only occasional nucleated red cells are found

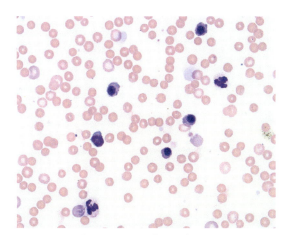

Fig 13.17a Metarubricytes (×1000)

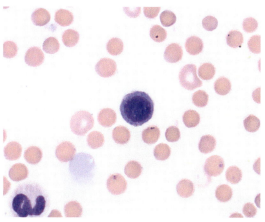

Fig 13.17b Rubricyte (larger and bluer than metarubricytes) (×1000)

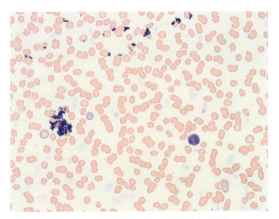

Fig 13.18 Rouleaux (feline blood film) (×500)

therefore repel each other. Cats have smaller erythrocytes than dogs, with lower negative charges, and so are more prone to rouleaux. Anything which reduces or neutralises the negative charge of erythrocytes also makes rouleaux more likely – the most common clinical cause of this is hyperglobulinaemia (usually due to inflammation, occasionally paraneoplastic).

When rouleaux is very marked, the rows of cells can curl back upon themselves and appear similar to agglutination (see below) – consequently, agglutination should be diagnosed with care in patients with very high globulin (this is why in-saline agglutination tests are performed at increasing dilutions – true agglutination will resist dilution much more than rouleaux).

Agglutination

Unlike rouleaux, which involves simple stacking of red blood cells, agglutination involves the immune-mediated adhesion of red blood cells due to immunoglobulins bound to the surface membranes. Although it can resemble rouleaux, agglutination involves the formations of irregular clumps of erythrocytes, somewhat resembling bunches of grapes, rather than the neat stacks observed in rouleaux. The presence of agglutination confirms immune mediated aetiology, although the absence of it does not exclude the possibility.

High power assessment – red cell morphology

After examination for regeneration and adhesion, individual red blood cells are assessed at high power for any morphological abnormalities. Again, this needs to be performed in the monolayer, as many red cells can resemble spherocytes when assessed in thicker areas of the film. Details on the most common and clinically relevant morphological changes are below.

Individual red cells displaying morphological changes are unlikely to be clinically relevant. The number of changes considered relevant varies slightly, but in general when more than one or two cells with the same morphology are found per high power field (×500), it is likely to be of significance.

Normal morphology (FIGS 13.19, 13.20)

Red blood cells have a distinctive biconcave shape, much like an incompletely-holed doughnut. On cytological specimens, red cells are usually laid on their side, and so appear as a small round ring with a pale centre (called *central pallor*). Cats, however, have much smaller erythrocytes and the area of central pallor is much harder to appreciate. Most cat red blood cells appear as small round red discs (and can easily be confused with spherocytes; see below).

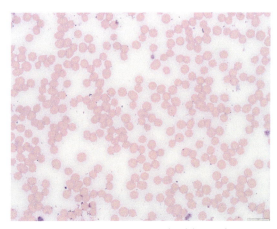

Fig 13.19 Normal erythrocytes (cat) (×1000)

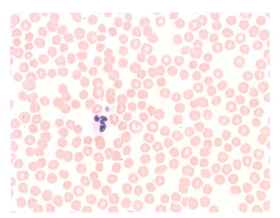

Fig 13.20 Normal erythrocytes (dog) (×1000)

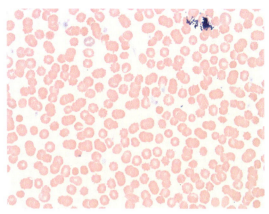

Fig 13.21 Echinocytes (×1000)

Nucleated red blood cells (nRBCs)

As red cells mature, they get smaller (due to cell division), redder (due to haemoglobin production) and, as they approach maturity, they extrude their nucleus. Early nucleated red blood cells can find their way into the circulation for various reasons. They comprise *rubricytes* – larger cells with bluer cytoplasm, dense round nuclei and chromatin with a cracked appearance, slightly similar to plasma cells – and the later stage *metarubricytes* – smaller cells with redder cytoplasm, smaller nuclei with denser (but still 'cracked' chromatin).

Both types can cause confusion both to analysers (which may misclassify them as leukocytes) and to cytologists (as they resemble lymphocytes). The distinctive cracked chromatin and the colour of the cytoplasm is usually enough to distinguish them, however.

Occasional nRBCs are often found in blood films (usually metarubricytes). They are found in increased numbers in regenerative anaemia and, inappropriately, in cases of heatstroke or lead poisoning (see page 291, above). Splenectomised dogs also have higher numbers of circulating nRBCs due to reduced clearance.

Echinocytes (FIG 13.21)

This is the most commonly noted RBC morphological change on blood films. Echinocytes are mostly important to recognise for their usual lack of clinical importance. Echinocytes (sometimes called 'burr cells') are crenated (crinkled) red cells which have a serrated or spiculated, rather than rounded, appearance. They represent changes to the surface membrane of the red cell, but usually occur in vitro. They are very common in blood smears made from older blood samples.

The spikes on these serrated red cells are symmetrical and uniform. Red cells with irregular spikes are more likely to be acanthocytes (see below).

Spherocytes (FIG 13.22)

Spherocytes are red cells that have lost their biconcave shape due to membrane damage; they are spherical and therefore appear perfectly round on blood films. They are wider than normal RBCs and therefore appear denser cytologically; spherocytes appear smaller, rounder and redder than normal red blood cells.

Despite this apparently clear-cut distinction, spherocytes can be difficult to spot and easily over diagnosed, especially when films are examined away from the monolayer. Spherocytes are most easily identified when adjacent to typical red blood cells with clear central pallor (see page 293, Fig 13.20). They can be very hard if not impossible to appreciate in cats (which have very little visible central pallor in erythrocytes), or in cases where

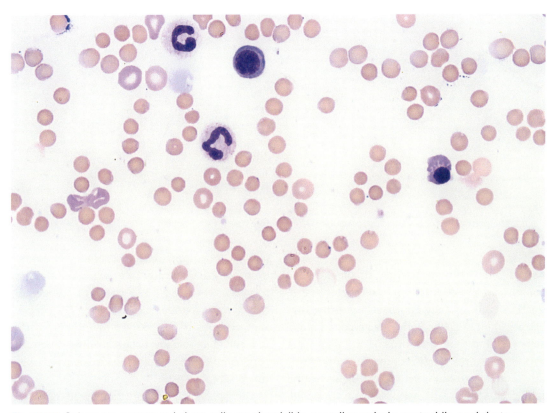

Fig 13.22 Spherocytes; scattered ghost cells are also visible, as well as polychromatophils, a rubricyte, a metarubricyte and hyposegmented neutrophils (×1000)

very high numbers of spherocytes are present (meaning that there are very few cells with central pallor to compare them with).

It is frustrating that they can be difficult to identify, as spherocytes are highly clinically relevant – they are most commonly associated with immune-mediated destruction of red blood cells, and high numbers of spherocytes on a blood film raise significant suspicion of IMHA, especially with other compatible features (such as strongly regenerative anaemia; see page 290, Fig 13.15 for a typical IMHA pattern). They usually represent extra-vascular haemolysis (i.e. red cells removed from the circulation for destruction, rather than destroyed whilst circulating).

Spherocytes are not pathognomonic for IMHA, however. Low numbers are sometimes seen in severe GI disease. Rare cases of hereditary spherocytosis have been reported, and they can also form in high numbers after snake envenomation or bee stings.

Anisocytosis, microcytosis and hypochromasia

Anisocytosis is not a single morphological change; rather, it is a visual assessment of the variation in size of the red blood cells (also measured by analysers, and reported as the *Red cell Distribution Width*, or RDW). Regenerative anaemia, with the appearance of larger polychromatophils, is the most common cause of increased anisocytosis.

Microcytosis and hypochromasia are similar in that they are visual assessments of the size and haemoglobin concentration of red cells (measured by analysers as MCV and MCH/MCHC respectively). Notably small red blood cells are recorded as microcytes, and notably pale red cells are recorded as evidence of hypochromasia. Visual judgement of these features is challenging unless the red cells are very small and/or very pale – this is a common finding with iron deficiency, the typical pattern of which is discussed later (see page 312).

Ghost red cells (FIG 13.23)

Rather as they sound, these cells are pale imitations of their former red-blooded selves. They represent cells which were lysed (ruptured) prior to sampling, and cytologically they resemble very pale (and often barely visible) red or bluish discs.

The presence of ghost cells is suggestive of intravascular haemolysis, typically a more severe form of haemolysis than extra-vascular haemolysis, usually associated with more severe anaemia and clinical disease. When Heinz bodies (see page 296, Fig 13.24) are the cause of the haemolysis, they can sometimes be seen attached to ghost cells.

Schistocytes and acanthocytes

Schistocytes are the result of red cell shearing injuries – erythrocytes that have been sheared into fragments by irregular blood or inflamed blood vessels. They appear, as one may expect, as fragments or fractions of red blood cells, with sharp edges where the shearing occurred. They can be found in patients with inflamed blood vessels (especially DIC) or vessel wall neoplasia (haemangiosarcoma). They are also more common in patients with iron deficiency (see page 312).

Acanthocytes are another form of 'spiky' blood cell, similar to echinocytes (see page 293, Fig 13.21), except that the spikes are irregular, and the cells often appear more like a splat than a cell. They represent lipid changes within the red cell membrane and are caused by similar blood vessel wall changes to schistocytes. Liver disease is also a consideration for these cells (due to abnormal fat metabolism) and, again, they are more common in patients with iron deficiency.

Heinz bodies/eccentrocytes (FIG 13.24)

Heinz bodies are small, condensed clumps of haemoglobin, and they appear cytologically as small dense red droplets. They can be seen within red blood cells (where they are often challenging to spot but appear as a slightly paler circle within the cytoplasm of the cell, similar to central pallor, but irregularly placed) or, because their presence triggers lysis of the cell, as free small round red fragments.

They can also sometimes be found attached to ghost red blood cells (see page 295, Fig 13.23). The presence of high numbers of erythrocytes with Heinz bodies in cats can sometimes be mistaken for normal erythrocytes with central pallor.

Eccentrocytes are also red cells containing condensed clumps of haemoglobin. In these cells, the haemoglobin has concentrated on one side of the cell, leaving a pale largely haemoglobin-free loose membrane, appearing somewhat like the handle of a bucket or a pale crescent attached to an irregular dense erythrocyte.

Both types of red cell are cause by oxidative damage. Heinz bodies are more common in cats, whereas eccentrocytes are more commonly found in dogs. Cats are particularly prone to oxidative damage to red blood cells due to

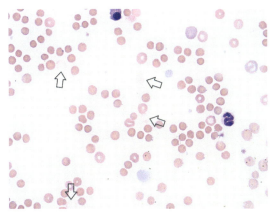

Fig 13.23 Ghost red blood cells (open arrows); note that spherocytes are also present (canine IMHA case) as well as polychromatophils and a metarubricyte (top centre of image) (×1000)

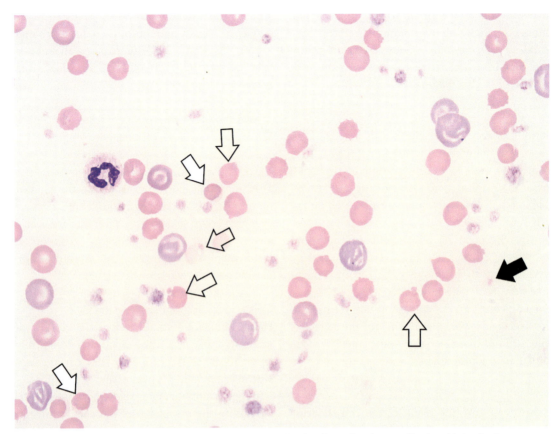

Fig 13.24 Heinz bodies (open arrows) attached to red blood cells and a ghost cell; a free Heinz body (detached from the RBC) is also visible (black arrow) as well as several eccentrocytes (white arrows) (×1000)

the structure of their haemoglobin molecules and their idiosyncratic biochemical pathways. Consequently low numbers of Heinz bodies can be found in cats with any disease or, occasionally, in clinically normal cats. High numbers of Heinz bodies or eccentrocytes, however, are suggestive of primary oxidative damage such as garlic, onion or paracetamol toxicity.

Howell-Jolly bodies (FIG 13.25)

These are small fragments of nucleus retained within mature red blood cells. They are often of little clinical significance, but it is worth recognising them to avoid confusion with other pathological processes. They are more common in splenectomised patients (as with nucleated red blood cells) and in regenerative anaemia.

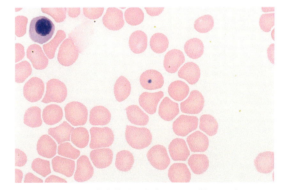

Fig 13.25 Howell-Jolly body (centre of image) (×1000)

High power assessment – infectious agents

Infectious agents within erythrocytes are rare in some parts of the world (such as the UK) but relatively common in others; climate change is affecting disease prevalence all over the world. Many infectious agents of RBCs trigger an immune response, and some directly destroy erythrocytes. Either way, most infectious agents of RBCs cause haemolysis (intra or extravascular) and therefore tend to produce strongly regenerative anaemia.

A few infectious agents are detailed below – this list is not exhaustive.

Mycoplasma (FIG 13.26)

The haemotropic mycoplasmas – also called *haemoplasmas* (previously known as haemobartonella) – are the most commonly found infectious agents of RBCs in the UK. They are also found in most other parts of the world, including North America, Europe, and Southern Africa, and Australia. They are small bacteria which attach to the surface membrane of the erythrocyte, difficult to spot because of their size. Although they can be found in dogs, they have not currently been reported to cause clinical disease. In cats, they are the cause of feline infectious anaemia (FIA).

Several species are found in cats, the most common of which is *Mycoplasma haemofelis*. Although there are some differences in size and shape, the species of mycoplasma cannot be reliably differentiated visually, and further testing (such as PCR, as the haemoplasmas are very difficult to grow on culture) is generally required to identify them.

The haemoplasmas (in common with other mycoplasma species) are much smaller than other bacteria and appear as small basophilic (blue to black) dots or rings, usually at the

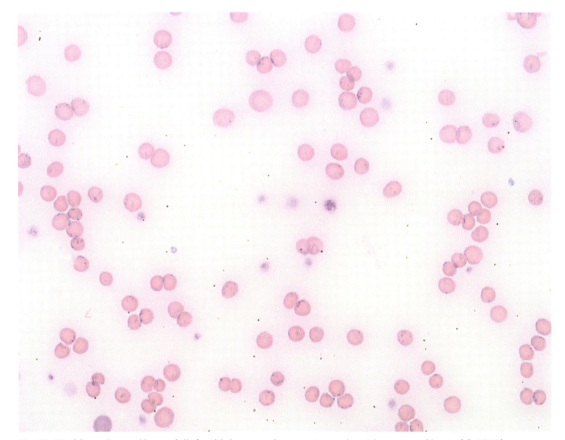

Fig 13.26 *Mycoplasma Haemofelis* (multiple examples, most prominent in centre of image) (×1000)

periphery of red cells. When present as dots, they are cytologically very similar to stain precipitate debris (see page 50, Fig 3.29) and are very challenging to identify. One way to distinguish them is that when found in profile they slightly indent the surface of the erythrocyte. Ring forms are also easier to spot. Unless the condition is severe, only a few organisms are likely to be found on a blood film.

Placing blood into EDTA tends to dislodge the organisms from the surface of the erythrocyte and makes finding them extremely challenging – assessment for mycoplasma organisms should be carried out on fresh blood films.

Babesia (FIG 13.27)

This is a disease with a worldwide distribution, found across Africa, Asia, Australia, Europe (including a few reported cases in the UK) and the Americas. They are protozoan organisms, spread by ticks. Again, a few different species can infect the domestic species, although clinical disease is only reported in dogs.

Babesia canis is a large organism with a teardrop shape, appearing somewhat similar to an apple pip, and is usually found in pairs in infected cells. Other babesia species, smaller and less common, appear more similar to the ring form of mycoplasma.

Distemper

Distemper is now very rare in many countries, thanks to vaccination, but infections can cause viral inclusions to form within red cells during the viraemic stage of the infection. Unusually, these inclusions are more visible using aqueous

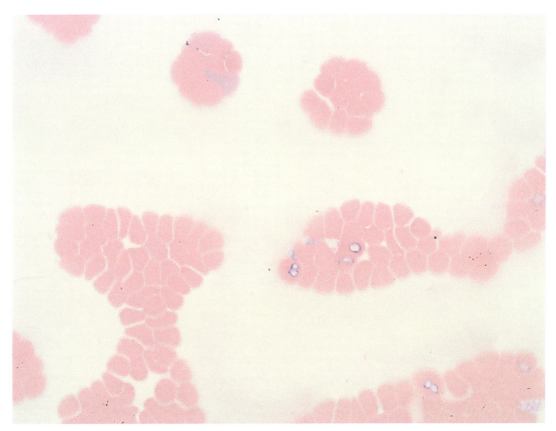

Fig 13.27 *Babesia Canis* in canine red blood cells (prominent pair in centre of image, also elsewhere both singly and in pairs) (×1000)

Romanowsky stains (such as *Diff-Quik*) (see page 27).

With aqueous Romanowsky stains, the inclusions appear as rounded large red inclusions, roughly the size of a platelet. With methanol Romanowsky, the inclusions are similar in shape and size but are a much fainter blue-grey colour.

> **Key points**
>
> **Erythrocytes**
> - One or more polychromatophils per ×1000 HPF in cats, and two or more in dogs, indicate regeneration
> - Agglutination and rouleaux should be assessed in the monolayer
> - The presence of significant numbers of nRBCs in the absence of regeneration is unusual (inappropriate rubricytosis)
> - Spherocytes are very difficult, if not impossible, to identify in cats
> - Cats are more prone to oxidative damage of RBCS and low numbers of Heinz bodies can be seen with many conditions

Leukocytes

Low power assessment – leukocyte numbers
(FIG 13.28)

Leukocyte numbers can be broadly assessed at low power. It can be more challenging to form an estimate of WBC numbers because they are unevenly and slightly unpredictably distributed (the distribution depends not only on leukocyte numbers but their size, any anaemia or alterations in blood viscosity or protein levels). In some cases, most leukocytes can be found in the tail of the film, with only scattered cells present in the body. In others, leukocytes are spread evenly throughout the body and the tail, and in others small groups of leukocytes are seen.

Regardless, experience can help roughly estimate whether the white cell count (WCC)

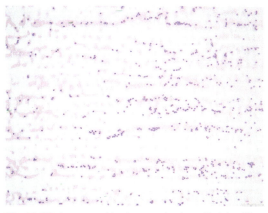

Fig 13.28 Increased leukocytes in the tail of the film (×100)

reported by an analyser is accurate or not – common causes of error in analyser reported WCCs include high numbers of nucleated red blood cells, or, less commonly, small platelet clumps or red cell agglutination.

A rough quantitative estimate can be performed by averaging the number of cells per ×10 low power field and multiplying by 100–150 – this gives a value per micro litre. To convert this to the more typical $×10^9/l$, divide this figure by 1,000. Note that this is a very rough estimate, rarely performed by the author, and is mostly useful to check analyser leukocyte numbers.

High power assessment – differential count

At high power, manual differential counts can be performed – identifying and tallying each leukocyte by type (many programmes and phone apps are available to assist). Manual differential counts are recommended when there is some doubt about analyser differentials, most commonly due to the presence of band neutrophils, nucleated red blood cells or atypical cells – the presence of more than a few of any of these cells should trigger the cytologist to perform a manual differential leukocyte count.

In all cases, the leukocyte proportions are less important than the absolute cell counts – it is less useful to know that 75% of the leukocytes present are neutrophils than there are only three neutrophils observed in total on the blood film. Therefore, leukocyte proportions must also be considered in conjunction with the total white cell count.

With significant leukocytosis, more cells should be counted as part of a manual differential count. If only 100 cells are counted each time, the proportionate value of each cell counted increases, and important information such as significant neutropenia can be lost when a large population of atypical cells are found. A useful rule of thumb is that the differential should comprise 100 cells per $10\times10^9/l$ WCC; therefore for most situations, counting 100 cells is adequate, but as WCC creeps into the 20s and 30s, 200 or 300 cell differentials should be performed.

High power assessment – morphology

As well as identifying cells, at high power the morphology of leukocytes can be assessed, and any abnormalities noted. The most common clinically relevant abnormalities for each leukocyte are noted below.

Neutrophils (FIG 13.29)

The workhorses of the immune system, neutrophils usually comprise the majority of leukocytes in dogs and cats, and are primarily involved in the defence against bacteria, amongst numerous other functions and defences. They have distinctive morphology with an elongated segmented nucleus. As neutrophils mature, the nuclear segmentation becomes more distinct and the band connecting these segments grows thinner.

Neutrophils contain cytoplasmic granules but these are indistinct and barely visible cytologically, particularly when using aqueous Romanowsky stains such as *Diff-Quik*.

> Note: the changes below (band neutrophils and toxic change) are best assessed on fresh blood films – neutrophils in older samples quickly swell and start to display cytoplasmic changes resembling toxic change. Even in films made only 24 hours after sampling, it can be challenging to distinguish between true band cells/toxic change and ageing artefact.

Band neutrophils (FIG 13.30)

Band neutrophils are neutrophils released early into the circulation, usually in response to increased demand. These early neutrophils have had less time to form the distinct nuclear segmentation seen in more mature cells; instead,

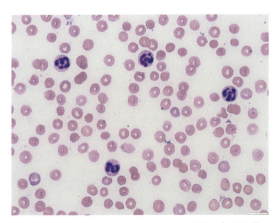

Fig 13.29 Neutrophils in canine blood film (×1000)

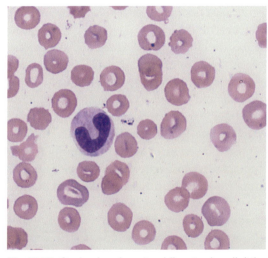

Fig 13.30 Canine band neutrophil; note also slightly increased basophilia (blueness) in cytoplasm (×1000)

their nucleus appears as a linear 'band' with parallel sides.

Inter-observer agreement is often poor between 'true' band neutrophils (which, technically, can have no area of the nucleus less than two thirds the width of any other part of the nucleus) and merely 'hyposegmented' cells, but the presence of poorly-segmented neutrophils is an indication of marked inflammation, and should trigger a manual differential count to confirm the reported analyser differential.

Metamyelocytes are even earlier neutrophils which have rounder nucleus, with only a slight indentation to suggest where future segmentation will occur (Fig 13.31). Metamyelocytes usually indicate very marked inflammation.

Other diseases which cause band neutrophils to appear in the circulation are far rarer than inflammation, but include chronic myeloid leukaemia, leukocyte adhesion deficiency and Pelger-Huët anomaly.

Toxic Change

The term 'toxic change' is confusing, as these changes do not indicate exposure of neutrophils to toxins. Rather, they are visual artefacts due to rushed production of neutrophils through the bone marrow. They range from mild to severe, as listed below (and, as with band neutrophils, these changes are often subjective with limited inter-observer agreement, even amongst professionals). These changes can be found in both mature and band neutrophils.

Mild toxic change – foamy cytoplasm (FIG 13.32)
These cells have 'foamy'-appearing cytoplasm due to the formation of high numbers of microvacuoles. This is a common and mild form of toxic change.

Moderate toxic change – Döhle bodies
(FIGS 13.33, 13.34)
Döhle bodies are remnants of endoplasmic reticulum. Cytologically, they appear as faint bluish-grey small irregular angular structures within the cytoplasm. Note that cat neutrophils from healthy cats often contain low numbers

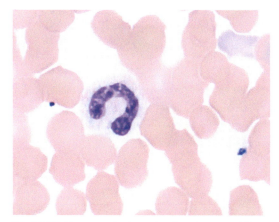

Fig 13.32 Foamy cytoplasm in a band neutrophil (×1000)

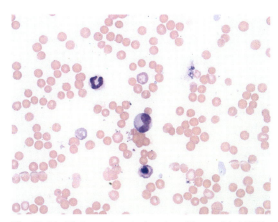

Fig 13.31 Metamyelocyte (centre of image) (×1000)

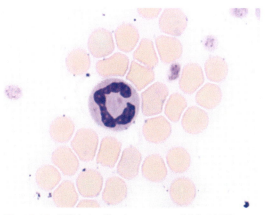

Fig 13.33 Döhle bodies in a neutrophil (×1000)

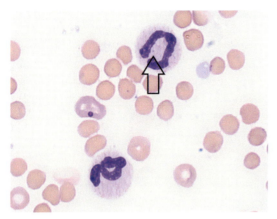

Fig 13.34 More subtle Döhle body in a neutrophil (open arrow) (×1000)

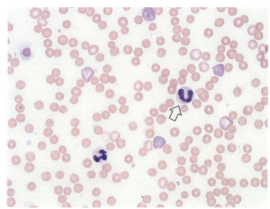

Fig 13.36 Basophilic cytoplasm in a band neutrophil (open arrow) (×1000)

of structures strongly resembling Döhle bodies (Fig 13.35), and toxic change must be interpreted cautiously in cats.

Moderate to marked toxic change – basophilic cytoplasm (FIG 13.36)

This is caused by retention of more endoplasmic reticulum, leading to a bluer cytoplasm than typical. The combination of bigger, blue and hyposegmented nuclei can make it difficult to distinguish them from monocytes on occasion. The pattern of the cytoplasm (which tends to be smoother in neutrophils and patchier in monocytes) is the easiest way to tell them apart, although it remains challenging even for experienced cytologists.

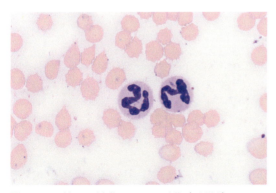

Fig 13.35 Normal feline neutrophils (×1000)

Marked toxic change – toxic granulation

This is a very rare form of toxic change in dogs and cats. These neutrophils retain granules from very early stages of maturation – the granules are small and reddish purple. Their presence indicates very severe toxaemia.

Lymphocytes

Lymphocytes have a variety of functions within the immune system, including regulation, antibody production and cell-mediated immunity.

Lymphocyte numbers

In adult dogs inflammation typically causes neutrophilia and lymphopenia in adults; the presence of lymphocytosis with other signs of inflammation should raise some concerns for other disease. Cats, however, are less predictable; although many cats with inflammation follow the typical pattern, others can have mild ($5-8 \times 10^9$/l) or (rarely) moderate lymphocytosis ($9-20 \times 10^9$/l) (depending upon the degree of inflammation).

In younger patients (less than one year) lymphocyte numbers are often slightly higher, occasionally slightly elevated (lymphocytosis). Patients with Addison's disease often also have mild lymphocytosis due to the lack of corticosteroids (corticosteroids increase circulating neutrophils and decrease lymphocytes), although in both cases circulating lymphocyte numbers rarely exceed $10 \times 10^9/l$.

Moderate to marked lymphocytosis (greater than $10 \times 10^9/l$) in dogs is more typically associated with lymphoproliferative disease – stage V lymphoma or leukaemia (see below). This is more challenging in cats but even here, the larger the lymphocytosis, the more confident the cytologist can feel about lymphoproliferative disease. Lymphocyte counts greater than $50 \times 10^9/l$ are unlikely to be anything other than a neoplastic population, even in cats.

Nevertheless, a blood film should always be examined to investigate lymphocytosis reported by analysers, as other cells (most commonly band neutrophils) are often misclassified as lymphocytes.

Lymphocyte morphology (FIG 13.37)

As is the case in lymph nodes, in normal circumstances most circulating lymphocytes are small (smaller than a neutrophil), with only a few intermediate (same size as a neutrophil) and rare large lymphocytes (larger than a neutrophil). Similar principles apply to circulating lymphocytes as those within lymph nodes; that is, a few larger or unusual-appearing lymphocytes are of limited clinical interest, but when many or the majority of lymphocytes share unusual size or morphological features, a neoplastic population may be suspected.

Reactive lymphocytes (FIG 13.38)

In the presence of inflammation, occasional circulating reactive lymphocytes are found. These are intermediate or large lymphocytes, often with a larger amount ('expanded') of cytoplasm, often more deeply blue than normal lymphocytes. They can have indented or convoluted nuclear shapes. These cells can often be mistaken for atypical lymphocytes and can be challenging to distinguish from them.

Reactive lymphocytes do not usually contain nucleoli except with extreme inflammation (in this case they may in fact be myeloblasts, which resemble large lymphocytes), and they are usually accompanied by many more small lymphocytes.

Granular lymphocytes (FIG 13.39)

Lymphocytes containing low numbers of small magenta granules are a relatively common and usually nonspecific finding on blood films, indicating CD8 or natural killer lymphocytes, although the presence of granules in the majority of lymphocytes observed can be an atypical feature (see below).

Atypical lymphocytes

'Atypical' lymphocytes are lymphocytes with appearances other than 'normal' small, intermediate or large lymphocytes. Atypical features are similar to those observed in neoplastic

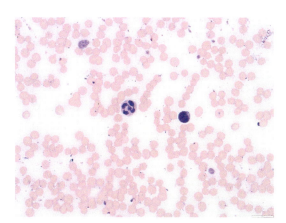

Fig 13.37 Circulating small lymphocyte (×1000)

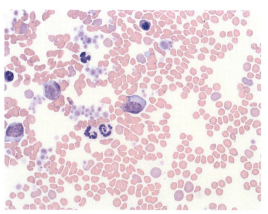

Fig 13.38 Reactive lymphocytes (×1000)

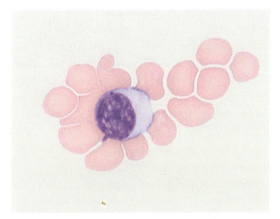

Fig 13.39 Small red granules in a circulating lymphocyte (×1000)

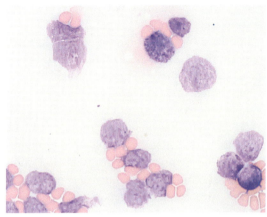

Fig 13.40 Basket cells (×1000)

lymphocytes within lymph nodes and include the presence of nucleoli, irregular granules, increased size, unusual nuclear features or multinucleation.

Cells with nucleoli are a highly unusual finding on blood films; whilst rare large cells with nucleoli can be found in patients with very marked inflammation, the presence of nucleoli in many cells, or few cells without obvious inflammation, raises significant concern for neoplasia (especially acute leukaemia – see page 308, Figs 13.50 and 13.51).

Many atypical lymphocytes can be extremely challenging to distinguish from other atypical circulating cells (such as neoplastic myeloid precursors). Although the morphology can be useful in suggesting an origin, flow cytometry is often required to definitively identify circulating atypical cells.

Atypical cells are generally large, and therefore are more commonly found in the tail of the film. They are also often more fragile than normal cells and are more likely to rupture during blood film preparation. The presence of high numbers of bare nuclei (which often appear like burst balloons or wicker baskets, hence the term 'basket cells') in the tail of the film raises some concern for neoplasia (Fig 13.40).

For further discussion of atypical cells and types of leukaemia, see below (page 308).

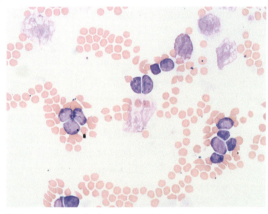

Fig 13.41 Circulating atypical lymphocytes; faint structures resembling nucleoli are present in the lymphocytes at the centre of the image, and most lymphocytes are monomorphic large lymphocytes; basket cells are also present (×1000)

Monocytes (FIG 13.42)

Monocytes are cells destined to develop into macrophages and dendritic cells. They are large, slightly blue, and have 'U' or 'L' shaped central nuclei, similar to band neutrophils, although the chromatin pattern is often slightly patchy. As with neutrophils, their numbers often increase with inflammation (although not usually to the same degree). Although a less reliable and less clinically relevant finding than band or toxic neutrophils, monocytes are often found with vacuolated cytoplasm in patients with marked inflammation (although

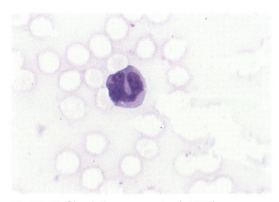

Fig 13.42 Circulating monocytes (×1000)

they can also be vacuolated in the absence of inflammation).

Monocytes are large cells and are therefore most commonly found in the tail of a blood film.

Monocytosis without neutrophilia, band neutrophils or toxic change is an unusual finding which may be associated with a neoplastic population.

Atypical monocytes (FIG 13.43)

'Atypical' monocytes are very difficult to distinguish from atypical lymphocytes. In general, they are more likely to have indented nuclei and will often be accompanied by unusual-appearing more mature monocytes and neutrophils, but these features are difficult to identify and not reliable; flow cytometry is much more accurate at identifying the origin of atypical cells.

Eosinophils (FIGS 13.44, 13.45)

Eosinophils are distinctive and are often associated with more unusual diseases such as hypersensitivity or parasitism (although eosinophil numbers do not generally increase with intestinal parasites except in cases of aberrant migration).

The characteristic eosinophilic (red) granules from which eosinophils derive their name have species-specific morphology: dogs have round granules, whereas cats have linear rod-shaped granules (this can be a useful check of species in cases where slides have become mixed up).

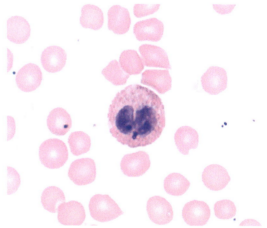

Fig 13.44 Circulating canine eosinophil (×1000)

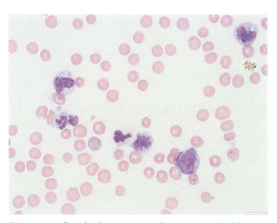

Fig 13.43 Atypical monocytes in acute myeloid leukaemia (×1000)

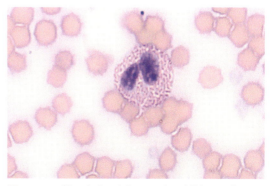

Fig 13.45 Circulating feline eosinophil (×1000)

Grey eosinophils (FIG 13.46)

Some breeds of dog have much lower amounts of peroxidase within their granules, and this leads to pale, washed out or 'grey' eosinophils, easily mistaken for neutrophils by both analysers and cytologists. The granules are visible but much paler than usual, although the patients do not seem to have any compromise of immune function. They are most commonly found in sight hounds but have also been reported in some other dog breeds. They have not been reported in cats.

Band eosinophils (FIG 13.47)

Although they are much less common than band neutrophils, overwhelming demand for eosinophils will lead to their early release and, similar to band neutrophils, these early-released eosinophils have less well-defined nuclear segmentation than mature eosinophils.

Basophils (FIG 13.48)

Basophils are closely related to mast cells, although they have segmented nuclei similar to (but less segmented than) neutrophils. Canine basophils have low numbers of purple granules, similar to mast cell granules but many fewer in number, whereas feline basophils are usually

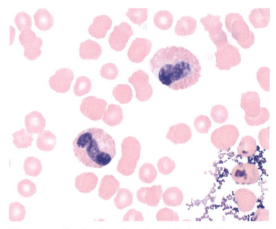

Fig 13.47 Canine band eosinophils (×1000)

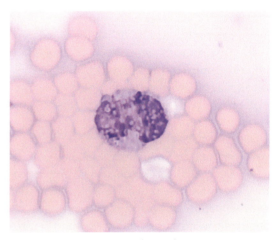

Fig 13.48 Feline basophil (×1000)

filled with pale lavender granules. Basophils are rare in dogs and cats and are usually found accompanying eosinophilic inflammation. They are only rarely of clinical significance.

Mast cells (FIG 13.49)

Circulating mast cells are also rare in dogs and cats but are of more clinical relevance than basophils. In cats, the presence of circulating mast cells (mastocythaemia) is almost always associated with mast cell neoplasia. In dogs, circulating mast cells can also be found in patients with very marked inflammation.

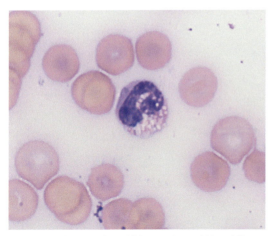

Fig 13.46 Grey eosinophil in greyhound blood film (centre of image) (×1000)

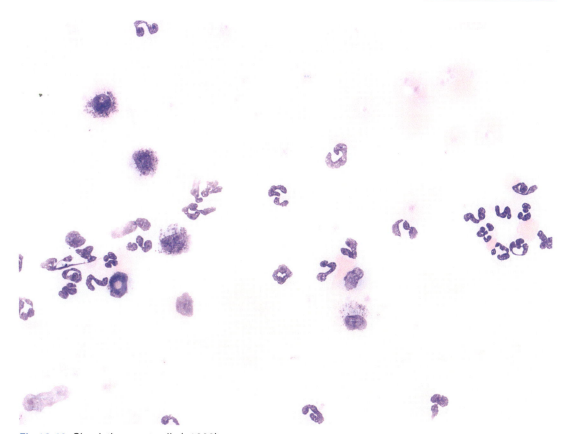

Fig 13.49 Circulating mast cells (×1000)

Leukaemia and circulating neoplastic cells

Most circulating neoplastic cells are due to leukaemia or stage V lymphoma; mast cells are occasionally found (see above), but other circulating neoplasms are very rare.

Lymphoma forms solid masses within lymph nodes and other tissues, but stage V lymphoma cases have circulating neoplastic lymphocytes (see 'atypical lymphocytes' (page 303) for discussion of morphology). Leukaemia does not usually cause solid masses within the tissues but comprises neoplastic cells within the bone marrow and circulation.

> Note: the distinction between lymphoma and leukaemia is not entirely clear cut. For instance, chronic lymphoid 'leukaemia' in dogs often originates in the spleen, rather than the bone marrow, and it can be challenging (and ultimately not especially clinically informative) to distinguish between stage V lymphoma which has infiltrated the bone marrow and leukaemia which has infiltrated lymph nodes or viscera. Many of the terms regarding leukaemia and lymphoma have been inherited from human medicine, some of which can be confusing when applied to the domestic species.

There are several classifications of leukaemia, but the most useful clinical distinctions are those between acute and chronic leukaemia, and those between myeloid and lymphoid leukaemia (these distinctions are not exclusive) – for instance, acute leukaemias can comprise lymphoid (ALL) or myeloid (AML) cells, as can chronic leukaemia (CLL and CML, respectively).

Acute and chronic leukaemia

Again, these are slightly confusing clinical terms, but refer to the fact that 'acute' leukaemia is a much more severe form of disease; patients are typically unwell and, without treatment, deteriorate rapidly. 'Chronic' leukaemia, by contrast, is often an incidental finding in otherwise clinically well patients. Chronic leukaemia typically has a much more indolent course and can be present for years before clinical problems occur.

Acute leukaemia involves very early leukocyte precursors (myeloid or lymphoid). The cells present in leukaemia are large (larger than a neutrophil) and often contain nucleoli – the presence of high numbers of circulating atypical cells containing obvious nucleoli raises significant suspicion for acute leukaemia (although stage V lymphoma is also possible) (Figs 13.50–13.53). The bone marrow is often affected by acute leukaemia, and so there are likely to be one or more cytopenic cell lines present (non-regenerative anaemia, thrombocytopenia, neutropenia).

Chronic leukaemia, however, involves the neoplastic proliferation of mature cells. Patients with chronic lymphoid leukaemia (CLL), for instance, have high (often very high) numbers of circulating unremarkable small lymphocytes (Fig 13.54). Chronic myeloid leukaemia (CML) is much rarer; patients typically have very high

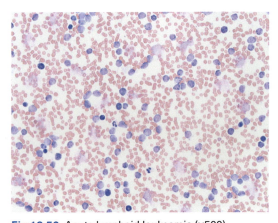

Fig 13.50 Acute lymphoid leukaemia (×500)

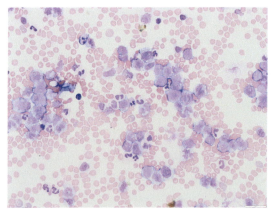

Fig 13.52 Acute myeloid leukaemia; note the difficulty distinguishing from lymphoid cells, but they are more varied and often indented; these cytological features are not reliable in distinguishing between myeloid and lymphoid disease however (flow cytometry or immunocytochemistry are required for this) (×500)

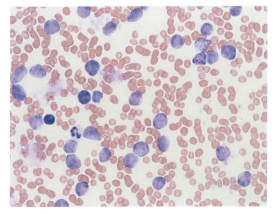

Fig 13.51 Acute lymphoid leukaemia (×1000)

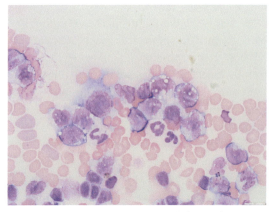

Fig 13.53 Acute myeloid leukaemia (×1000)

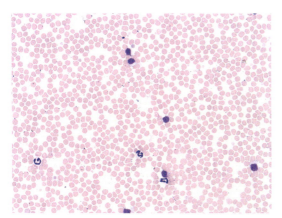

Fig 13.54 Chronic lymphoid leukaemia (×500)

numbers of circulating neutrophils (often present as band neutrophils), although other even rarer forms have excessive eosinophils, monocytes or basophils.

Polycythaemia vera (or primary erythrocytosis) is thought to be a form of chronic leukaemia, which produces high numbers of mature red blood cells. Patients with chronic leukaemia are usually diagnosed incidentally due to the presence of high numbers of lymphocytes (or other cells) on blood smears or in multiple aspirates.

Canine chronic lymphoid leukaemia is more common than feline. There is a common form of canine CLL involving CD8 T-lymphocytes. With this form of CLL, the lymphocytes are intermediate, rather than large (approximately the size of neutrophil), due to slightly increased amounts of cytoplasm, and most of the cells contain small magenta cytoplasmic granules. Nucleoli are not present within the cells (distinguishing them from acute lymphoid leukaemia).

Acute leukaemia is more responsive to chemotherapy but is a much more aggressive disease; chronic leukaemia is challenging to treat medically but progresses more slowly, although it can eventually transform into a much more severe disease, similar to acute leukaemia.

Lymphoid and myeloid leukaemia

Lymphoid leukaemia – that is, leukaemia involving lymphocytes and lymphocyte precursors – is much more common than myeloid leukaemia. Although 'myeloid' can be a confusing term, in this context it refers to haemopoietic cells not of lymphoid origin – i.e. the cells which produce neutrophils, monocytes, eosinophils or basophils (or, very rarely, red blood cells). Myeloid leukaemia most commonly involves neutrophils, monocytes, or both.

The reason this distinction is useful is because, typically, myeloid leukaemia is less responsive to chemotherapy than lymphoid.

Infectious agents of leukocytes

Distemper

Distemper inclusions (see page 298) can be found in leukocytes as well as erythrocytes and, as with erythrocytes, they are more easily visualised with aqueous Romanowsky stains (such as *Diff-Quik*).

Ehrlichia and anaplasma (FIG 13.55)

These are Rickettsiae – a group classified as bacteria but actually somewhat intermediate between bacteria and viruses. They are obligate intracellular organisms, and infect various different leukocytes (or, in the case of *Anaplasma platys*, platelets). They form tightly packed clusters of organisms within cells called *morulae*, which appear cytologically as pale greyish-blue rounded structures, usually present during the acute phase of infection.

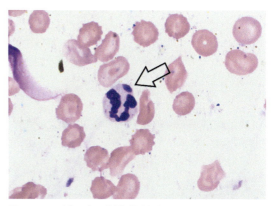

Fig 13.55 Morule of *Ehrlichia* in a canine neutrophil (open arrow) (×1000)

They are most commonly found within neutrophils, monocytes or, occasionally, eosinophils (largely depending on the species of the bacteria). They cause varying diseases from mild fever to severe illness, most commonly in dogs. Haematologically they most often cause severe thrombocytopenia. They also typically cause lymphopenia, but rarely can trigger an immune response that produces a marked lymphocytosis. This can potentially be mistaken for lymphoma or lymphoid leukaemia and should be considered in cases where exposure to the organism is a possibility.

Further testing (such as PCR) is usually required to identify the organisms.

Hepatozoon

These are Protozoal parasites found within the cytoplasm of circulating neutrophils in infected dogs (they are not reported to cause clinical disease in cats), usually in temperate and tropical parts of the world.

Once seen, never forgotten, the gamonts resemble large tablets embedded adjacent to the nucleus. Two species, *H. canis* and *H. americanum*, are known to affect dogs. Of the two species, *H. americanum* causes much more severe disease, but this is rarely found in circulating blood – when gamonts are found on a blood film, they are almost always *H. canis*, which usually causes very mild disease.

Bacteria and other oddities

Rarely, other organisms can be found in circulating blood, including a variety of bacteria (with sepsis) or fungi (with disseminated disease). Mycobacterial organisms are rarely in circulating neutrophils, although they are challenging to spot (see page 114). Monocytes or neutrophils containing phagocytosed mast cell granules can occasionally be found with circulating mast cell neoplasia.

If there has been a delay between sampling and creating the blood film, it is worth considering the possibility that any organisms found may be contaminants, especially if the symptoms of the patient are not consistent with the cytological finding. Context, once again, is important.

> **Key points**
>
> **Leukocytes**
> - The presence of more than a few nucleated red blood cells, band neutrophils or atypical cells should trigger the cytologist to perform a manual differential leukocyte count
> - Band neutrophils and toxic change are best assessed on fresh blood films
> - 'Normal' feline neutrophils often contain structures resembling Döhle bodies
> - A blood film should always be examined to investigate lymphocytosis reported by analysers
> - Younger patients (<one year) and patients with Addison's disease can have mild lymphocytosis
> - Grey eosinophils are found in sight hounds and several other dog breeds
> - In cats, the presence of circulating mast cells (mastocythaemia) is almost always associated with mast cell neoplasia
> - Circulating cells with nucleoli are unusual and should be investigated or monitored
> - Acute leukaemia is generally a severe disease; chronic leukaemia is often indolent and frequently found as an incidental finding

Some 'classic' patterns

Blood film examination can reveal a great deal about a patient, and whilst a detailed examination is always recommended, there are several patterns which are quickly recognisable and clinically very useful. Some common examples are discussed below.

Regenerative anaemia (FIG 13.56)

Although this has been discussed above, it is worth summarising the most noticeable changes here; blood films with regenerative anaemia have higher numbers of polychromatophils (larger blue erythrocytes) – at least one per ×100 HPF for cats, or one to two in dogs, are sufficient to suspect anaemia is regenerative.

Strongly regenerative anaemia usually also contains nucleated red blood cells (nRBCs) – the stronger the regenerative pattern, the more nRBCs present (see page 291). Erythrocytes may also contain small blue flecks of iron ('basophilic stippling'), although this is less common in dogs and cats than other species.

Very strongly regenerative patterns are often associated with retention of iron – clinically, this means that haemolysis and internal haemorrhage usually have a much stronger regenerative response than external blood loss (note that GI haemorrhage usually involves loss of iron and represents 'external' blood loss in this context).

Immune mediated haemolytic anaemia (IMHA) (FIG 13.57)

'Classic' immune mediated haemolytic anaemia combines a number of distinctive features on a blood film. There is typically a strong regenerative response, accompanied with neutrophilia, monocytosis and (often) a neutrophilic left shift.

Spherocytes may be present in high numbers (always check for spherocytes in the monolayer), and agglutination may be evident on the film (distinguish from rouleaux – see page 290).

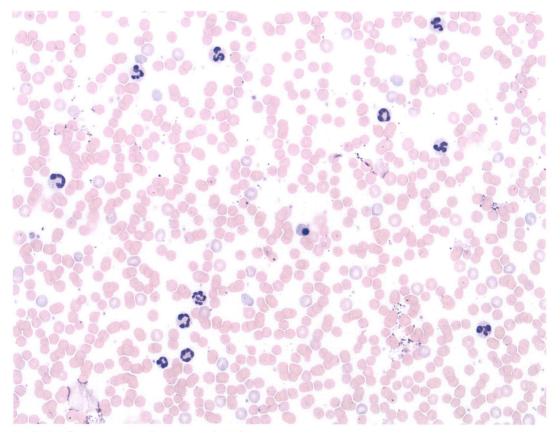

Fig 13.56 Canine regenerative anaemia (×500)

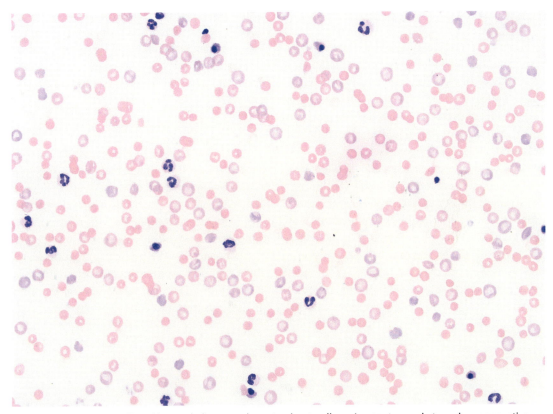

Fig 13.57 Immune-mediated haemolytic anaemia; note ghost cells, spherocytes and strongly regenerative anaemia (×500)

A combination of all of these features is strongly suggestive of immune mediated haemolysis. The absence of some features does not exclude the possibility, although IMHA is unlikely in the absence of regenerative anaemia (although PIMA – precursor immune mediated anaemia – can produce a severe non-regenerative anaemia. Definitive diagnosis of this requires bone marrow examination).

Coombs' test is a standardised assessment of autoagglutination – there is no need to perform Coombs' test if agglutination is already evident on the blood film (or if an in-saline agglutination test is strongly positive).

Iron deficiency (leptocytes) (FIG 13.58)

Iron deficiency only rarely occurs due to dietary deficiencies. It is much more commonly due to chronic iron loss, usually because of chronic GI haemorrhage.

As iron stores are depleted, red cells are retained longer within the bone marrow in order to achieve the same concentration of haemoglobin. Consequently, they often undergo more cell division, leading to smaller red blood cells (microcytes) and reduced mean corpuscular volume as measured by analysers (MCV). Red cells are often paler (hypochromasia, or decreased MCHC) and more fragile than usual.

Blood films from patients with iron deficiency have an evident non-regenerative anaemia. The erythrocytes may appear smaller or, most commonly, paler, with a larger area of central pallor than typical erythrocytes; this is often evident at low power. The fragility of the erythrocytes leads to the presence of red cell fragments – schistocytes and acanthocytes are relatively

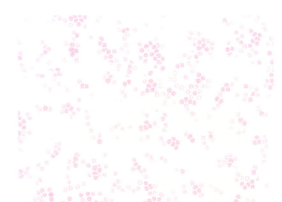

Fig 13.58 Iron deficiency anaemia; red cells are smaller, paler and have larger areas of central pallor (×500)

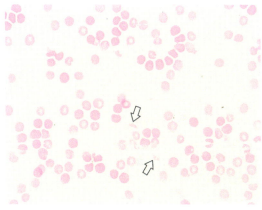

Fig 13.59 Iron deficiency anaemia; the fragile leptocytes are sometimes ruptured into schistocytes (open arrows) (×1000)

common, and the fragile pale red cells are sometimes seen folded over upon themselves (collectively, the thin, fragile and sometimes folded cells are termed 'leptocytes').

Chapter 13 – take home messages

- Platelet clumps make assessment of numbers difficult, but also make clinically significant thrombocytopenia very unlikely.
- The presence of one or more polychromatophils per ×1000 high power field in cats, or two or more in dogs, is consistent with regeneration.
- In cats, the presence of circulating mast cells (mastocythaemia) is almost always associated with mast cell neoplasia.
- Haemolysis and internal haemorrhage usually have a much stronger regenerative response than external blood loss.

Part three

Further thoughts on cytology

Chapter 14

'Edge cases'

When looking at the pictures in textbooks (including this one), the amateur cytologist can easily be fooled into thinking that every case presents a beautiful and distinctive pattern, and that all one needs to do is recognise the pattern to reach a diagnosis.

Whilst this is sometimes the case, it is worth remembering that the most beautiful and most distinctive patterns are the ones that send cytologists scrambling for their digital cameras to get into textbooks. Unfortunately, a good proportion of the average cytologist's time is spent looking at samples of much lower quality. These are cases which are potentially diagnostic but are in some way compromised – the cellularity may be low and comprise a few scattered, different cells, or the cells may be slightly badly preserved, making identification difficult but not impossible. They may be heavily haemodiluted, making searching for nucleated cells a chore amongst the hordes of erythrocytes.

These are 'edge cases' – not absolutely non-diagnostic, but difficult to make sense of and challenging to be definitive about. They are, in short, cases that usually do not make it into a textbook. This chapter discusses some common situations which make cases challenging, and suggests some approaches to them (or, at least, offers solidarity to those experiencing them).

General thoughts

Ideas on how to approach these edge cases are necessarily subjective, hence the term 'thoughts' rather than tips here. Exactly how far one is willing to push a suspicion when faced with a suboptimal sample is largely a matter of personal choice and experience. With that in mind, some general advice follows – *from here, the author will revert to the pronouns 'I' and 'you' to emphasise that these ideas are subjective personal opinions*.

I think it is important to be aware of the limitations of a preparation, and to make others who may be relying upon your diagnosis to be aware of this also. In short – *show your working*.

As part of this process, it is helpful to take a step back and ask yourself everything that you can state for certain faced with the sample under your microscope (e.g. 'there are very few cells here, mostly neutrophils with a few scattered large irregular poorly preserved cells'). It is then useful to consider the case in entirety, as the clinical context can help greatly with these difficult cases (e.g. 'I can't really tell what those big cells are, but this is a young dog, and there's inflammation present – it's likely that they're either reactive fibroblasts or, maybe, macrophages').

If you are examining a case for a colleague, or writing a report, then explain your difficulties in the report, and make it clear where you are certain and where you are unsure and have made an educated guess. Not only does this clarify your position, it means that if it becomes clear later that you have made an incorrect assumption, this can quickly be corrected and a new course taken. If you are examining a case for yourself, potentially months later, personal notes can help you understand how you arrived at the conclusion you did.

- Try to differentiate the cases where there is clearly nothing useful to be gleaned (e.g. completely acellular samples; blood only) from those where there may be some clues (e.g. a few scattered macrophages interspersed with the blood; very low numbers of mixed cells which taken together could suggest an inflammatory response; a mixed cellular harvest; necrosis or degenerate cells).
- Consider the context of the case, and whether repeat sampling is likely to produce the same result or if steps can be taken to improve sample quality (e.g. rapid drying of the slides, sampling from a more peripheral area of the lesion, sample without suction) and, where necessary, communicate this to the clinician.

'Possible' and 'Probable'

Whether examining preparations for one's own cases or reporting for another clinician, it is worth considering how confident you feel about your opinion. Some cytologists list this as a percentage (i.e., lymphoma, 75% confidence). Personally, I feel that this is misleadingly precise and leads to an impression of confidence, when the report is actually attempting to communicate a *lack* of confidence in their diagnosis.

I find the adjectives 'possible' and 'probable' more useful for myself and for the clinicians I am communicating with. I use 'probable' when I think a particular diagnosis is likely but there is some room for doubt (i.e. 'probable lymphoma' when there is a greatly increased population of large lymphocytes, but there are just enough other mixed lymphocytes present to leave the possibility open of a very unusual pattern of reactivity).

I use 'possible' where I am unsure of a diagnosis but the material on the slide is at least suggestive (i.e. 'possible mast cell tumour' where there a few scattered ruptured cells surrounded by a few granules resembling mast cell granules in a reddened cutaneous mass).

Specific edge cases

Poorly cellular samples (FIG 14.1)

Samples with very low cellularity are challenging because it is hard to know whether the preparations are representative of the sampled tissue as a whole. If there are a few scattered mixed lymphocytes in one corner of a sample taken from an enlarged lymph node, can they be taken as an indication of the entire lymphoid population? If the only cells present on an aspirate are a few adipocytes, or ruptured mast cells, is that enough to diagnose a lipoma, or a mast cell tumour?

The answer, as with much in cytology, is that the clinical context must be considered. Do the few cells you have make sense in the clinical context? If there are adipocytes present, does the lesion appear grossly like a lipoma? If there are mast cells, was mast cell tumour a suspicion? If the clinical context is appropriate, then the cytologist can note their suspicion as a possibility.

The most common lesions which exfoliate poorly are mesenchymal masses – fibrous tissue and sarcomas; knowing this helps the cytologist judge whether the samples may be representative or not.

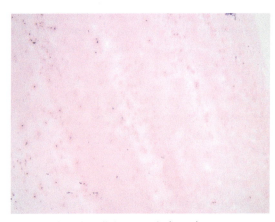

Fig 14.1 Poorly cellular sample (×100)

Poorly preserved samples (FIG 14.2)

Sometimes the first challenge with these preparations is to recognise that the material on the aspirates is poorly preserved; in particular, when cells are apoptotic or necrotic, they can appear to be relatively bland epithelial cells (Fig 14.3). Some clues to poor preservation include the presence of haemoglobin crystals (associated with drying artefact; see page 334, Fig 15.2), a greenish colour to erythrocytes (associated with formalin fumes; see page 333, Fig 15.1), high numbers of ruptured cells or 'basket cells', very irregular and moth eaten chromatin, and marked cellular pleomorphism (some of the features of poor preservation, especially in cells which have spent more than a few hours within fluid, and most especially urine).

Poorly preserved cells are a frustrating diagnostic challenge, and very often no diagnosis or attempt at a diagnosis can be made, but even in completely ruptured cells there are occasional small clues to their origin.

- 'Lymphoglandular bodies' (see page 39) are not specific but often indicate the presence of lymphocytes.
- Free purple granules could reflect mast cells (although gels such as local anaesthetic cream appear very similar) (Fig 14.4).
- Free red granules could indicate the presence of eosinophils (rod-shaped in cats, round in dogs) (Fig 14.5).
- Patches of extracellular matrix (see page 81) could reflect a mesenchymal component.
- High numbers of bare nuclei with occasional small clusters can be a feature of neuroendocrine cells.
- Necrosis is more commonly associated with underlying neoplasia than infection (Fig 14.6).

Mixed cellularity

A very mixed cellular pattern can make it difficult to decide what the underlying disease

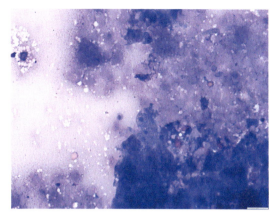

Fig 14.2 Poorly preserved cells and necrosis from a carcinoma; cytological details are very hard to assess (×1000)

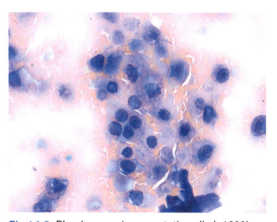

Fig 14.3 Bland-appearing apoptotic cells (×1000)

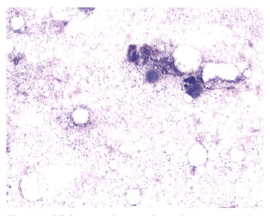

Fig 14.4 High power image of mostly ruptured cells from a mast cell tumour, showing high numbers of mast cell granules in the background alongside bare nuclei (×1000)

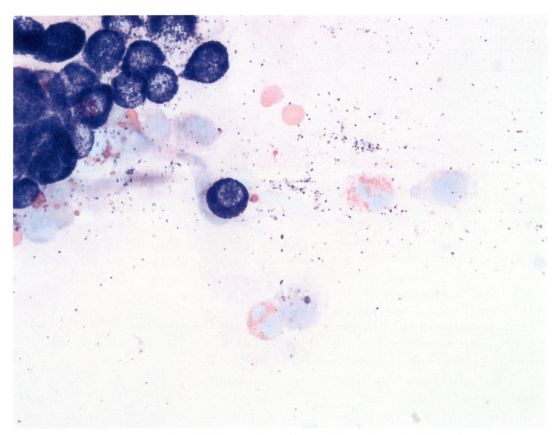

Fig 14.5 Free red granules mixed with higher numbers of mast cell granules; a single intact but poorly-preserved eosinophil is present (×1000)

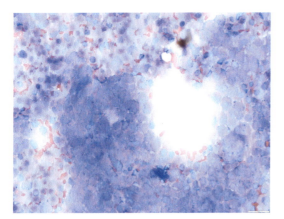

Fig 14.6 Necrosis and ruptured cells; the cells are mostly not intact but they appear to be present in cohesive clusters (×1000)

process is, especially (as is often the case) when combined with low cellularity and suboptimal preservation. Some common patterns of mixed cells include the following.

- Mixed inflammation – most commonly neutrophilic/macrophagic (pyogranulomatous); in these cases the most numerous leukocytes are likely to be the most relevant but the presence of significant numbers of eosinophils (which could indicate a degree of hypersensitivity or parasitism) or lymphocytes (which could represent aspiration of an inflamed lymph node/nodule or may be evidence of immune stimulation) can also be relevant. See page 69 for more details on mixed inflammation (Fig 14.7).

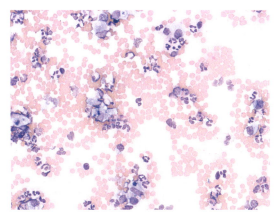

Fig 14.7 A very mixed inflammatory pattern; neutrophils, macrophages, eosinophils and small lymphocytes are all present (×500)

- Inflamed tumours (Fig 14.8) – some tumours are often accompanied with inflammation, most commonly squamous cell carcinomas (neutrophilic inflammation – see page 328, Fig 14.22 and below), histiocytomas (lymphocytic inflammation – see page XX) and mast cell tumours (eosinophilic inflammation; they often also contain pleomorphic mesenchymal cells – see page 135).
- Fibroadnexal hamartomas – these are benign neoplasms which generally exfoliate very poorly; samples often contain low numbers of very mixed cells including basal epithelium, mesenchymal cells, mast cells and collagen;

they are often accompanied with small amounts of mixed inflammation.

Additionally, many cutaneous masses are prone to trauma and can contain low-grade mixed inflammation, usually neutrophils and macrophages.

As with other edge cases, context is important – if the mass has been present for years, but has recently grown in size, then causes beyond inflammation should be considered; if a young puppy recently ran into a door at full speed, the inflammation is likely more relevant than pleomorphic mesenchymal cells, however atypical they appear.

Very bloody samples

Sometimes, no matter how small a needle is used, even without pressure, samples contain lots of peripheral blood. Scanning at low power is most useful for these samples to assess for islands of other cells surrounded by blood, but close examination at high power is also recommended, frustrating though it may be. Slides which appear to consist entirely of peripheral blood can, on closer inspection, reveal the presence of low numbers of macrophages, which have no business in the circulation.

If the macrophages contain phagocytosed erythrocytes or dark pigment resembling haemosiderin, a haemorrhagic lesion such as a vascular hamartoma or haemangioma may be suspected. In the author's experience, macrophages are often found around the periphery or at the edge of these smears, presumably because of their larger size (Fig 14.9).

With extremely bloody samples, estimation of inflammation becomes challenging, partially because the blood dilutes any leukocytes already present, and partially because it is impossible to tell whether the leukocytes were blood-derived or present in the lesion (exceptions to this include macrophages and plasma cells, neither of which should be found circulating in normal circumstances).

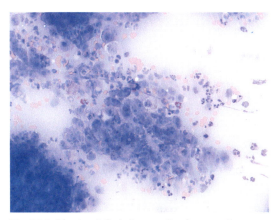

Fig 14.8 Neutrophilic inflammation in a carcinoma (×500)

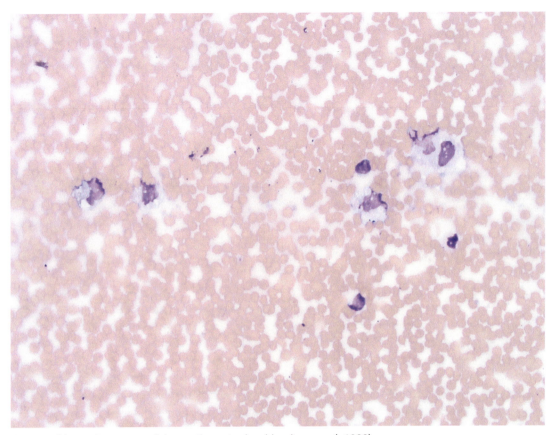

Fig 14.9 Macrophages containing erythrocytes in a bloody smear (×1000)

In these cases, it helps to imagine examining a blood film, and asking yourself if you would consider the white cell count to be significantly elevated – if so, then inflammation is possible (although circulating leukocytosis is also possible). If leukocytes are found clumped in groups rather than evenly distributed throughout the preparations, then inflammation may also be more likely than mere haemodilution (Fig 14.10).

The dreaded Ms

Here we come to the dreaded 3 'm's – cells that frequently fool the unwary inexperienced cytologist, as well as many wary experienced ones: mesenchymal cells, macrophages and mesothelial cells. All three cell types can appear significantly atypical, even when they are part of a benign reactive or inflammatory process. More specific notes for each cell type are below.

Mesenchymal cells – atypical or reactive
(FIG 14.11)

As discussed before (see page 69), mesenchymal cells can proliferate either as a reactive process (fibroplasia) or neoplasia (sarcomas), and it can be extremely difficult to distinguish between these possibilities, especially when cellularity is low and inflammation is present. With significant trauma, fibroblasts (the cells involved in reactive fibroplasia) display many features of malignancy – marked pleomorphism, anisocytosis, anisokaryosis, multinucleation, multiple nucleoli.

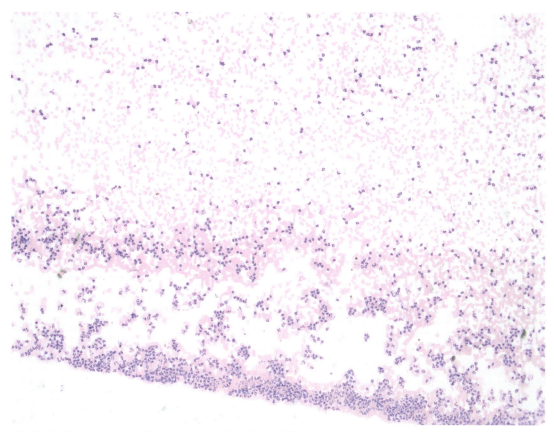

Fig 14.10 Bloody smear with increased neutrophils (×100)

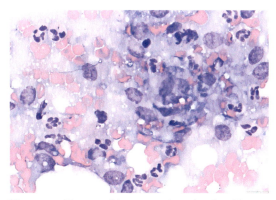

Fig 14.11 Pleomorphic mesenchymal cells with inflammation (×1000)

This is also the case when present alongside neoplasia (especially mast cell tumours). As mentioned previously, great care must be taken when diagnosing a sarcoma or atypical mesenchymal cells when inflammation is present (this also applies to macrophages – see below).

Ultimately, the distinction is likely to require histopathology, but much can be gleaned from a thorough history (did the mass appear suddenly? Is there a history of trauma? How long has it been present?).

Macrophages versus atypical cells

Macrophages are extremely versatile cells, plastic – under the influence of chemical markers, they can cling together like epithelial cells (*epithelioid macrophages*) or spawn multiple nuclei (Figs 14.12, 14.13); they can become deeply basophilic when highly active and appear highly pleomorphic with significant inflammation. In short, activated macrophages were

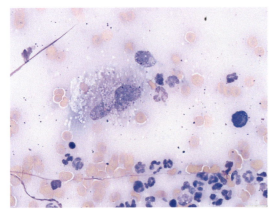

Fig 14.12 Multinucleate macrophage (×1000)

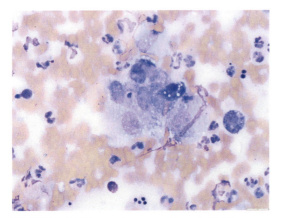

Fig 14.13 Multinucleate macrophage (×1000)

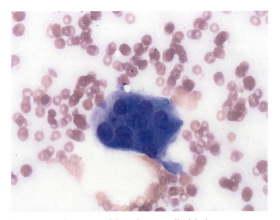

Fig 14.14 Large multinucleate cell; this is an osteoclast (bone-dwelling macrophages) – note the similar-size nuclei (×1000)

almost perfectly designed to fox and befuddle unlucky cytologists.

No method of attempting to distinguish between macrophages and atypical cells is entirely foolproof, but perhaps the most reliable method is to examine the nuclei closely. As a general rule, macrophages can display marked shape variation (pleomorphism) and size variation (anisocytosis) but only relatively mild nuclear size variation (anisokaryosis). That is, no matter how dramatically transformed macrophages may appear, they typically still have relatively small oval nuclei, roughly 10–15µm in diameter (about 1.5–2 erythrocytes). They have coarsely stippled or coarse chromatin (see page 38) and usually only have one to two nucleoli. Populations of cells with marked nuclear size variation are unlikely to be macrophages, especially when combined with high numbers of nucleoli.

Similarly, multinucleate macrophages can have many nuclei (in some cases 20 or more) but usually the nuclei are very similar sizes (Fig 14.14). Cells with marked anisokaryosis within the same cell are unlikely to be macrophages.

Nuclear to cytoplasmic ratio is also helpful here – for many neoplastic cells, one of the first features of malignancy is an increase in size of the nucleus with respect to the rest of the cell – the nuclear:cytoplasmic ratio increases. For most activated macrophages, the opposite is true – the cytoplasm expands without a significant increase in nuclear size, leading to a reduction in the nuclear to cytoplasmic ratio.

Perhaps the most difficult distinction a cytologist is likely to face is attempting to differentiate between marked macrophagic (granulomatous) inflammation, and well-differentiated histiocytic sarcoma (neoplastic macrophages or dendritic cells). Close examination of these cells often reveals occasional cells that have gone 'too far' – cells whose features appear too extreme for macrophages. Nevertheless, this remains subjective and sometimes a clear distinction cannot be made.

A final reminder: take great care diagnosing the presence of atypical cells where significant inflammation is present. In particular, macrophages often appear highly pleomorphic in the presence of keratin (i.e. a ruptured follicular cyst) or injected material (i.e. injection site reaction) (Figs 14.15–14.17).

Mesothelium versus atypical cells (FIG 14.18, 14.19)

The final cell type in the cytologist's trifecta of traps, mesothelial cells disobey most of the rest of the rules discussed previously, especially in the section discussing 'General features of malignancy' (see page 92). Reactive mesothelial cells can display marked pleomorphism (variation in shape), anisocytosis and anisokaryosis (cell size and nuclear size variation). They can

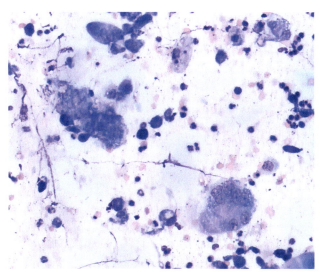

Fig 14.15 Ruptured cyst with neutrophilic/macrophagic inflammation and a multinucleate macrophage (×500)

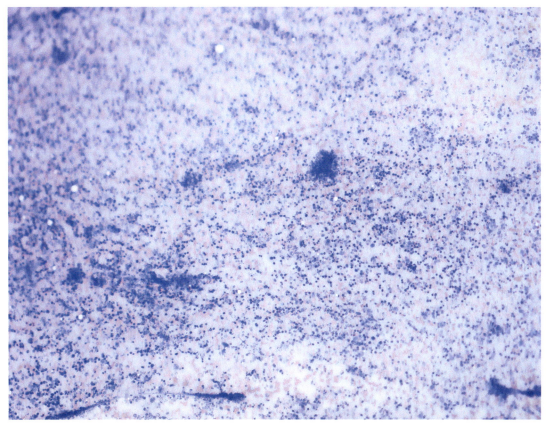

Fig 14.16 Vaccine reaction (×100)

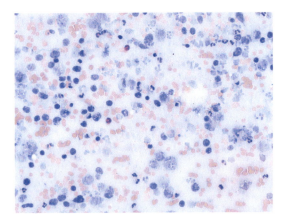

Fig 14.17 Vaccine reaction; the macrophages often contain greyish-blue vaccine adjuvant (×500)

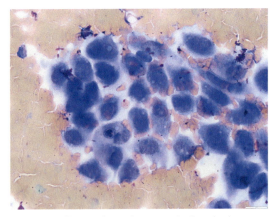

Fig 14.18 Sheet of reactive mesothelium in the spleen (×1000)

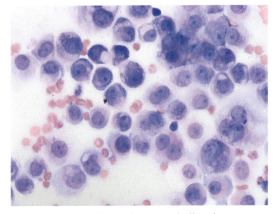

Fig 14.19 Sheet of reactive mesothelium in pericardial effusion (×1000)

have multiple nucleoli and even macronucleoli – there are few recognisable features to distinguish between marked reactive mesothelium and neoplasia.

They are particularly prevalent, and particularly atypical-appearing, in pericardial effusions; be very careful before diagnosing neoplasia based on a pericardial effusion. Sheets of mesothelium line the pleural, peritoneal and pericardial spaces, and even non-reactive mesothelium can cause headaches for cytologists (as they can be mistake. for epithelial cells).

Sheets of non-reactive mesothelium are not uncommonly harvested during sampling of thoracic and abdominal organs.

Mesenchymal versus epithelial cells and poorly differentiated neoplasia

Although the distinction between mesenchymal and epithelial cells may seem clear (see page 72, Table 4.2), it can be difficult with poorly differentiated neoplasia; as epithelial tumours evolve, the selective pressure to reduce cohesion between epithelial cells (leads to easier metastasis) leads to a phenomenon known as 'epithelial-mesenchymal transition'; as malignancy develops, the epithelial cells start to resemble mesenchymal cells (Fig 14.20). Poorly differentiated carcinomas often form loose aggregates, instead of tight dense clusters. Individual cells become more pleomorphic and somewhat fusiform (spindle-shaped).

Consequently, it can be difficult to cytologically distinguish between poorly differentiated carcinomas and poorly differentiated sarcomas (although the presence of a malignant neoplasm is usually not in doubt). The context, as ever, is helpful – the biological behaviour and clinical appearance can help to narrow down the possibilities (for example, a poor differentiated neoplasm metastasised to a lymph node is much more likely to be a carcinoma than a sarcoma).

Cytologists often describe such lesions as a 'poorly differentiated malignancy' or similar. Best

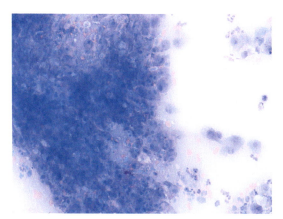

Fig 14.20 Carcinoma resembling mesenchymal cells (×1000)

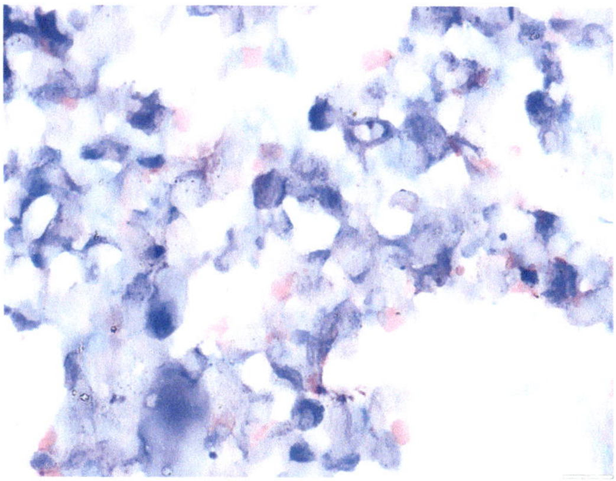

Fig 14.21 Degenerative material aspirated from a feline cutaneous mass; note the lack of inflammation (×1000)

guesses can often be made; where this is done, my advice is as above: *show your working*. Make it clear where there is doubt in your interpretation.

Myoepithelium

A related and similarly confusing tissue to examine cytologically is *myoepithelium* – this is epithelial tissue with some contractile ability, similar to muscle. It is most commonly found within mammary aspirates, usually mammary tumours (see page 164), although similar-appearing material can sometimes be found in aspirates from salivary carcinomas (see page 167). They are also present in sweat glands but are very rarely found in non-mammary, non-salivary samples.

Myoepithelium generally appears as typical cuboidal epithelium in the centre of the clusters – tightly cohesive and generally well-ordered cells – but at the periphery, the cells develop a more fusiform shape and the overall impression is of a somewhat jagged or feathery edge, as opposed to the much rounder border observed in more typical epithelial clusters.

Degeneration* versus necrosis (FIG 14.21)

When applied to cytological specimens, these terms are generally used to refer to different processes. When discussing 'degenerate material', cytologists usually mean non-cellular material which has lost its typical cytological appearance and is now visually degenerate and hard to identify. This is most commonly seen with keratin, which can lose its distinct angular appearance and even deep blue colour to appear as amorphous pale blue to grey sludge. In this form, degenerate material can be challenging to distinguish from necrosis (see page 96).

The distinction is important because, clinically, degenerate material is rarely associated with serious disease, and usually represents a benign process, whereas necrosis is more often associated with neoplasia, often malignant neoplasia, or severe inflammation.

Cytologically, the main difference is the presence of *necrotic cell ghosts*. Patches of necrosis usually contain faded grey structures, hard to assess as they are often blurry, but of similar size and shape to cells or nuclei; they are, indeed, the remnants of necrotic cells. Although they are found more easily in early necrosis, at least a few can usually be found in more advanced necrotic processes.

Additionally, necrosis triggers inflammation, whereas degeneration usually doesn't. Patches of necrosis usually contain low or moderate numbers of neutrophils and activated macrophages embedded within it. Degenerate material does not usually contain inflammatory cells, although in some cases (ruptured keratin cysts, for example) significant inflammation may be present around and sometimes within the material. Once again, the context is important and, once again, when in doubt it is important to acknowledge this.

> *Note that this is distinct from the more typical use of the term 'degeneration' which refers to cells that have been damaged but not irretrievably so, such as hydropic degeneration in the hepatocytes, which leads to the cytological appearance of indiscrete vacuolation.

Squamous cell carcinomas versus inflammation and keratin (FIGS 14.22, 14.23)

Squamous cell carcinomas are often accompanied with significant neutrophilic inflammation (see page 171) and can also contain moderate amounts of keratin. Ruptured keratin cysts and inflamed skin aspirates also contain keratin, high numbers of leukocytes and occasional nucleated squamous epithelial cells, making distinguishing between them frustrating on occasion.

Cytologically obvious squamous cell carcinomas contain relatively little keratin, and highly atypical keratinised cells, including 'tadpole cells' (see page 140); they also often contain atypical appearing denser clusters of more basal epithelium. These present little cytological challenge, but some cases have more keratin, no obvious basal epithelial clusters, and low numbers of nucleated squames, and these are the 'edge cases', hard to distinguish from inflamed cysts and other skin inflammation.

As a general rule, a diagnosis of squamous cell carcinoma should be made with care in the absence of dense clusters of atypical epithelium, unless the degree of atypia displayed by the squamous epithelial cells is very marked.

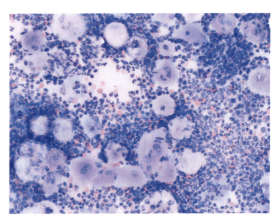

Fig 14.22 Squamous cell carcinoma with marked neutrophilic inflammation; note the increased numbers of nucleated squamous cells (occasionally binucleate) (×1000)

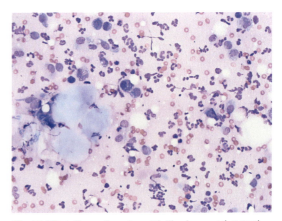

Fig 14.23 Inflamed ruptured follicular cyst (×1000)

Similarly, but conversely, the possibility of a squamous cell carcinoma should never be completely excluded when more than a few scattered nucleated squamous epithelial cells are present.

Squamous cell carcinomas versus papillomas (FIG 14.24)

For similar reasons to above, the distinction between these lesions can sometimes be difficult, especially when papillomas are inflamed. Overall, however, although both lesions comprise atypical nucleated squamous epithelial cells, those within papillomas (*koilocytes*)

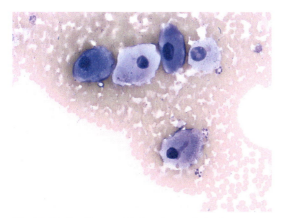

Fig 14.24 Papilloma with free bacteria in the background and within koilocytes (×1000)

are quite distinctive (see page 146, Fig 6.28). Keratinocytes have nuclei that appear moth eaten, or which appear to be disintegrating, and nucleoli are rare and often small. Their cytoplasm often contains distinctive laminar purple striations (rather like an onion cut in half), or sometimes a slightly bubbly appearance. The cells usually display far less pleomorphism than those found within squamous cell carcinomas.

Cysts (FIG 14.25)

Aspirates from cystic structures are not a diagnostic challenge, in that they are readily identifiable. The problem is that they *all look the same*, and so it is very difficult to distinguish between the possible causes of the cyst. It is effectively impossible cytologically to distinguish between a 'true' cyst and a cystic area within a larger neoplasm. Cystic fluid has a stippled background, usually containing scattered red blood cells, low numbers of activated macrophages (organising and removing the fluid), and occasionally low numbers of neutrophils.

As ever, the context of the lesion is helpful to further evaluate cystic structures, but 'pure' cystic fluid (i.e. cystic fluid without other evidence of inflammation, and into which none of the surrounding cells have exfoliated (which they rarely do)) is generally unhelpful cytologically, and further information will usually require histopathological examination of the wall of the structure.

Joint fluid versus myxoma/myxosarcoma (FIG 14.26)

Joint fluid has a distinctive cytological background – it is stippled, pink, and often has protein clefts. It also sometimes has a 'cracked' appearance. It often contains windrowing cells (see page 52), mononuclear or sometimes slightly mesenchymal in appearance.

So, annoyingly, do myxomas and myxosarcomas; these are mesenchymal neoplasms that

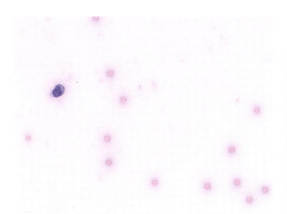

Fig 14.25 Typical appearance of cystic fluid; pale pink stippled background with scattered erythrocytes and macrophages (×1000)

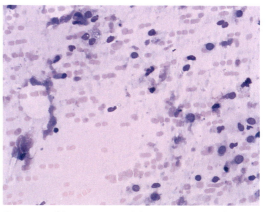

Fig 14.26 Myxoma resembling synovial fluid (×500)

produce a mucous-like substance that strongly resembles joint fluid cytologically. It can be very difficult to distinguish between these possibilities when lesions are present close to or attached to joint capsules.

The context and history are useful (of course) but ultimately histopathology is often required to distinguish between these possibilities.

> **Chapter 14 – take home messages**
>
> - Context is extremely important to help distinguish between lesions that have a similar cytological appearance.
> - 'Show your working' – where there is doubt in an interpretation, acknowledge this and clearly understand where supposition and guesswork has occurred (and show this to the clinician if it is not your case).

Chapter 15

Submitting to an external lab

Cytology is a varied and often challenging skill. Cytologists who spend their working lives examining specimens encounter new, interesting and often confusing cases daily. There is no shame and a great deal of wisdom in asking for help. At the very least, it can be reassuring to discover that even highly experienced pathologists are as confused by your case as you are. At best, it can greatly help in the interpretation of difficult cases.

Pathologists in an external laboratory do not have all of the facts of the case at their fingertips and rely upon the submitting clinician to help them interpret the specimens. What follows is some advice on how best to improve the chances of diagnosis when submitting to external labs.

Labelling samples

External laboratories process hundreds of slides a day. Accurate labelling is essential to reduce the risk of the specimens getting lost during processing, and to save time for the pathologist when a case is presented to them.

- Label the submitted slides with the patient's name, surname, and brief description of the sample location.
- **Label each slide individually** – unlabelled slides in labelled slide holders are impossible to identify if the slides get mixed up (although label the slide holders too).

Felt pen on slides will often be erased during the staining process; ink pen occasionally will be too. Sticky labels can also be lost during processing. Pencil written on frosted glass is preferable and unlikely to be lost. Scratching details onto a slide with an engraving tool is also a possibility, although time consuming for the clinician.

Fluids

If fluid specimens are included, make sure they are again labelled on every sample tube with the patient's name and site of the sample (especially important when multiple fluids are submitted, or fluid is submitted alongside blood). The date of sampling is also useful for fluid samples to help assess deterioration since sampling (Fig 15.2). Where possible (i.e. where there is enough sample), submitting direct fresh in-house smears can be useful (although this is largely unhelpful for poorly cellular fluids such as CSF or respiratory samples).

When in-house smears are included with a specimen, clearly label whether the preparation was smeared directly from the sample (direct) or whether the sample was concentrated prior to preparing the smear (concentrated). This makes it much easier for the pathologist to assess the cellularity of the sample.

Submission form

Pathologists in external labs understand the demands of practice, and how it can be challenging to find a few moments to fill in a form amongst the chaos, but missing out important details can lead to delays in reporting as the laboratory tries to clarify ambiguities or uncover missing information. The author has received submissions from practices missing any (or all!) of the information discussed below, and in each case the reporting of the sample has been slower as a consequence.

Patient and practice details

Include all salient details of the patient with the submission form – this includes name, age, species, breed, date of sampling, sex and neutering status – as well as the submitting practice and the clinician involved.

Where some details are ambiguous or have recently changed (for instance, a sample taken from a patient that was neutered at the same time as sampling) then briefly explain this in the history section.

History

A concise and relevant history is extremely important for submissions. As demonstrated previously, cytology is a highly subjective discipline, and the context in which samples are taken and examined is highly important.

Omitting any history at all is much more likely to lead to an equivocal and less helpful report (or, at least, a phone call from the lab requesting more details, delaying the report). Almost as unhelpful is including unedited clinical notes for patient's last few weeks, months or years – the pathologist is much more likely to miss relevant details sandwiched between pages of clinical notes, flea treatment and wormer sales.

The most helpful details to include with a submission are as follows.

- *Precise* location of sites sampled (see below for some notes on anatomy).
- Reason for sampling (e.g. lesions found on imaging, persistent enlargement, history of neoplasia elsewhere).
- Gross appearance (or appearance on imaging/features on palpation for internal masses) (e.g. hairless, diffuse versus discrete mass, hyper/hypoechoic, colour, texture, attached versus mobile).
- Other relevant clinical findings (e.g. marked hyperglobulinaemia, hypercalcaemia, masses elsewhere not sampled).
- Details from previous history which may be relevant (e.g. previous mast cell tumour, currently on chemotherapy, bouts of pancreatitis, history of trauma in the sample location).

It can also be useful to include the differential diagnoses you are most suspicious of or ask any clinical questions that you are particularly interested in, which can help focus the pathologist on the details most relevant to your case (e.g. 'Concerned for mast cell tumour'; 'Is this swelling a lymph node?'; 'Suspect hepatic nodular hyperplasia but want to rule out neoplasia' etc.).

Some notes on anatomy

Medical terminology, as well as providing extremely useful face-saving terms such as 'idiopathic' and 'iatrogenic', furnishes clinicians with detailed ways of describing the precise location of lesions. It is a shame to allow these elegant terms to go to waste by instead using ambiguous language which can lead to confusion and misinterpretation. Listed below are some terms best avoided or that require further clarification.

Neck

This may seem like a precise term, but it actually covers everywhere from the thoracic inlet to the submandibular region, and says nothing about whether a lesion is dorsal, ventral, or lateral. 'Neck lump' could represent anything from a thyroid carcinoma to a sarcoma involving the spinous processes of the cervical vertebrae.

Throat

Again, this may seem like a precise location, but actually covers a wide anatomical area, and, in isolation, does not make it clear whether a lesion is present within the oropharynx, larynx, or subcutaneous or cutaneous tissues surrounding them.

Rump
This is another term which can refer to large areas of a patient, from the dorsal pelvis, pelvic limbs, tail base or anal mass.

Bum
The author feels we should be able to do better than this.

Abdominal/thoracic
Remember to include details of whether lesions are *intra*abdominal/thoracic, or *extra*abdominal. 'Abdominal mass' is more ambiguous than it appears at first.

Cervical
Frustratingly, despite the author waxing lyrical above about the elegance of anatomical terms, 'cervical' can actually refer to two separate anatomical locations: the cervical spine, or the cervix (it comes from the Latin for 'neck' but is often applied to general narrowing of tissues). Regardless, remember to clarify which location you are referring to with submissions.

Subcutaneous versus cutaneous
These *are* precise terms (as are their synonyms *dermal* and *subdermal*) but are often misused, especially as it can be challenging to tell the difference in some diffuse or invasive lesions. See page 130 for a further discussion, but 'cutaneous' masses are usually visible on the skin's surface or are clearly palpable just underneath it – if the skin is lifted, then a cutaneous mass lifts as well. In contrast, 'subcutaneous' masses are present beneath the surface of the skin and are only visible when they deform the overlying skin. The skin is generally mobile over subcutaneous masses except for lesions which have invaded the cutaneous layer, and when the skin is lifted, a subcutaneous mass should remain in its original position.

For lesions where it is not entirely clear whether the mass is cutaneous or subcutaneous, record this difficulty in classifying on the submission form.

Packaging
Even when the sample has been successfully taken, labelled, and a concise and relevant history has been included, mistakes in packaging can significantly affect the quality of specimens and the chance of diagnosis. Here are the most common situations to avoid:

Packing cytology with histopathology (FIG 15.1)
Unfortunately, cytology specimens are very sensitive to formalin fumes; even limited exposure has a significantly deleterious effect on the quality and preservation of samples. Cytology exposed to formalin has a washed-out appearance, with erythrocytes and many nucleated cells often stained a nauseating greenish colour. This can ruin an otherwise diagnostic sample. To avoid the risk of this, submit histopathology and cytology specimens separately.

Packaging wet (FIG 15.2)
When slides are placed into slide holders before they are fully dry, the condensation results in 'drying artefact' – it leads to rupture of many

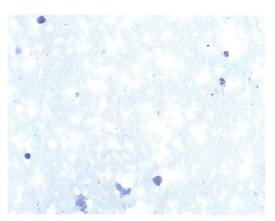

Fig 15.1 Greenish-blue material from a preparation affected by formalin fumes (×500)

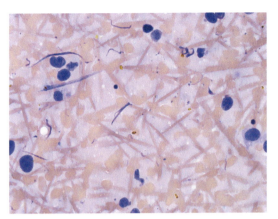

Fig 15.2 Drying artefact (×1000)

cells and markedly reduces the quality of samples. The telltale sign of drying artefact is red cells reduced to spiky haemoglobin crystals and this can, again, ruin a perfectly good sample. To avoid, ensure that slides are completely dry before packaging. For some samples (such as synovial fluid preparations), using a hairdryer on low heat or cool settings can help to speed up the drying process.

Prestaining slides

It is perfectly understandable that, after a sample is procured, the clinician will want to examine the specimens. Unfortunately, pathologists are creatures of habit and ritual, and are likely to be accustomed to the stain used in their particular lab. Although pre-staining will not ruin preparations, it alters the staining properties of the slides and can make certain conditions more challenging to identify for cytologists used to a certain stain. As with many things in life, prestaining is fine in moderation, but it is helpful to leave some cellular slides unstained to increase the chances of a diagnosis.

Chapter 15 – take home messages

- Label individual slides as well as slide holders, ideally with pencil on frosted glass.
- A concise and relevant history will help speed up the process and improve chances of a diagnosis.
- Use precise anatomical terms (avoid 'neck', 'throat', 'bum').
- Package cytological and histological specimens separately.
- Do not package slides when they are still wet.

Chapter 16

Digital and remote cytology

Digital cytology – the ability to scan parts or the entirety of cytological specimens, and then upload them so that the image can be sent elsewhere – is gaining rapid ground in both human and veterinary medicine. The current limitations (internet speeds, size and storage of digital files) are diminishing quickly and digital cytology (and histology) are likely to represent the bulk of future work for pathologists very soon.

The many benefits of digital cytology include the ability to work from anywhere with a computer (or, in the future, a tablet or even a phone), rapid sharing with colleagues for extra opinions, and being able to show (rather than attempt to describe) pathological changes to the client.

For those who examine their own slides in house, the benefits are less obvious but they remain – simple or clear cases can be examined in house, whereas more complex or confusing cases can be shared with specialists for an opinion or a detailed report.

Quality of digital samples

Scan speed and quality are rapidly improving, and very soon (if not already) will be as good quality as glass slide preparations, even at high magnifications. Software exists to correct for thick smears present in multiple focal planes.

Digital cytology does not create samples better than those originally taken, however – at least currently, the preparations still need to be stained before they are uploaded. Poorly cellular or poorly preserved samples will remain so digitally, and issues with stain or drying will also be visible on digital samples. Future iterations of digital software will probably be able to correct for some stain or preservation issues, but the author's mother's phrase, taught to them long ago, remains as true for digital work as it does for British prime ministers: *'You can't polish a turd!'*

Sampling method for digital samples

Procuring a sample for digital work remains (at the time of writing) identical to taking a sample for in-house or external submission (see Chapter 2). The sample may need to be prepared differently after staining, however – most digital scanners currently require cover slips to be used. The original glass sample is not consumed in the process and remains accessible for further examination.

Scanning

After the sample is prepared, samples are scanned via a digital scanner. These vary from small scale machines, which scan one or low numbers of slides at a time, to large machines used in labs. which scan hundreds of slides at once. The scanning time (and image size) varies depending on the scanner and the maximum magnification required.

Histopathologists can often work successfully at lower magnifications, as they are more concerned with architecture than individual cell morphology, but cytology specimens usually require more detailed high power sample. Consequently, cytology digital samples may take longer to scan and may produce larger files, although this is becoming less of an issue as technology progresses.

Examination

Once scanned, the images are as they sound – cytology preparations stored digitally. They can be examined (with the right software) just as a glass slide, with a few extra bells and whistles – artificial intelligence algorithms can rapidly count cells and display all suspected examples of a certain cell type, for instance. The examination process is and principles of cytology remain as described in the previous chapters of this book, however.

The principal advantage of the digital image is its mobility. The image can now be shared (internet speed permitting) with anyone around the world with access to the software, and second opinions rapidly sought.

Remote cytology

This is an alternative technique for remote viewing of cytology samples. Rather than converting the image to a digital file and uploading it, this technique gives remote access and control of the microscope to a cytologist elsewhere. The slide is placed on a remote-controlled microscope with a camera attached – the remote cytologist can then log into this machine and examine it as they would a preparation in the same room. The technique has a number of advantages (no cumbersomely large files, no need to scan the slides) but limitations too (only one person can view the image at once, or at least control the microscope at once, requires a constant stable internet connection).

Artificial intelligence and the future of cytology

As a child who grew up watching the *Terminator* films, the author has a healthy respect for digital sentience and would like to be the first to salute their new robot overlords. This aside, however, artificial intelligence remains (at the time of writing) a blunt and inconsistent tool. It is very good at recognising patterns and can make what seem to us surprising logical leaps, depending upon how much data are fed into it. Cytology is, however, (as hopefully this book has made clear) often a subjective science, highly dependent upon context.

Artificial intelligence has the potential to greatly augment cytological examination, and to pick up on patterns not immediately apparent to the cytologist. It may even replace human examination in some standardised areas of cytological examination (such as blood film assessment). Even for these samples, however, a human is likely to remain necessary in at least the medium term to examine cases which the AI has flagged up as unusual.

For non-standardised cases (i.e. most of the rest of cytology), humans will remain essential to assess the whole context of the case and to make educated guesses where details are scarce. This is likely to remain the case until digital intelligence surpasses that of human and, at this stage, humanity will have larger problems than a few unemployed pathologists.

Chapter 16 – Take home messages

- Digital cytology is advancing rapidly and the information here is likely to already be out of date.
- Taking a good sample remains very important; digital tools cannot currently correct for poor samples.

Appendix A

Summary of cell examination and description

Low power

- **Number of cells** (low; moderate; high)
- **Preservation** (poor; moderate; good)
- **Cohesion** (individual cells; loose aggregates; tight clusters)
- **Pattern** (papillary; honeycomb; pavement; trabecular etc.)

High power – nucleus

- **Size** (compared to RBCs or neutrophils)
- **Shape** (round; oval; indented; polygonal etc.)
- **Position** (central; paracentral; eccentric)
- **Chromatin pattern** (hyperchromatic; coarse; stippled; lacy etc.)
- **Nucleoli** (number; shape; size (macronucleoli = larger than RBC)
- **Number** (mononuclear; binucleate; multinucleate)

High power – cytoplasm

- **Amount** (scant; low; moderate; abundant)
- **Colour** (basophilic; eosinophilic; pink; pale)
- **Vacuolation** (amount; size)
- **Granulation** (amount; size; colour)
- **N:C ratio**

Appendix B

Decoding pathology reports – a cytological glossary

Many terms in a pathology report are seldom seen in the outside world, and many phrases and words have subtly different meanings. Below are the terms most commonly used or, occasionally, abused, in a pathology report, with attempts to explain what the pathologist is likely to be trying to indicate.

Aggregate: loosely connected cells (usually refers to mesenchymal cells)
Amorphous: a pool or splat of usually smooth material
Amphophilic: pink/purple (affinity for both basic and acidic stains)
Anisocytosis: variation in cell size
Anisokaryosis: variation in nuclear size
Atypical: unusual – not necessarily neoplastic; could also refer to dysplasia (secondary to inflammation)
Azurophilic: purple or reddish (very confusing term given that 'azure' is a blue colour)
Basophilic: blue (affinity for the basic stain, i.e. an acidic substance such as DNA, which is why most nuclei are blue)
Cluster: tightly connected cells (usually refers to epithelial cells)
Concern for: similar to 'probable' but with a lesser degree of certainty
Crowded: cells more tightly packed than normal; usually an atypical feature in epithelium
Disorganised: cells irregularly grouped together; usually an atypical feature in epithelium

Eosinophilic: red or pinkish red (affinity for the eosin stain, which is acidic, and therefore has affinity for basic substances such as the major basic protein in eosinophil granules)
Flocculent: cloud-like (looks fluffy with irregular staining, often refers to mucous or similar material)
Hypocellular: a few cells may be present, but too few for an interpretation
Metachromic: something which has stained an unusual colour given its chemical components (most commonly applied to mast cell granules)
Monomorphic: all appearing the same; in the context of bacteria, infection is more likely than contamination; in the context of lymphocytes, lymphoma is more likely than a reactive population
Nuclear:cytoplasmic ratio: the size of the nucleus compared to the overall size
Pleomorphic: variation in shape
Polygonal: an irregular shape, not especially oval or round
Possible: code for 'I am not sure (because of low cellularity, preservation or something weird) but I think it might be this thing...'
Poorly-differentiated: cells that have diverged from their original morphology and so are now hard to identify (usually associated with higher-grade tumours)
Probable: code for 'I don't want to say for absolute definite (because of low cellularity, preservation or something weird) but this is the most likely thing...'

Proliferation: code for 'there are a lot of these things but I'm not entirely sure if they are inflammatory, hyperplastic or neoplastic'

Stroma: connective tissue; cytologically refers to mesenchymal cells with scattered other cells (such as lymphocytes); most commonly refers to the spleen

Suspicious of: similar to 'possible', although usually with less certainty

Well-differentiated: appearing as expected – synonym for 'normal'

Appendix C

Backgrounds

Table A.1

Colour	Texture/pattern	Possibilities
Eosinophilic	Smooth	Haemodilution
Pink/amphophilic	Stippled, protein clefts	Seroma or other proteinaceous fluid
Pink to deeply pink	Stippled to 'cracked', protein clefts, windrowing present	Synovial fluid
Deeply basophilic	Smooth	Histiocytoma
Basophilic to deeply basophilic	Stippled	Hyperglobulinaemia
Clear	Fat droplets	Adipose tissue

Appendix D

Common crystals (FIGS A.1–4)

Note: these are specifically crystals observed on cytological samples rather than urine sediment examination

Table A.2

Crystal	Colour	Shape	Significance
Cholesterol	Clear	Square-rectangular	Due to cell wall degeneration; most commonly found in epidermal inclusion cysts (see page 179)
Haematoidin	Golden-brown/ orange	Rhomboid	Due to red cell degeneration; often indicates prior haemorrhage (see page 98) (although cytologically appear very similar/identical to bilirubin crystals*
Bilirubin	Golden-brown/ orange	Rhomboid/ linear	Presence of bilirubin (appears very similar/ identical to haematoidin)*
Calcium oxalate monohydrate	Clear	Variable – classic shapes are 'picket fence' and 'dumbbell'	Raise significant concern for ethylene glycol toxicity when found on renal aspirates

*Haematoidin and bilirubin are the same chemical; the difference is subjective due to their suspected derivation – haematoidin is usually seen following haemorrhage, bilirubin is usually seen in bile

342 Decoding pathology reports – a cytological glossary

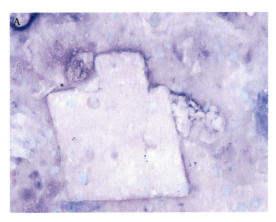

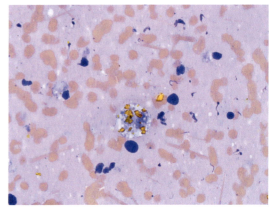

Fig A.2 Haematoidin crystals (×500)

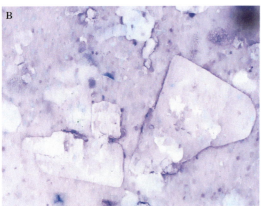

Fig A.1a, b Cholesterol crystals (×1000)

Appendix E

Species/sex/breed predispositions

This is not an exhaustive list of all disease predispositions in dogs and cats; rather, it is a reference for the breeds most commonly affected by certain conditions – that is, if a cytologist is examining samples from one of the breeds below, they should be more alert to the possibility of certain diseases.

Amyloidosis: Shar Pei; Abyssinian, Rex, and Siamese cats

Mast cell tumour: Boxer; Staffordshire bull terrier; Labrador retriever

Histiocytic sarcoma: Flat-coat retriever; Bernese mountain dog; Rottweiler; miniature schnauzer

Urothelial (transitional cell) carcinoma: Castrated male dogs

Appendix F

Further staining and extra tests

Many extra stains and tests can be used with cytological specimens. Here are a few of the most common:

Ziehl-Neelsen stain (ZN, acid-fast stain): this stain is used to highlight bacteria that stain poorly with Romanowsky stain. In particular, it is used to highlight *Mycobacterium sp.*
Periodic acid Schiff stain (PAS): the stain highlights polysaccharides, and is used to highlight mucous, as well as the glycoproteins in the wall of fungal organisms
Grocott's methenamine silver stain (GMS): highlights fungal organisms (a broader stain than PAS)
Congo red stain: used for confirmation of the presence of amyloid
PCR for Antigen Receptor Rearrangement (PARR): this is a PCR test that implies the unique T- or B-cell receptor DNA fragments; it detects whether many of the 'unique' receptors are, in fact, the same – i.e. it tests for clones; clonal lymphocytes are likely to be neoplastic (although, rarely, infectious diseases such as *Ehrlichia sp.* can trigger a clonal response)
Immunocytochemistry (ICC): staining cytological specimens for cellular markers (protein sequences that bind to dyes); can be used to identify many cells including epithelium, mesenchymal cells, T-lymphocytes, B-lymphocytes, cells of histiocytic origin, melanocytes and many others

Appendix G

Mitotic figures (FIG A.5)

Mitotic figures appear when cells are dividing, and therefore low numbers of mitotic figures are occasionally found in most tissues, but when mitotic figures are found in increased amounts (this is subjective but finding more than one or two, even on relatively cellular samples, is unusual) or when they are atypical, they raise concern for malignancy.

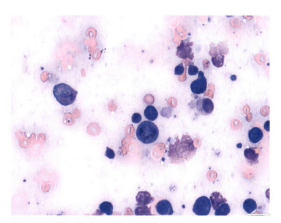

Fig A.3 Mitotic figure (×1000)

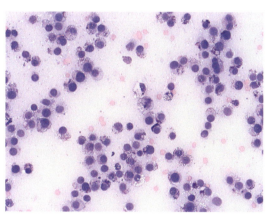

Fig A.4 Mitotic figure in mast cell tumour (×500)

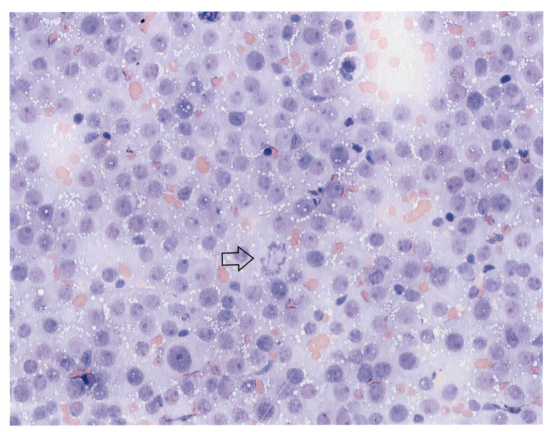

Fig A.5 Mitotic figure in histiocytic sarcoma (open arrow); the individual dots are 'lag' chromosomes, lagging behind the normal spindle formation; this is an atypical feature in mitosis (×500)

Appendix H

Pathology jokes

- Two neutrophils walk into a bar. The barman points at the youngest one and says, 'Hey, you can't come in here, you're band!'
- I was going to pretend that I saw *Ehrlichia* within a neutrophil, but I realised it would have been morulae wrong.
- I had to give up my job of judging the quality of microscope lenses – I found it very difficult to give an objective opinion.
- Cytologists can't work with broken microscopes. They find it hard to focus.
- Cytologists don't trust glass slides; they can see right through them.
- There's no cell quite like one that's been phagocytosed by a bone-based macrophage – they're in an osteoclast of their own.
- Where do you usually find mitosis? On the end of my foot, sis.

Bibliography

Textbooks

Barger, A. M., MacNeill, A. L., & Bain, P. J. (2017). *Small animal cytologic diagnosis*. CRC Press, Taylor et Francvis Group.

Cowell, R. L., & Valenciano, A. C. (2020). *Cowell and Tyler's diagnostic cytology and hematology of the dog and cat*. Elsevier.

Elliott, P. (2019). *Improve international manual of clinical small animal internal medicine*. 5m Publishing.

Greene, C. E. (2012). *Infectious diseases of the dog and cat*. Elsevier/Saunders.

Harvey, J. W. (2012a). *Veterinary hematology: A diagnostic guide and color atlas*. Elsevier, Saunders.

Harvey, J. W. (2012b). *Veterinary hematology: A diagnostic guide and color atlas*. Elsevier, Saunders.

Latimer, K. S. (2011). *Duncan and Prasse's Veterinary Laboratory Medicine: Clinical Pathology, 5th*. John Wiley & Sons.

Meuten, D. J. (2017). *Tumors in domestic animals*. John Wiley & Sons, Inc.

Raskin, R., & Meyer, D. J. (2016). *Canine and feline cytology: A Color Atlas and interpretation guide*. Elsevier.

Stockham, S. L., & Scott, M. A. (2008). *Fundamentals of veterinary clinical pathology*. Blackwell Publishing.

Papers

Abdollahi, A., & Nozarian, Z. (2016). Diagnostic value of measurement specific gravity by refractometric and dipstick method in differentiation between transudate and exudate in pleural and peritoneal fluid. *Iranian Journal of Pathology*, *11*(4), 363–369.

Adewoyin, A. S., & Nwogoh, B. (2014). Peripheral blood film – A review. *Annals of Ibadan Postgraduate Medicine*, *12*(2), 71–79.

Al-Abbadi, M. A. (2011). Basics of cytology. *Avicenna Journal of Medicine*, *1*(1), 18–28. https://doi.org/10.4103/2231-0770.83719

Allen, S. W., Prasse, K. W., & Mahaffey, E. A. (1986). Cytologic differentiation of benign from malignant canine mammary tumors. *Veterinary Pathology*, *23*(6), 649–655. https://doi.org/10.1177/030098588602300601

Allison, D. B., Simner, P. J., & Ali, S. Z. (2018). Identification of infectious organisms in cytopathology: A review of ancillary diagnostic techniques. *Cancer Cytopathology*, *126*(Suppl. 8), 643–653. https://doi.org/10.1002/cncy.22023

Bau-Gaudreault, L., & Grimes, C. N. (2019). Effect of time and storage on toxic or pseudo-toxic change in canine neutrophils. *Veterinary Clinical Pathology*, *48*(3), 400–405. https://doi.org/10.1111/vcp.12755

Bavle, R. M. (2014). Lymphoglandular bodies. *Journal of Oral and Maxillofacial Pathology*, *18*(3), 334–335. https://doi.org/10.4103/0973-029X.151308

Camus, M. S., Priest, H. L., Koehler, J. W., Driskell, E. A., Rakich, P. M., Ilha, M. R., & Krimer, P. M. (2016). Cytologic criteria for mast cell tumor grading in dogs with evaluation of clinical outcome. *Veterinary Pathology*, *53*(6), 1117–1123. https://doi.org/10.1177/0300985816638721

Cannon, C. M., Knudson, C., & Borgatti, A. (2015). Clinical signs, treatment, and outcome in cats with myeloma-related disorder receiving systemic therapy. *Journal of the American Animal Hospital Association*, *51*(4), 239–248. https://doi.org/10.5326/JAAHA-MS-6216

Caserto, B. G. (2013). A comparative review of canine and human rhabdomyosarcoma with emphasis on classification and pathogenesis. *Veterinary Pathology*, *50*(5), 806–826. https://doi.org/10.1177/0300985813476069

Conboy, G. (2009). Cestodes of dogs and cats in North America. *Veterinary Clinics of North America. Small Animal Practice*, *39*(6), 1075–1090. https://doi.org/10.1016/j.cvsm.2009.06.005

Dolka, I., Czopowicz, M., Gruk-Jurka, A., Wojtkowska, A., Sapierzyński, R., & Jurka, P. (2018). Diagnostic efficacy of smear cytology and Robinson's cytological grading of canine mammary tumors with respect to histopathology, cytomorphometry, metastases and overall survival. *PLOS ONE*, *13*(1), e0191595. https://doi.org/10.1371/journal.pone.0191595

Dyachenko, V., Pantchev, N., Gawlowska, S., Vrhovec, M. G., & Bauer, C. (2008). Echinococcus multilocularis infections in domestic dogs and cats from Germany and other European countries. *Veterinary Parasitology*, *157*(3–4), 244–253. https://doi.org/10.1016/j.vetpar.2008.07.030

Elliott, J. W., Cripps, P., Blackwood, L., Berlato, D., Murphy, S., & Grant, I. A. (2016). Canine oral mucosal mast cell tumours. *Veterinary and Comparative Oncology*, *14*(1), 101–111. https://doi.org/10.1111/vco.12071

Eosinophilic granuloma complex in cats and dogs. (2003). In *Congress Proceedings*: 28 TH World Congress the World Small Veterinary Association. Bangkok. World Small Animal Veterinary Association.

Evaluation of the blood smear. (2004). In *2004 world congress: 29th World Small Animal Veterinary Congress. WSAVA*, 10th european Congress, FECAVA, 7th Hellenic Congress, HVMS: October 6, *7* p. 8, 9. Rhodes. Acharnes, Greece: Produced and printed by Alta Grafico S.A.

Evans, S. J. M., Connolly, S. L., Schaffer, P. A., Vieson, M. D., Stiles, A., & Moore, A. R. (2018). Basal cell enumeration does not predict malignancy in canine perianal gland tumor cytology. *Veterinary Clinical Pathology*, *47*(4), 634–637. https://doi.org/10.1111/vcp.12671

Faletti, T., Seguin, B., Selmic, L. E., Lapsley, J., Worley, D., Griffin, M., & Tremolada, G. (2022). Potential seeding from fine-needle aspiration of an axial osteosarcoma: A case report. *Frontiers in Veterinary Science*, *9*, 847933. https://doi.org/10.3389/fvets.2022.847933

Fernandez, N. J., Gilroy, C. V., Wagg, C. R., Kwong, G. P. S., & Roy, M. F. (2019). Intra- and inter-rater agreement for the detection of band neutrophils and toxic change in horses. *Veterinary Clinical Pathology*, *48*(4), 668–676. https://doi.org/10.1111/vcp.12811

Finotello, R. et al. (2017). Feline large granular lymphocyte lymphoma: An Italian society of veterinary oncology retrospective study. *Veterinary and Comparative Oncology*, *16*(1), 159–166. https://doi.org/10.1111/vco.12325

Garrett, L. D. (2014). Canine mast cell tumors: Diagnosis, treatment, and prognosis. *Veterinary Medicine*, 5, 49–58. https://doi.org/10.2147/VMRR.S41005

Genchi, C., & Kramer, L. (2017). Subcutaneous dirofilariosis (Dirofilaria repens): An infection spreading throughout the Old World. *Parasites and Vectors*, *10*(Suppl. 2), 517. https://doi.org/10.1186/s13071-017-2434-8

Goldfinch, N., & Argyle, D. J. (2012). Feline Lung–Digit syndrome: Unusual metastatic patterns of primary lung tumours in cats. *Journal of Feline Medicine and Surgery*, *14*(3), 202–208. https://doi.org/10.1177/1098612×12439267

Griffin, M. A., Culp, W. T. N., & Rebhun, R. B. (2021). Canine and feline haemangiosarcoma. *Veterinary Record*, *189*(9), e585. https://doi.org/10.1002/vetr.585

Haematological changes associated with tick-borne diseases. (2004). In *2004 world congress: 29th World Small Animal Veterinary Congress. WSAVA*, 10th european Congress, FECAVA, 7th Hellenic Congress, HVMS: October 6, *7* p. 8, 9. Rhodes. Acharnes, Greece: Produced and printed by Alta Grafico S.A.

Hassan, B., B., A. Abdelrahman, H., Samir, A., & R. Mousa, M. (2021). Cutaneous tumors in dogs: A retrospective epidemiological and histological study of 112 cases. *Advances in Animal and Veterinary Sciences*, *10*(1). https://doi.org/10.17582/journal.aavs/2022/10.1.170.182

Hayakawa, S., Spangler, E. A., Christopherson, P. W., & Boudreaux, M. K. (2016). A novel form of macrothrombocytopenia in Akita dogs. *Veterinary Clinical Pathology*, *45*(1), 103–105. https://doi.org/10.1111/vcp.12331

Henry, C., & Herrera, C. (2013). Mast cell tumors in cats: Clinical update and possible new treatment avenues. *Journal of Feline Medicine and Surgery*, *15*(1), 41–47. https://doi.org/10.1177/1098612×12470343

Hooi, K. S., Defarges, A. M., Jelovcic, S. V., & Bienzle, D. (2019). Bronchoalveolar lavage hemosiderosis in dogs and cats with respiratory disease. *Veterinary Clinical Pathology*, *48*(1), 42–49. https://doi.org/10.1111/vcp.12698

Jegatheeson, S., Dandrieux, J. R., & Cannon, C. M. (2020). Suspected pancreatic carcinoma needle tract seeding in a cat. *JFMS Open Reports*, *6*(1), 2055116920918161. https://doi.org/10.1177/2055116920918161

MacWilliams, P. S., & Friedrichs, K. R. (2003). Laboratory evaluation and interpretation of synovial fluid. *Veterinary Clinics of North America. Small Animal Practice*, *33*(1), 153–178. https://doi.org/10.1016/s0195-5616(02)00083-9

Masserdotti, C., & Drigo, M. (2012). Retrospective study of cytologic features of well-differentiated hepatocellular carcinoma in dogs. *Veterinary Clinical Pathology*, *41*(3), 382–390. https://doi.org/10.1111/j.1939-165X.2012.00436.x

Mellor, P. J., Haugland, S., Murphy, S., Smith, K. C., Holloway, A., Archer, J., Powell, R. M., Polton, G. A., Tasker, S., McCormick, D., Tempest, M. E., McNeil, P. E., Scase, T. J., Knott, C. D., Bonfanti, U., Villiers, E. J., Argyle, D. J., Herrtage, M. E., & Day, M. J. (2006). Myeloma-related disorders in cats commonly present as extramedullary neoplasms in contrast to myeloma in human patients: 24 cases with clinical follow-up. *Journal of Veterinary Internal Medicine*, *20*(6), 1376–1383. https://doi.org/10.1892/0891-6640(2006)20[1376:mdiccp]2.0.co;2

Monti, P., Barnes, D., Adrian, A. M., & Rasotto, R. (2018). Synovial cell sarcoma in a dog: A misnomer—Cytologic and histologic findings and review of the literature. *Veterinary Clinical Pathology*, *47*(2), 181–185. https://doi.org/10.1111/vcp.12590

Moore, P. F. (2014). A review of histiocytic diseases of dogs and cats. *Veterinary Pathology*, *51*(1), 167–184. https://doi.org/10.1177/0300985813510413

Palić, J., Heier, A., & Wohlsein, P. (2022). Cytologic features of an acanthomatous Ameloblastoma in a dog. *Veterinary Clinical Pathology*, *51*(2), 258–262. https://doi.org/10.1111/vcp.13080

Pey, P., Diana, A., Rossi, F., Mortier, J., Kafka, U., Veraa, S., Groth, A., MacLellan, M., Marin, C., & Fracassi, F. (2020). Safety of percutaneous ultrasound-guided fine-needle aspiration of adrenal lesions in dogs: Perception of the procedure by radiologists and presentation of 50 cases. *Journal of Veterinary Internal Medicine*, *34*(2), 626–635. https://doi.org/10.1111/jvim.15743

Piccione, J., Levine, G. J., Duff, C. A., Kuhlman, G. M., Scott, K. D., & Esteve-Gassent, M. D. (2016). Tick-borne relapsing fever in dogs. *Journal of Veterinary Internal Medicine*, *30*(4), 1222–1228. https://doi.org/10.1111/jvim.14363

Piccione, J., Levine, G. J., Duff, C. A., Kuhlman, G. M., Scott, K. D., & Esteve-Gassent, M. D. (n.d.). *Tick-borne relapsing fever in dogs*, Journal of veterinary internal medicine. https://pubmed.ncbi.nlm.nih.gov/27353196/Retrieved September 30, 2023

Ragetly, G. R., Bennett, R. A., & Ragetly, C. A. (2011). Septic peritonitis: Etiology, pathophysiology, and diagnosis. *Compendium*, *33*(10), E1–6; quiz E7.

Sapierzyński, R., Jankowska, U., Jagielski, D., & Kliczkowska-Klarowicz, K. (2015). Large granular lymphoma in six cats. *Polish Journal of Veterinary Sciences*, *18*(1), 163–169. https://doi.org/10.1515/pjvs-2015-0021

Simon, D., Schoenrock, D., Nolte, I., Baumgärtner, W., Barron, R., & Mischke, R. (2009). Cytologic examination of fine-needle aspirates from mammary gland tumors in the dog: Diagnostic accuracy with comparison to histopathology and association with postoperative outcome. *Veterinary Clinical Pathology*, *38*(4), 521–528. https://doi.org/10.1111/j.1939-165X.2009.00150.x

Thrift, E., Greenwell, C., Turner, A. L., Harvey, A. M., Maher, D., & Malik, R. (2017). Metastatic pulmonary carcinomas in cats ('feline lung–digit syndrome'): Further variations on a Theme. *JFMS Open Reports*, *3*(1), 2055116917691069. https://doi.org/10.1177/2055116917691069

Torous, V. F., Dodd, L. G., McIntire, P. J., & Jiang, X. S. (2022). Crystals and crystalloids in cytopathology: Incidence and importance. *Cancer Cytopathology*, *130*(10), 759–770. https://doi.org/10.1002/cncy.22602

Trappler, M. C., Popovitch, C. A., Goldschmidt, M. H., Goldschmidt, K. H., & Risbon, R. E. (2014). Scrotal tumors in dogs: A retrospective study of 676 cases

(1986–2010). *Canadian Veterinary Journal*, *55*(1), 1229–1233.

van der Steen, F. E. M. M., Grinwis, G. C. M., Weerts, E. A. W. S., & Teske, E. (2021). Feline and canine Merkel cell carcinoma: A case series and discussion on cellular origin. *Veterinary and Comparative Oncology*, *19*(2), 393–398. https://doi.org/10.1111/vco.12672

Valli, V. E., San Myint, M., Barthel, A., ... Vernau, W. (2011). Classification of canine malignant lymphomas according to the World Health Organization criteria. *Veterinary pathology*, *48*(1), 198–211. https://doi.org/10.1177/0300985810379428

Warland, J., & Dobson, J. (2013). Breed predispositions in canine mast cell tumour: A single centre experience in the United Kingdom. *Veterinary Journal*, *197*(2), 496–498. https://doi.org/10.1016/j.tvjl.2013.02.017

Zhai, W., Wu, F., Zhang, Y., Fu, Y., & Liu, Z. (2019). The immune escape mechanisms of mycobacterium tuberculosis. *International Journal of Molecular Sciences*, *20*(2), 340. https://doi.org/10.3390/ijms20020340

Zhu, B. Y., Johnson, L. R., & Vernau, W. (2015). Tracheobronchial brush cytology and bronchoalveolar lavage in dogs and cats with chronic cough: 45 cases (2012–2014). *Journal of Veterinary Internal Medicine*, *29*(2), 526–532. https://doi.org/10.1111/jvim.12566

Websites

'Big blue' cells. (2021). *eClinpath*. https://eclinpath.com/hematology/morphologic-features/white-blood-cells/big-blue-cells/ Retrieved September 30, 2023

Branam, E., & D. (2022). *Common neoplastic skin lesions in dogs and cats*: Cytologic diagnosis and treatment options, Today's Veterinary Practice. https://todaysveterinarypractice.com/dermatology/common-neoplastic-skin-lesions-dogs-catscytologic-diagnosis-treatment-options/ Retrieved September 30, 2023

Garrett, L. D. (2014). *Canine mast cell tumors*: Diagnosis, treatment, and prognosis: VMRR, *Veterinary Medicine*: *Research and Reports*. https://www.dovepress.com/canine-mast-cell-tumors-diagnosis-treatment-and-prognosis-peer-reviewed-fulltext-article-VMRR Retrieved September 30, 2023

Homepage. (2023). *MedVet*. https://www.medvetforpets.com/idexx-diagnostic-challenge-dog-vague-gi-signs/ Retrieved September 30, 2023

Overview of anatomic and clinical pathology. (n.d.). https://documents.cap.org/documents/overview-anatomic-clinical-pathology-medical-students.pdf Retrieved September 30, 2023

Peregrine, A. S. (2023). *Tapeworms in dogs and cats – Digestive system*, *MSD Veterinary Manual*. https://www.msdvetmanual.com/digestive-system/gastrointestinal-parasites-of-small-animals/tapeworms-in-dogs-and-cats Retrieved September 30, 2023

Setting up cytology in Your practice (proceedings). (n.d.). *DVM360*. https://www.dvm360.com/view/setting-cytology-your-practice-proceedings Retrieved September 30, 2023

Shaun, O. (2022). *Oral melanomas in dogs*: Atlantic Veterinary Internal Medicine, Atlantic Veterinary Internal Medicine and Oncology. https://avim.us/oral-melanomas-in-dogs/ Retrieved September 30, 2023

SOS equipment for veterinary cytologists. (2022). *Veterinary Cytology*. https://veterinarycytology.org/equipment Retrieved September 30, 2023

Staff, A. V. E. (2021). *Performing in-house cytology: What equipment do I need?*. *DVM360*. https://www.dvm360.com/view/performing-in-house-cytology-what-equipment-do-i-need Retrieved September 30, 2023

Using a microscope. (n.d.). https://www.bristol.ac.uk/media-library/sites/vetscience/documents/clinical-skills/Using%20a%20Microscope.pdf Retrieved September 30, 2023. University of Bristol.

Webpathology. (n.d.). *Webpathology.com. A collection of surgical pathology images*. https://www.webpathology.com/image.asp?case=768&n=27#:~:text=Flame%20cells%20are%20atypical%20plasma,as%20well%20as%20reactive%20plasmacytosis Retrieved: September 30, 2023.

What is Epulis in dogs? Symptoms, causes and treatment options. (n.d.). *Carecredit*. https://www.carecredit.com/well-u/pet-care/epulis-in-dogs/ Retrieved September 30, 2023

Index

Page numbers followed by an *f* indicates figures; *t* indicates tables

A
abdominal lymph nodes 200, 202–3
acanthocytes 295
acellular debris 29, 48–52
acellular lesions 97–104
adenocarcinomas 71, 95*f*
adenomas 71
adipocytes 133–4, 133–4*f*, 150–1*f*
agglutination 292
alcohol swab 16
amyloid 101, 103*f*
amyloidosis 101, 103*f*, 180, 343
anaemia 288–90, 289–90*f*, 311–12*f*, 311–13
anaesthetic cream 16
anal sac apocrine gland adenocarcinomas 161–2, 163*f*
anal sac apocrine glands 43*f*, 78*f*
anal sac impaction 163–4, 164*f*
anatomic pathology 4
anisocytosis 35*f*, 44, 294
anisokaryosis 34, 35*f*, 44
apocrine cysts 98, 99*f*, 180
apoptotic cells 96
artefacts 47–8
artificial intelligence (AI) 336
automated stainers 11–12, 12

B
babesia 298, 298*f*
bacilli 110–11, 111*f*
backgrounds 57, 59, 59*f*, 340
bacteria 51–2, 61, 106–10*f*, 107–16, 178
bacteriuria 211
bare nuclei 31–3, 32*f*, 47*f*
basal cell tumour 138, 139*f*
basal epithelium 132, 132*f*
basophilic cytoplasm 302, 302*f*
basophils 306

benign tumours 85, 92, 92*f*
bile peritonitis 279, 279*f*
biliary carcinoma 195
biliary epithelium 187
bilirubin 270, 341
binocular lenses 7
binocular microscope 6*f*
bladder
    masses 15
    neoplastic lesions 212–13
    samples 24
blood cells 131, 131*f*, 186
blood collection tubes 18, 21
blood contamination *see* haemodilution
blood films
    evaluation and examination 285–313
    preparation and procedure 282–5, 282–5*f*
bone 261–5
bone marrow 263
bone remodelling 261–2, 263*f*
bony lesions 15, 18
broncho-alveolar lavage (BAL) 23–4, 23*f*, 219–21, 223*t*, 224–5*f*
buffy coat preparation 22, 22*f*

C
carcinomas 71, 95*f*
    see also carcinomas by name
catheterisation 24, 24*f*
cell borders 42, 43*f*
cell count 269, 270*f*
cell shape 42
cellularity 55–7, 56*f*
cestodes 124
cholesterol 270, 341
chondroma 157–9
chondrosarcoma 157*f*
chromatin 31, 33, 35, 38–9*f*, 39, 55, 94–5

chylous effusions 277, 278f
clinical pathology 4
cocci 110–11, 110f
cohesion 44–5, 45f
collagen 101, 101–2f, 131, 131f
Conchiformibius 111, 112f, 182, 183f
condenser lens 9–10, 9
conjunctiva 15
contact gel 48, 49f
context, for specimens 4
Coombs' test 312
cornea 25
cover slips 10f, 28
creatinine 270
crystals 103, 341, 342f
cutaneous lymphoma 86, 145, 145f
cutaneous mass 129–30, 130f
cutaneous neoplasia 134–50
cysts 14, 179–80, 198, 329
cytocentrifuges 12, 13f, 21–2
cytological artefacts 47–8
cytology specimen, clarity of 4, 5f
cytoplasm 29, 31–3, 31f, 39–42, 40–2f, 95
cytoplasmic fragments 39–40, 40f

D
digital cytology 335–6
distemper 298–9, 309
drying samples 26
dysplasia 177–8
dystrophic mineralisation 98, 100, 100f

E
ear canals 15, 26
ear swabs 180
eccentrocytes 295–6, 296f
echinocytes 293, 293f
edge cases 317–29
EDTA (Ethylenediaminetetraacetic acid) tubes 18, 21
effusions 15
  see also fluid specimens
eosinophilic inflammation 61f, 62, 63–4f, 175–6, 175f, 223–4, 226f
eosinophilic lymphadenitis 246, 247f
eosinophils 47f, 305–6, 305–6f
epidermal inclusion cyst 179
epithelial cells 129, 132f, 187, 204, 204f
epithelial dysplasia 177–8
epithelial tumours 71–6, 72–7f, 137–41, 137–41f, 146–7
epulis 183–4
equipment 4, 6–13

erythrocytes 34t, 47, 47f, 52, 288–99, 289–98f, 290f
exfoliation 29, 30f
external laboratories 5, 331–4
extracellular matrix 102, 103f
extra-medullary haematopoiesis (EMH) 191, 249–50, 251f, 252
exudates 275–6, 275f

F
facial lymph nodes 232, 232f
fat cells 101, 101f, 129, 133, 133–4f, 150–1
fenestration *see* non-suction technique
fibrinocellular aggregates 50, 50f
fibroblasts 69–70, 105
fibromas 153–5, 154–5f
fine needle aspirate biopsy (FNAB) 4, 16–18, 17–18f
fingerprints 48, 50f, 97
flame cells 69
fluid specimens 14, 21f
  analysis 269–74
  backgrounds 270–2, 271f
  classification 274–80
  labelling 331
  preparation techniques 21–5
formalin-fixed specimens 4
formalin fume damage 5f
frosted slides 11
fungal spores 51–2, 51f
fungi 116–19, 117–21f, 178, 179f
fusiform cells 43f

G
gastrointestinal system 198–9
  abdominal lymph nodes 200, 202–3
  liver 186–98
  oral cavity 182–6
  pancreas 200
gel contamination 17f
genitourinary system
  bladder 212–13
  kidneys 204–9
  prostate 213–14
  urine 209–12
ghost red cells 295, 295f
glomeruli 204
glucose 270
granules 40–2, 41–2f

H
haemangiosarcoma 147–8, 148f, 156–7, 156f, 193, 194f, 252–3, 253f, 261
haematoidin 341

haematomas 98, 180, 253–4
haemodilution 49–50, 50*f*, 53–4, 53*f*, 265–6, 266*f*, 321–2
haemoglobin crystals 47, 47*f*
haemorrhagic effusions 276–7, 276–7*f*
hair clipping 16
hair fragment 48*f*
hard masses 15
  see also bony lesions
Heinz bodies 295–6, 296*f*
hepatic carcinoid 196
hepatic splenosis 197
hepatocellular adenoma 193–4
hepatocellular carcinoma 193–4, 195*f*
hepatocytes 186–91, 187–91*f*, 230
hepatoid gland tumours 161, 161–2*f*
hepatozoon 310
histiocytic sarcoma 88–90, 91*f*, 94*f*, 136, 155, 155*f*, 343
histiocytoma 85–6, 86*f*, 136, 136–7*f*
histology specimen, clarity of 4*f*
histopathology 4, 14
Howell-Jolly bodies 296, 296*f*
hyperplasia 96, 96*f*
hyphae 116–17, 117*f*
hypochromasia 294–5

I
immersion oil 10
immune mediated haemolytic anaemia (IMHA) 311
impression smears 14, 25, 25*f*, 130–1
infection 106
  bacterial 107–16, 178
  fungal 116–19, 178, 179*f*
  and inflammation 106–7, 107*f*
  parasitic 122–6, 178
  protozoa 119–22
  viral 126
inflammation 59, 104
  anal sac 163–4
  eosinophilic 61*f*, 62, 63–4*f*, 175–6, 175*f*
  estimating 53–4
  and infectious agents 106–7, 107*f*
  kidneys 209
  liver 196–7, 197*f*
  lungs 229
  lymph nodes 244–5
  lymphocytic 66–8, 67–9*f*, 176–7, 177*f*
  macrophagic 62–3, 64–7*f*, 65, 172–5, 173–6*f*
  mast cells 82–3
  mixed 69, 177
  mononuclear 266–7, 267*f*

muscle 261
  neutrophilic 59–62, 60–1*f*, 171–2, 172*f*, 267, 267*f*
  plasma cells 68–9, 70–1*f*
  plasmacytic 177
  prostate 214
  respiratory system 222–6
  spleen 256–7
  synovial fluid 266–7
  urine 211
in-house laboratories 5
iron deficiency 312

J
joints see synovial fluid

K
keratin 48, 48*f*, 97–8, 97–8*f*, 132, 132*f*
kidneys
  inflammation 209
  neoplastic lesions 206–9
  normal appearance 204, 204–5*f*

L
labelling 27–8, 331
laboratories
  external 5, 331–4
  in-house 5
leiomyoma 160, 160*f*, 261, 261*f*
leiomyosarcoma 261, 261*f*
lesions see cysts; neoplasia; tumours
leukaemia 307–10, 308–9*f*
leukocytes 48, 53, 204–5, 299–310, 299*f*, 309
light source 10
lipoma 150–1
liposarcoma 159, 159*f*
liver
  cystic lesions 198
  hepatic splenosis 197
  inflammation 196–7, 197*f*
  neoplastic lesions 191–6, 192–6*f*
  normal appearance 186–8, 186–8*f*
lungs 227–30
  inflammation 229
  neoplastic lesions 228–9
  normal appearance 228
lungworm 122–3, 226*f*
lymph nodes 167, 231–48
  abdominal 200, 202–3, 202*f*
  facial 232, 232*f*
  inflammation 244–5
  normal findings 232–4
  reactive 236, 236*f*, 237*f*

sampling 231–2
see also lymphoma
lymphocytes 31, 33, 33*f*, 38*f*, 131, 186–7, 232–4, 234*f*, 302–4, 303–4*f*
lymphocytic inflammation 66–8, 67–9*f*, 176–7, 177*f*
lymphoid hyperplasia 252, 252*f*
lymphoma 44, 66–8, 145*f*, 160, 236–7, 239–42, 239–42*f*, 307–8
   cutaneous 86, 145
   kidneys 206
   large cell 87, 88*f*, 160, 160*f*, 239–40, 240*f*
   liver 193, 194*f*
   oral cavity 184
   small cell 87, 89*f*, 160, 240, 240*f*
   spleen 254–5, 254*f*
lymphorrhagic effusions 277, 278–9*f*

M

macrophagic (granulomatous) lymphadenitis 246–8, 248*f*
macrophagic inflammation 62–3, 64–7*f*, 65, 172–5, 173–6*f*
magnification 8–9
malignant epithelial neoplasms 147, 147*f*
malignant tumours 87–90, 92–5, 93*f*, 105, 141, 147, 185
mammary masses 164–7, 165–6*f*
mammary tumours 14, 18–19, 105
mast cell tumours 30*f*, 39*f*, 41*f*, 82–4, 83–5*f*, 135–6, 135–6*f*, 153, 153*f*, 155*f*, 185, 306, 307*f*, 343
matrix 102, 103*f*
Melamed-Wolinska bodies 212, 212*f*
melanin 101, 102*f*, 236
melanocytic tumours 87, 89–90*f*, 141–2, 141–2*f*, 185
mesenchymal tumours 72*t*, 78–82, 79–82*f*, 147–8, 150–3, 153–61, 322–3
mesothelial cells 187, 272, 272–3*f*
metaplasia 178
metastatic neoplasia 148–9, 148*f*, 191, 192*f*, 193, 206, 228, 255, 255*f*
microcytosis 294
microhaematocrit reader 12, 13*f*
microscopes 6–10, 7*f*
mitotic figures 345, 345–6*f*
mixed cellularity 319–21
monocular lenses 7
monocytes 304–5, 305*f*
mononuclear inflammation 266–7, 267*f*
Mott cells 69, 70–1*f*
mucinosis 180

mucosae 15, 26
muscle 259–61, 259–61*f*
Mycobacterium 113–14*f*, 114, 229
mycoplasma 114–15, 115*f*, 297–8
myelolipoma 256, 256*f*
myoepithelium 327
myxoma 155–6, 156*f*, 329

N

nasal flushes 24, 24*f*
nasal masses 15
   see also nose
necrosis 62, 96–7, 96*f*, 180, 327–8
needle biopsy *see* fine needle aspirate biopsy (FNAB)
needles 10–11
negative staining 113–14*f*, 114
nematodes 122–3, 125*f*
neoplasia 62, 70–1
   bladder 212–13
   bone 263–4
   cutaneous 134–50
   effusions 280
   kidneys 206–9
   liver 191–6
   lungs 228–9
   muscle 259–61
   nose 218–19
   oral cavity 183–5
   prostate 214
   respiratory system 221
   spleen 252
   subcutaneous 150–61
   thymus 257–8
   urine 211–12
   see also tumours
neoplasms 31*f*, 71, 72*t*, 280
nephroblastoma 208–9, 208–9*f*
neuroendocrine tumours 72*t*, 76–8, 77–8*f*
neutrophilic inflammation 59–62, 60–1*f*, 171–2, 172*f*, 267, 267*f*
neutrophilic lymphadenitis 246, 247*f*
neutrophils 34*t*, 300–1, 300*f*
non-neoplastic lesions 163–4, 168, 169*f*, 179–80, 179*f*
non-nucleated cells 47
non-suction technique 17–18, 17*f*
nose
   nasal masses 218–19
   normal appearance 217–18
nuclear moulding 45, 46*f*
nuclear to cytoplasmic ratio (N:C) 43–4, 44*f*
nucleated cells 29, 31–46

nucleated red blood cells (nRBCs) 290–3, 290f
nucleoli 31–2, 31f
nucleus 29, 31–2, 31f, 34–9, 36–7f

O
objective lenses 8–9, 8–9f
ocular lenses 7–8, 7f
oral cavity
    inflammation 185–6
    neoplastic lesions 183–5, 184–5f
    normal oral material 182–3, 182f
oral contamination 51
oropharyngeal contamination 221, 222f
osteoblasts 262, 262f
osteoclasts 262, 262f
osteomyelitis 264
osteosarcoma 263–4, 263–4f

P
packing specimens 5, 333–4
palpation 129–30
pancreas 200, 201f
papilloma 146, 146–7f
parasites 122–6, 125f, 178
pathology 4
perianal region 161
plant material 52, 52f
plasma cells 68–9, 70–1f, 86, 86–7f
plasma cell tumour 195–6, 196f
plasmacytic inflammation 177
plasmacytoma 142–4, 143–4f, 185
platelets 286–8, 286–9f
pleomorphism 44
polychromasia 289–90
preservation 55–7, 57f
prestaining 334
primary pulmonary carcinoma 228, 229f
prostate 15, 25, 213–14
    inflammation 214
    neoplastic lesions 214, 215f
    normal appearance 213–14, 213–14f
    squamous metaplasia 214–15, 215f
prostatic wash 25
proteinaceous fluids 59
protein content 270
protozoa 119–22, 122–5f
pseudochylous effusions 277, 279

R
ragocytes 267
red blood cells 290–5
regenerative anaemia 311

remote cytology 336
renal carcinoma 206, 207f
renal epithelial cells 204, 204f
renal sarcoma 206–8, 208f
re-sampling 55
respiratory system 217
    infectious agents 226–7
    inflammation 222–6
    lungs 227–30
    nose 217–19
    respiratory tract 15, 22–4, 219–27, 220f
rhabdomyoma 259–61
rhabdomyosarcoma 160–1, 259–60
Rickettsiae 309
risks 15–16
rolled cells 34, 34f
rolled swabs 26, 26f
Romanowsky stains 11–12, 27, 39, 82, 101, 114, 116, 299
round cell tumours 43f, 72t, 82–91, 135–7, 142–4, 149

S
saliva contamination 51f
salivary lesions 167–8, 167–8f
sampling
    digital cytology 335–6
    labelling 27–8, 331
    methods 14–15, 15t
    re-sampling 55
    sites 14
    techniques 16–27
    see also specimens
schistocytes 295
scraping 25–6, 26f
sebaceous epithelium 132–3, 133f
sebaceous proliferation 137–8, 137f
septic diseases 61
seromas 98, 180
Shar Pei fever 180
Simonsiella see Conchiformibius
sinus tracts 15
skeletal muscle 134, 134f
skin, normal 129–30, 130f
skin lesions 129–31
    common cytological findings 131–4
    cutaneous 134–50
    infectious diseases 178–80
    inflammatory lesions 171–8
    mammary masses 164–7
    perianal region 161–4
    subcutaneous 150–61
    see also neoplasia

slides 11
  preparation techniques 19–21, 19–21*f*
  see also blood films
soft masses 15
soft tissue sarcoma 151–3, 152–3*f*
specimens 4
  backgrounds 57, 59, 59*f*
  evaluation and examination 55–9, 58*t*, 104–5
  labelling 27–8, 331
  packing 5, 333–4
  see also sampling
spherocytes 293–4, 294*f*
spirochaetes 111, 112*f*, 114
spleen 248–57
  inflammation 256–7
  neoplastic lesions 252
  normal appearance 249, 249–50*f*
splenitis 256–7, 256*f*
squames 48, 97, 97*f*, 130–1, 131*f*
squamous cell carcinoma 138, 140–1, 140–1*f*, 184–5, 184*f*, 328–9
staining 5, 27, 114, 334
stain precipitate 48, 50*f*, 108–9, 109*f*
stains 5, 11, 27, 39, 116, 344
Staphylococcus 107, 178
storage 27–8
streaming chromatin 33–4, 34*f*, 47*f*
Streptococcus 178
stromal sarcoma 255–6, 255*f*
subcutaneous mass 129–30, 130*f*
subcutaneous neoplasia 150–61
submission form 331–3
suction technique 17, 18, 18*f*
surgical biopsy 15, 25
synovial fluid 22, 50, 265–7, 329–30
  inflammation 266–7
  normal appearance 265, 265–6*f*
syringes 11

T
thymic carcinoma 257–8
thymoma 257–8, 258*f*
thymus 257–8
thyroid gland 76–8
thyroid tumour 168, 170–1*f*
tonsils 182–3, 184–5
toxic change 301–2
transmissible venereal tumour 90, 91*f*, 149, 149*f*
trans-tracheal wash (TTW) 23, 219
transudates 274–5, 274*f*
traumatic catheterisation 24, 24*f*
trematodes 124
triglycerides 270
tumours
  benign 85, 92, 92*f*
  characteristics 72*t*
  epithelial 71–6, 72–7*f*, 72*t*, 129, 137–41, 137–41*f*, 146–7
  grading 104–5
  histiocytoma 85–6, 86*f*, 136, 136–7*f*
  malignant 87–90, 92–5, 93–5*f*, 105, 141, 147, 185
  mast cells 82–4, 83–5*f*, 135–6, 135–6*f*, 153, 153*f*, 155*f*, 185, 306, 307*f*, 343
  melanocytic 87, 89–90*f*, 141–2, 141–2*f*, 185
  mesenchymal 72*t*, 78–82, 79–82*f*, 147–8, 150–3, 153–61
  neuroendocrine 72*t*, 76–8, 77–8*f*
  round cell 72*t*, 82–91, 135–7, 142–4, 149
  see also lymphoma; neoplasia
turbidity 269

U
ulcerated lesions 25
ultrasound contact gel 16
urea 270
urine
  analysis 209–12
  inflammation 211
  normal appearance 210–11
uroabdomen 279–80
urothelial carcinoma 212, 212*f*, 343

V
vacuolation 41*f*
vascular hamartoma 144–5, 144*f*
vascular lesions 17
viruses 126
viscosity 269
viscous fluid 15
visible examination 129

W
Wilde, Oscar 5
windrowing 52–3, 52*f*

Y
yeasts 51, 117–19, 119–21*f*

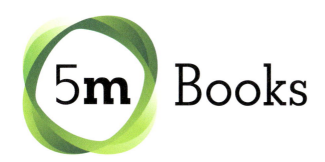

£100 FREE BOOKS?

Tell us about how you came to this book and we'll enter you in our next draw to win £100 of our books.

Scan the QR code to start or visit
https://forms.office.com/e/97P5QTyZmk

We at 5m are passionate about improving the health and happiness of the animals we farm and live with and of the environment we farm in.

Our mission is to publish the highest quality books in veterinary and animal sciences, agriculture and aquaculture.

Join us at www.5mbooks.com or follow our social media channels to be part of our community and to find out more about our books and authors.

We welcome proposals for new books in the areas in which we publish. We would be delighted to hear from you, please email us: hello@5mbooks.com

www.5mbooks.com

@5mBooks | @5m_Books | @5m_Books
linkedin.com/company/5mbooks

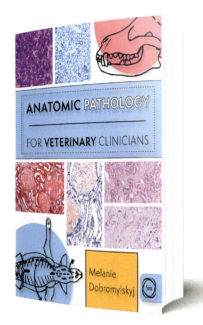

Anatomic Pathology for Veterinary Clinicians

Melanie Dobromylskyj

This book is a concise guide for practising vets on anatomic pathology that will aid the reader's understanding of pathology, thus allowing optimisation of diagnostic tests.

Anatomic Pathology for Veterinary Clinicians will teach practitioners how to:

• Take quality biopsy samples to get better results

• Understand histopathology reports

• Know when additional tests are warranted and are likely to give clinically useful information

Jul 2023 | ISBN 9781789182378
£55 | $85 | €66 | 220p PB

Diagnostic Radiology in Small Animal Practice 2nd Edition

Silke Hecht

This reference book covers using digital radiology and medical imaging procedures such as ultrasound, MRI and scintigraphy in veterinary practice. The approach is a step-by-step guide, with tips and techniques to ensure optimal X-rays and advice on how to improve radiation protection. All commonly kept pets are included: small mammals, birds, amphibians and reptiles.

Dec 2020 | ISBN 9781789180930
£150 | $235 | €180 | 532p HB

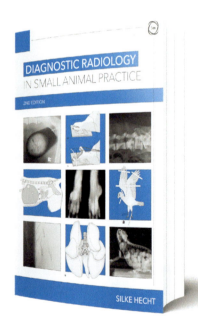

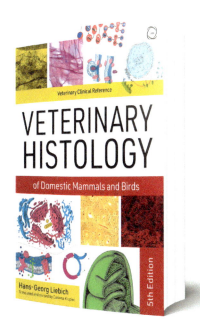

Veterinary Histology of Domestic Mammals and Birds 5th Edition
Textbook and Colour Atlas

Edited by Hans-Georg Liebich

A full colour atlas of veterinary histology images with accompanying text, covering domestic mammals and birds. It provides a peerless collection of diagrams, schematics, colour micrographs and electron microscope images, plus online access to a further 900 colour images. The author presents information from both a structural and functional perspective. This applied approach highlights the importance of understanding histology as a basis for identifying disease.

Oct 2019 | ISBN 9781789180091
£150 | $235 | €180 | 504p HB

Avian Anatomy 2nd Edition
Textbook and Colour Atlas

Edited by Horst E. König

Containing very high quality photographs, including histological and radiographic images and schematic diagrams, this edition focuses on ornamental birds and poultry. Among the various species examined are chickens, ducks and geese, as well as budgerigars, psitaccines and many others. In addition, wild bird species such as the common buzzard and falcon are taken into account and raptors are featured in a dedicated new chapter.

Dec 2016 | ISBN 9781910455609
£150 | $235 | €180 | 360p HB

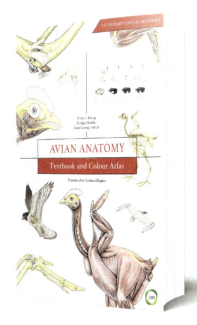

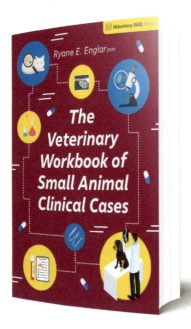

The Veterinary Workbook of Small Animal Clinical Cases

Ryane Englar

This workbook is intended to be a bridge between classroom learning and clinical training; to improve patient care and clinician confidence in practice. Common presentations in small animal practice are presented as real-world case studies while the reader is guided through work-up, critical thinking and problem solving to run the consultation efficiently.

Aug 2021 | ISBN 9781789181296
£55 | $85 | €66 | 700p PB

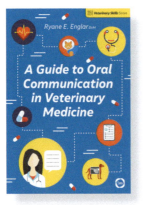

9781789180954
Jul 2020
250p
PB
£34.95
$55.00
€42.00

A Guide to Oral Communication in Veterinary Medicine

Ryane Englar

This guide covers why communication skills are important, the structure of typical communications and suggested approaches, veterinary specific communication pathways and sample scripts between vet and client.

 Veterinary Skills Series

The Veterinary Skills Series provides practical advice for students and professionals in study and research skills, and techniques for written and oral communication in veterinary medicine.

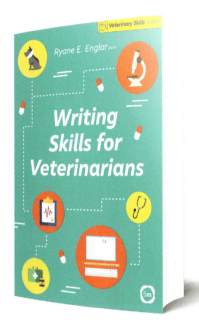

Writing Skills for Veterinarians

Ryane Englar

Communicating ideas in veterinary medicine is a fundamental part of continuing veterinary research and building a career as a clinician.

The purpose of this book is to help increase efficiency and effectiveness in writing professional documents, e.g. writing a concise yet thorough discharge statement to avoid repeated client call-backs to clarify medical recommendations. The book also aims at improving the reader's confidence in writing skills through guided and well-thought out "homework" or practice exercises.

Feb 2019 | ISBN 9781789180350
£24.95 | $39.95 | €29.95 | 280p PB

Research and Study Skills for Veterinary Nurses

Jane Davidson

Aimed at veterinary nurses and technicians this book will guide the reader through the various research and study disciplines required of them. Research and Study Skills for Veterinary Nurses discusses why these academic skills are now required of the veterinary nurse, different types of source material, how to complete written assignments, how to reference properly, how to approach different test questions, exam preparation, how to respond to oral exams, how to complete OSCEs, CPD training and work-based practical assessments.

Apr 2019 | ISBN 9781789180138
£24.95 | $39.95 | €29.95 | 272p PB

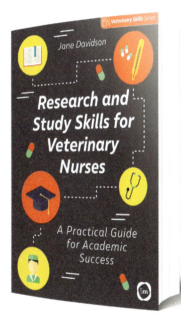